Brain Disorders
SOURCEBOOK

Fifth Edition

Fifth Edition

Brain Disorders

SOURCEBOOK

*Basic Consumer Health Information about Acquired
and Traumatic Brain Injuries, Brain Tumors, Cerebral
Palsy and Other Genetic and Congenital Brain Disorders,
Infections of the Brain, Epilepsy, and Degenerative
Neurological Disorders Such as Dementia, Huntington
Disease, and Amyotrophic Lateral Sclerosis (ALS)*

*Along with Information on Brain Structure and
Function, Treatment and Rehabilitation Options,
a Glossary of Terms Related to Brain Disorders, and
a Directory of Resources for More Information*

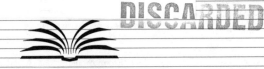

OMNIGRAPHICS

615 Griswold, Ste. 901, Detroit, MI 48226

Bibliographic Note

Because this page cannot legibly accommodate all the copyright notices, the Bibliographic Note portion of the Preface constitutes an extension of the copyright notice.

* * *

OMNIGRAPHICS
John Tilly, *Managing Editor*

17/18 Omni

***

Copyright © 2018 Omnigraphics

17-18

ISBN 978-0-7808-1620-6
E-ISBN 978-0-7808-1621-3

Library of Congress Cataloging-in-Publication Data

Names: Omnigraphics, Inc.

Title: Brain disorders sourcebook: basic consumer health information about acquired and traumatic brain injuries, brain tumors, cerebral palsy and other genetic and congenital brain disorders, infections of the brain, epilepsy, and degenerative neurological disorders such as dementia, huntington disease, and amyotrophic lateral sclerosis (als); along with information on brain structure and function, treatment and rehabilitation options, a glossary of terms related to brain disorders, and a directory of resources for more information.

Description: Fifth edition. | Detroit, MI: Omnigraphics, [2018] | Includes bibliographical references and index.

Identifiers: LCCN 2018002740 (print) | LCCN 2018003548 (ebook) | ISBN 9780780816213 (eBook) | ISBN 9780780816206 (hardcover: alk. paper)

Subjects: LCSH: Brain--Diseases--Popular works.

Classification: LCC RC351 (ebook) | LCC RC351.B735 2018 (print) | DDC 616.8--dc23

LC record available at https://lccn.loc.gov/2018002740

Table of Contents

Part III: Genetic and Congenital Brain Disorders

Part IV: Brain Infections

Part V: Traumatic and Acquired Brain Injuries

Part VI: Brain Tumors

Part VII: Degenerative Brain Disorders

Part VIII: Seizures and Neurological Disorders of Sleep

Part IX: Additional Help and Information

Preface

About This Book

Millions of Americans and their families experience the daily challenges of living with physical, mental, or emotional difficulties that result from brain disorders caused by heredity, infection, injury, tumors, or degeneration. For example, an estimated four million people are currently living with the effects of stroke, which is the leading cause of serious, long-term disability in adults. An estimated 5.5 million Americans are affected by Alzheimer disease, and each year 2.8 million Americans suffer a traumatic brain injury. Although damage to the brain may result in permanent disability, with appropriate treatment and follow-up care, many affected individuals are able to participate fully in life's activities.

Brain Disorders Sourcebook, Fifth Edition provides readers with updated information about brain function, neurological emergencies such as a brain attack (stroke) or seizure, and symptoms of brain disorders. It describes the diagnosis, treatment, and rehabilitation therapies for genetic and congenital brain disorders, brain infections, brain tumors, seizures, traumatic brain injuries, and degenerative neurological disorders such as Alzheimer disease and other dementias, Parkinson disease, and amyotrophic lateral sclerosis (ALS). A glossary of related terms is also included along with a directory of additional resources about brain disorders.

How to Use This Book

This book is divided into parts and chapters. Parts focus on broad areas of interest. Chapters are devoted to single topics within a part.

Part I: Brain Basics describes the human brain and how the aging process and the environment may contribute to brain disorders. Symptoms of brain disorders and details about identifying neurological emergencies are discussed. Facts about coma, other states of impaired consciousness, and brain death are also included.

Part II: Diagnosing and Treating Brain Disorders reviews common neurological tests and describes current treatments, including the use of steroids, chemotherapy, radiation therapy, and brain surgery. Information about cognitive recovery, measurements of brain function, and brain rehabilitation is also presented.

Part III: Genetic and Congenital Brain Disorders offers information about adrenoleukodystrophy, Batten disease, and other neurological conditions that create severe disability and often shorten the lifespan. It also reviews congenital disorders that affect brain function throughout life, but which are not always progressively debilitating. These include cerebral palsy, cephalic disorders, and other birth defects.

Part IV: Brain Infections describes inflammatory diseases caused by bacteria, viruses, or parasites that affect the brain and related structures. These ailments, which can cause severe illness—and even death—in otherwise healthy individuals, include encephalitis, meningitis, and cysticercosis.

Part V: Traumatic and Acquired Brain Injuries offers guidelines for identifying traumatic head injuries and offering first aid. Facts about concussions are provided, and detailed information about traumatic brain injury (TBI) is given to help individuals and families affected by it. Separate chapters present information about acquired (nontraumatic) brain injuries, including cerebral aneurysm, agnosia, hydrocephalus, and stroke.

Part VI: Brain Tumors describes the symptoms and treatments for primary, metastatic, pituitary, childhood and adult brain tumors as well as benign and tumor-associated brain cysts. It offers tips for managing treatment side effects, fatigue, cognitive changes, and work-related concerns.

Part VII: Degenerative Brain Disorders discusses neurological disorders that often lead to progressive deterioration of physical or mental functioning. These include Alzheimer disease and other dementias, amyotrophic lateral sclerosis (ALS), Creutzfeldt-Jakob disease, Friedreich ataxia, Huntington disease, multiple sclerosis (MS), Parkinson disease, and progressive supranuclear palsy (PSP).

Part VIII: Seizures and Neurological Disorders of Sleep describes epileptic and nonepileptic seizure disorders, myoclonus, restless legs syndrome, and narcolepsy.

Part IX: Additional Help and Information provides a glossary of terms related to brain disorders and a directory of organizations and resources for additional information.

Bibliographic Note

This volume contains documents and excerpts from publications issued by the following government agencies: Administration for Community Living (ACL); Agency for Toxic Substances and Disease Registry (ATSDR); Centers for Disease Control and Prevention (CDC); Child Welfare Information Gateway; *Eunice Kennedy Shriver* National Institute of Child Health and Human Development (NICHD); Genetic and Rare Diseases Information Center (GARD); Genetics Home Reference (GHR); National Aeronautics and Space Administration (NASA); National Cancer Institute (NCI); National Heart, Lung, and Blood Institute (NHLBI); National Institute of Biomedical Imaging and Bioengineering (NIBIB); National Institute of Mental Health (NIMH); National Institute of Neurological Disorders and Stroke (NINDS); National Institute on Aging (NIA); National Institute on Drug Abuse (NIDA); National Institutes of Health (NIH); *NIH News in Health*; U.S. Department of Health and Human Services (HHS); U.S. Department of Veterans Affairs (VA); U.S. Environmental Protection Agency (EPA); and U.S. Food and Drug Administration (FDA).

It may also contain original material produced by Omnigraphics and reviewed by medical consultants.

About the Health Reference Series

The *Health Reference Series* is designed to provide basic medical information for patients, families, caregivers, and the general public. Each volume takes a particular topic and provides comprehensive coverage. This is especially important for people who may be dealing with a newly diagnosed disease or a chronic disorder in themselves or in a family member. People looking for preventive guidance, information about disease warning signs, medical statistics, and risk factors for health problems will also find answers to their questions in the *Health Reference Series*. The *Series*, however, is not intended to serve as a tool for diagnosing illness, in prescribing treatments, or as a substitute for the physician/patient relationship. All people concerned about medical symptoms or the possibility of disease are encouraged to seek professional care from an appropriate healthcare provider.

A Note about Spelling and Style

Health Reference Series editors use *Stedman's Medical Dictionary* as an authority for questions related to the spelling of medical terms and the *Chicago Manual of Style* for questions related to grammatical structures, punctuation, and other editorial concerns. Consistent adherence is not always possible, however, because the individual volumes within the *Series* include many documents from a wide variety of different producers, and the editor's primary goal is to present material from each source as accurately as is possible. This sometimes means that information in different chapters or sections may follow other guidelines and alternate spelling authorities. For example, occasionally a copyright holder may require that eponymous terms be shown in possessive forms (Crohn's disease vs. Crohn disease) or that British spelling norms be retained (leukaemia vs. leukemia).

Medical Review

Omnigraphics contracts with a team of qualified, senior medical professionals who serve as medical consultants for the *Health Reference Series*. As necessary, medical consultants review reprinted and originally written material for currency and accuracy. Citations including the phrase, "Reviewed (month, year)" indicate material reviewed by this team. Medical consultation services are provided to the *Health Reference Series* editors by:

Dr. Vijayalakshmi, MBBS, DGO, MD
Dr. Senthil Selvan, MBBS, DCH, MD
Dr. K. Sivanandham, MBBS, DCH, MS (Research), PhD

Our Advisory Board

We would like to thank the following board members for providing initial guidance on the development of this series:

- Dr. Lynda Baker, Associate Professor of Library and Information Science, Wayne State University, Detroit, MI

- Nancy Bulgarelli, William Beaumont Hospital Library, Royal Oak, MI

- Karen Imarisio, Bloomfield Township Public Library, Bloomfield Township, MI

- Karen Morgan, Mardigian Library, University of Michigan-Dearborn, Dearborn, MI

- Rosemary Orlando, St. Clair Shores Public Library, St. Clair Shores, MI

Health Reference Series *Update Policy*

The inaugural book in the *Health Reference Series* was the first edition of *Cancer Sourcebook* published in 1989. Since then, the *Series* has been enthusiastically received by librarians and in the medical community. In order to maintain the standard of providing high-quality health information for the layperson the editorial staff at Omnigraphics felt it was necessary to implement a policy of updating volumes when warranted.

Medical researchers have been making tremendous strides, and it is the purpose of the *Health Reference Series* to stay current with the most recent advances. Each decision to update a volume is made on an individual basis. Some of the considerations include how much new information is available and the feedback we receive from people who use the books. If there is a topic you would like to see added to the update list, or an area of medical concern you feel has not been adequately addressed, please write to:

Managing Editor
Health Reference Series
Omnigraphics
615 Griswold, Ste. 901
Detroit, MI 48226

Part One

Brain Basics

Chapter 1

Brain Basics: Know Your Brain

The brain is the most complex part of the human body. This three-pound organ is the seat of intelligence, interpreter of the senses, initiator of body movement, and controller of behavior. Lying in its bony shell and washed by protective fluid, the brain is the source of all the qualities that define our humanity. The brain is the crown jewel of the human body.

For centuries, scientists and philosophers have been fascinated by the brain, but until recently they viewed the brain as nearly incomprehensible. Now, however, the brain is beginning to relinquish its secrets. Scientists have learned more about the brain in the last 10 years than in all previous centuries because of the accelerating pace of research in neurological and behavioral science and the development of new research techniques. As a result, Congress named the 1990s the *Decade of the Brain*. This chapter is a basic introduction to the human brain. It may help you understand how the healthy brain works, how to keep it healthy, and what happens when the brain is diseased or dysfunctional.

This chapter includes text excerpted from "Brain Basics—Know Your Brain," National Institute of Neurological Disorders and Stroke (NINDS), December 16, 2016.

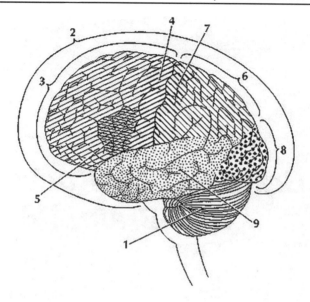

Figure 1.1. *Know Your Brain*

The Architecture of the Brain

The brain is like a committee of experts. All the parts of the brain work together, but each part has its own special properties. The brain can be divided into three basic units: the forebrain, the midbrain, and the hindbrain.

The hindbrain includes the upper part of the spinal cord, the brainstem, and a wrinkled ball of tissue called the **cerebellum** (1). The hindbrain controls the body's vital functions such as respiration and heart rate. The cerebellum coordinates movement and is involved in learned rote movements. When you play the piano or hit a tennis ball you are activating the cerebellum. The uppermost part of the brainstem is the midbrain, which controls some reflex actions and is part of the circuit involved in the control of eye movements and other voluntary movements. The forebrain is the largest and most highly developed part of the human brain: it consists primarily of the **cerebrum** (2) and the structures hidden beneath it.

When people see pictures of the brain it is usually the cerebrum that they notice. The cerebrum sits at the topmost part of the brain and is the source of intellectual activities. It holds your memories, allows you to plan, enables you to imagine and think. It allows you to recognize friends, read books, and play games.

4

The cerebrum is split into two halves (hemispheres) by a deep fissure. Despite the split, the two cerebral hemispheres communicate with each other through a thick tract of nerve fibers that lies at the base of this fissure. Although the two hemispheres seem to be mirror images of each other, they are different. For instance, the ability to form words seems to lie primarily in the left hemisphere, while the right hemisphere seems to control many abstract reasoning skills.

For some as-yet-unknown reason, nearly all of the signals from the brain to the body and vice-versa crossover on their way to and from the brain. This means that the right cerebral hemisphere primarily controls the left side of the body and the left hemisphere primarily controls the right side. When one side of the brain is damaged, the opposite side of the body is affected. For example, a stroke in the right hemisphere of the brain can leave the left arm and leg paralyzed.

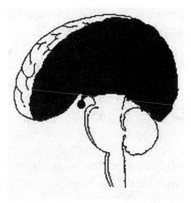

Figure 1.2. *The Forebrain*

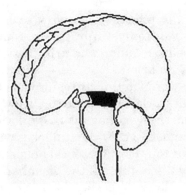

Figure 1.3. *The Midbrain*

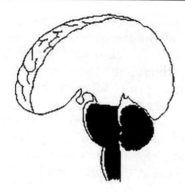

Figure 1.4. *The Hindbrain*

The Geography of Thought

Each cerebral hemisphere can be divided into sections, or lobes, each of which specializes in different functions. To understand each lobe and its specialty we will take a tour of the cerebral hemispheres, starting with the **two frontal lobes** (3), which lie directly behind the forehead. When you plan a schedule, imagine the future, or use reasoned arguments, these two lobes do much of the work. One of the ways the frontal lobes seem to do these things is by acting as short-term storage sites, allowing one idea to be kept in mind while other ideas are considered. In the rearmost portion of each frontal lobe is a **motor area** (4), which helps control voluntary movement. A nearby place on the left frontal lobe called **Broca area** (5) allows thoughts to be transformed into words.

When you enjoy a good meal—the taste, aroma, and texture of the food—two sections behind the frontal lobes called the **parietal lobes** (6) are at work. The forward parts of these lobes, just behind the motor areas, are the **primary sensory areas** (7). These areas receive information about temperature, taste, touch, and movement from the rest of the body. Reading and arithmetic are also functions in the repertoire of each parietal lobe.

As you look at the words and pictures provided, two areas at the back of the brain are at work. These lobes, called the **occipital lobes** (8), process images from the eyes and link that information with images stored in memory. Damage to the occipital lobes can cause blindness.

The last lobes on our tour of the cerebral hemispheres are the **temporal lobes** (9), which lie in front of the visual areas and nest under the parietal and frontal lobes. Whether you appreciate symphonies or rock music, your brain responds through the activity of these lobes.

At the top of each temporal lobe is an area responsible for receiving information from the ears. The underside of each temporal lobe plays a crucial role in forming and retrieving memories, including those associated with music. Other parts of this lobe seem to integrate memories and sensations of taste, sound, sight, and touch.

The Cerebral Cortex

Coating the surface of the cerebrum and the cerebellum is a vital layer of tissue the thickness of a stack of two or three dimes. It is called the cortex, from the Latin word for bark. Most of the actual information processing in the brain takes place in the cerebral cortex. When people talk about "gray matter" in the brain they are talking about this thin rind. The cortex is gray because nerves in this area lack the insulation that makes most other parts of the brain appear to be white. The folds in the brain add to its surface area and therefore increase the amount of gray matter and the quantity of information that can be processed.

The Inner Brain

Deep within the brain, hidden from view, lie structures that are the gatekeepers between the spinal cord and the cerebral hemispheres. These structures not only determine our emotional state, they also modify our perceptions and responses depending on that state, and allow us to initiate movements that you make without thinking about them. Like the lobes in the cerebral hemispheres, the structures described below come in pairs: each is duplicated in the opposite half of the brain.

The **hypothalamus** (10), about the size of a pearl, directs a multitude of important functions. It wakes you up in the morning, and gets the adrenaline flowing during a test or job interview. The hypothalamus is also an important emotional center, controlling the molecules that make you feel exhilarated, angry, or unhappy. Near the hypothalamus lies the **thalamus** (11), a major clearinghouse for information going to and from the spinal cord and the cerebrum.

An arching tract of nerve cells leads from the hypothalamus and the thalamus to the **hippocampus** (12). This tiny nub acts as a memory indexer—sending memories out to the appropriate part of the cerebral hemisphere for long-term storage and retrieving them when necessary. The **basal ganglia** (not shown) are clusters of nerve cells surrounding the thalamus. They are responsible for initiating and integrating movements. Parkinson disease, which results in tremors,

7

rigidity, and a stiff, shuffling walk, is a disease of nerve cells that lead into the basal ganglia.

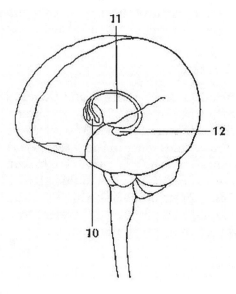

Figure 1.5. *Inner Brain*

Making Connections

The brain and the rest of the nervous system are composed of many different types of cells, but the primary functional unit is a cell called the neuron. All sensations, movements, thoughts, memories, and feelings are the result of signals that pass through neurons. Neurons consist of three parts. The **cell body** (13) contains the nucleus, where most of the molecules that the neuron needs to survive and function are manufactured. **Dendrites** (14) extend out from the cell body like the branches of a tree and receive messages from other nerve cells. Signals then pass from the dendrites through the cell body and may travel away from the cell body down an **axon** (15) to another neuron, a muscle cell, or cells in some other organ. The neuron is usually surrounded by many support cells. Some types of cells wrap around the axon to form an insulating **sheath** (16). This sheath can include a fatty molecule called myelin, which provides insulation for the axon and helps nerve signals travel faster and farther. Axons may be very short, such as those that carry signals from one cell in the cortex to another cell less than a hair's width away. Or axons may be very long, such as those that carry messages from the brain all the way down the spinal cord.

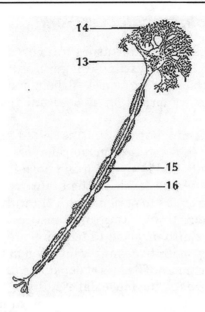

Figure 1.6. *Making Connections*

Scientists have learned a great deal about neurons by studying the synapse—the place where a signal passes from the neuron to another cell. When the signal reaches the end of the axon it stimulates the release of tiny **sacs** (17). These sacs release chemicals known as **neurotransmitters** (18) into the **synapse** (19). The neurotransmitters cross the synapse and attach to **receptors** (20) on the neighboring cell. These receptors can change the properties of the receiving cell. If the receiving cell is also a neuron, the signal can continue the transmission to the next cell.

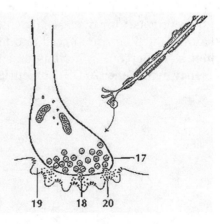

Figure 1.7. *Cell Body*

Some Key Neurotransmitters at Work

Acetylcholine is called an **excitatory neurotransmitter** because it generally makes cells more excitable. It governs muscle contractions and causes glands to secrete hormones. Alzheimer disease (AD), which initially affects memory formation, is associated with a shortage of acetylcholine.

GABA (gamma-Aminobutyric acid) is called an inhibitory neurotransmitter because it tends to make cells less excitable. It helps control muscle activity and is an important part of the visual system. Drugs that increase GABA levels in the brain are used to treat epileptic seizures and tremors in patients with Huntington disease (HD).

Serotonin is a neurotransmitter that constricts blood vessels and brings on sleep. It is also involved in temperature regulation. Dopamine is an inhibitory neurotransmitter involved in mood and the control of complex movements. The loss of dopamine activity in some portions of the brain leads to the muscular rigidity of Parkinson disease (PD). Many medications used to treat behavioral disorders work by modifying the action of dopamine in the brain.

Neurological Disorders

When the brain is healthy it functions quickly and automatically. But when problems occur, the results can be devastating. Some 50 million people in this country—one in five—suffer from damage to the nervous system. Some of the major types of disorders include: neurogenetic diseases (such as HD) and muscular dystrophy), developmental disorders (such as cerebral palsy (CP)), degenerative diseases of adult life (such as PD and AD), metabolic diseases (such as Gaucher disease), cerebrovascular diseases (such as stroke and vascular dementia), trauma (such as spinal cord and head injury), convulsive disorders (such as epilepsy), infectious diseases (such as acquired immune deficiency syndrome (AIDS) dementia), and brain tumors.

Chapter 2

Brain Development and Aging

Chapter Contents

Section 2.1

Brain Development in Childhood

This section includes text excerpted from "Understanding the Effects of Maltreatment on Brain Development," Child Welfare Information Gateway, April 27, 2015.

How the Brain Develops

What we have learned about the process of brain development has helped us understand more about the roles both genetics and the environment play in our development. It appears that genetics predisposes us to develop in certain ways. But our experiences, including our interactions with other people, have a significant impact on how our predispositions are expressed. In fact, research now shows that many capacities thought to be fixed at birth are actually dependent on a sequence of experiences combined with heredity. Both factors are essential for optimum development of the human brain.

The Newborn Brain

The raw material of the brain is the nerve cell, called the neuron. When babies are born, they have almost all of the neurons they will ever have, more than 100 billion of them. Although research indicates some neurons are developed after birth and well into adulthood, the neurons babies have at birth are primarily what they have to work with as they develop into children, adolescents, and adults.

During fetal development, neurons are created and migrate to form the various parts of the brain. As neurons migrate, they also differentiate, so they begin to "specialize" in response to chemical signals. This process of development occurs sequentially from the "bottom up," that is, from the more primitive sections of the brain to the more sophisticated sections. The first areas of the brain to fully develop are the brainstem and midbrain; they govern the bodily functions necessary for life, called the autonomic functions. At birth, these lower portions of the nervous system are very well developed, whereas the higher regions (the limbic system and cerebral cortex) are still rather primitive.

Newborns' brains allow babies to do many things, including breathe, eat, sleep, see, hear, smell, make noise, feel sensations, and recognize the people close to them. But the majority of brain growth and development takes place after birth, especially in the higher brain regions involved in regulating emotions, language, and abstract thought. Each region manages its assigned functions through complex processes, often using chemical messengers (such as neurotransmitters and hormones) to help transmit information to other parts of the brain and body.

The Growing Baby's Brain

Brain development, or learning, is actually the process of creating, strengthening, and discarding connections among the neurons; these connections are called synapses. Synapses organize the brain by forming pathways that connect the parts of the brain governing everything we do—from breathing and sleeping to thinking and feeling. This is the essence of postnatal brain development, because at birth, very few synapses have been formed. The synapses present at birth are primarily those that govern our bodily functions such as heart rate, breathing, eating, and sleeping.

The development of synapses occurs at an astounding rate during children's early years, in response to the young child's experiences. At its peak, the cerebral cortex of a healthy toddler may create 2 million synapses per second. By the time children are 3, their brains have approximately 1,000 trillion synapses, many more than they will ever need. Some of these synapses are strengthened and remain intact, but many are gradually discarded. This process of synapse elimination—or pruning—is a normal part of development. By the time children reach adolescence, about half of their synapses have been discarded, leaving the number they will have for most of the rest of their lives. Brain development continues throughout the lifespan. This allows us to continue to learn, remember, and adapt to new circumstances.

Another important process that takes place in the developing brain is myelination. Myelin is the white fatty tissue that insulates mature brain cells by forming a sheath, thus ensuring clear transmission across synapses. Young children process information slowly because their brain cells lack the myelin necessary for fast, clear nerve impulse transmission. Like other neuronal growth processes, myelination begins in the primary motor and sensory areas (the brainstem and cortex) and gradually progresses to the higher-order regions that control thought, memories, and feelings. Also, like other neuronal growth processes, a child's experiences affect the rate and growth of myelination, which continues into young adulthood.

By the age of 3, a baby's brain has reached almost 90 percent of its adult size. The growth in each region of the brain largely depends on receiving stimulation, which spurs activity in that region. This stimulation provides the foundation for learning.

Plasticity—The Influence of Environment

Researchers use the term plasticity to describe the brain's ability to change in response to repeated stimulation. The extent of a brain's plasticity is dependent on the stage of development and the particular brain system or region affected. For instance, the lower parts of the brain, which control basic functions such as breathing and heart rate, are less flexible than the higher functioning cortex, which controls thoughts and feelings. While cortex plasticity may lessen as a child gets older, some degree of plasticity remains. In fact, this brain plasticity is what allows us to keep learning into adulthood and throughout our lives.

The developing brain's ongoing adaptations are the result of both genetics and experience. Our brains prepare us to expect certain experiences by forming the pathways needed to respond to those experiences. For example, our brains are "wired" to respond to the sound of speech; when babies hear people speaking, the neural systems in their brains responsible for speech and language receive the necessary stimulation to organize and function. The more babies are exposed to people speaking, the stronger their related synapses become. If the appropriate exposure does not happen, the pathways developed in anticipation may be discarded. This is sometimes referred to as the concept of "use it or lose it." It is through these processes of creating, strengthening, and discarding synapses that our brains adapt to our unique environment.

The ability to adapt to our environment is a part of normal development. Children growing up in cold climates, on rural farms, or in large sibling groups learn how to function in those environments. But regardless of the general environment, all children need stimulation and nurturance for healthy development. If these are lacking—if a child's caretakers are indifferent or hostile—the child's brain development may be impaired. Because the brain adapts to its environment, it will adapt to a negative environment just as readily as it will adapt to a positive one.

Sensitive Periods

Researchers believe that there are sensitive periods for development of certain capabilities. These refer to windows of time in the developmental process when certain parts of the brain may be most susceptible to particular experiences. Animal studies have shed light on sensitive periods, showing, for example, that animals that are artificially blinded during the sensitive period for developing vision may never develop the capability to see, even if the blinding mechanism is later removed.

It is more difficult to study human sensitive periods. But we know that, if certain synapses and neuronal pathways are not repeatedly activated, they may be discarded, and the capabilities they promised may be diminished. For example, infants have the genetic predisposition to form strong attachments to their primary caregivers. But if a child's caregivers are unresponsive or threatening, and the attachment process is disrupted, the child's ability to form any healthy relationships during his or her life may be impaired.

While sensitive periods exist for development and learning, we also know that the plasticity of the brain often allows children to recover from missing certain experiences. Both children and adults may be able to make up for missed experiences later in life, but it may be more difficult. This is especially true if a young child was deprived of certain stimulation, which resulted in the pruning of synapses (neuronal connections) relevant to that stimulation and the loss of neuronal pathways. As children progress through each developmental stage, they will learn and master each step more easily if their brains have built an efficient network of pathways.

Memories

The organizing framework for children's development is based on the creation of memories. When repeated experiences strengthen a neuronal pathway, the pathway becomes encoded, and it eventually becomes a memory. Children learn to put one foot in front of the other to walk. They learn words to express themselves. And they learn that a smile usually brings a smile in return. At some point, they no longer have to think much about these processes—their brains manage these experiences with little effort because the memories that have been created allow for a smooth, efficient flow of information.

The creation of memories is part of our adaptation to our environment. Our brains attempt to understand the world around us and fashion our interactions with that world in a way that promotes our survival and, hopefully, our growth. But if the early environment is abusive or neglectful, our brains will create memories of these experiences that may adversely color our view of the world throughout our life.

Babies are born with the capacity for implicit memory, which means that they can perceive their environment and recall it in certain unconscious ways. For instance, they recognize their mother's voice from an unconscious memory. These early implicit memories may have a significant impact on a child's subsequent attachment relationships.

In contrast, explicit memory, which develops around age 2, refers to conscious memories and is tied to language development. Explicit memory allows children to talk about themselves in the past and future or in different places or circumstances through the process of conscious recollection.

Sometimes, children who have been abused or suffered other trauma may not retain or be able to access explicit memories for their experiences. However, they may retain implicit memories of the physical or emotional sensations, and these implicit memories may produce flashbacks, nightmares, or other uncontrollable reactions. This may be the case with very young children or infants who suffer abuse or neglect.

Section 2.2

The Adolescent Brain

This section includes text excerpted from "The Teen Brain: Still under Construction," National Institute of Mental Health (NIMH), 2011. Reviewed February 2018.

One of the ways that scientists have searched for the causes of mental illness is by studying the development of the brain from birth to adulthood. Powerful new technologies have enabled them to track the growth of the brain and to investigate the connections between brain function, development, and behavior. The research has turned up some surprises, among them the discovery of striking changes taking place during the teen years. These findings have altered long-held assumptions about the timing of brain maturation. In key ways, the brain doesn't look like that of an adult until the early 20s.

An understanding of how the brain of an adolescent is changing may help explain a puzzling contradiction of adolescence: young people at this age are close to a lifelong peak of physical health, strength, and mental capacity, and yet, for some, this can be a hazardous age. Mortality rates jump between early and late adolescence. Rates of death by injury between ages 15–19 are about six times that of the rate between ages 10–14. Crime rates are highest among young males and rates of alcohol abuse are high relative to other ages. Even though most adolescents come through this transitional age well, it's important to understand the risk factors for behavior that can have serious consequences. Genes, childhood experience, and the environment in which a young person reaches adolescence all shape behavior. Adding to this complex picture, research is revealing how all these factors act in the context of a brain that is changing, with its own impact on behavior.

The more we learn, the better we may be able to understand the abilities and vulnerabilities of teens, and the significance of this stage for life-long mental health. The fact that so much change is taking place beneath the surface may be something for parents to keep in mind during the ups and downs of adolescence.

The "Visible" Brain

A clue to the degree of change taking place in the teen brain came from studies in which scientists did brain scans of children as they grew from early childhood through age 20. The scans revealed unexpectedly late changes in the volume of gray matter, which forms the thin, folding outer layer or cortex of the brain. The cortex is where the processes of thought and memory are based. Over the course of childhood, the volume of gray matter in the cortex increases and then declines. A decline in volume is normal at this age and is in fact a necessary part of maturation

The assumption for many years had been that the volume of gray matter was highest in very early childhood, and gradually fell as a child grew. The more recent scans, however, revealed that the high point of the volume of gray matter occurs during early adolescence.

While the details behind the changes in volume on scans are not completely clear, the results push the timeline of brain maturation into adolescence and young adulthood. In terms of the volume of gray matter seen in brain images, the brain does not begin to resemble that of an adult until the early 20s.

The scans also suggest that different parts of the cortex mature at different rates. Areas involved in more basic functions mature first: those involved, for example, in the processing of information from the senses, and in controlling movement. The parts of the brain responsible for more "top-down" control, controlling impulses, and planning ahead—the hallmarks of adult behavior—are among the last to mature.

What's Gray Matter?

The details of what is behind the increase and decline in gray matter are still not completely clear. Gray matter is made up of the cell bodies of neurons, the nerve fibers that project from them, and support cells. One of the features of the brain's growth in early life is that there is an early blooming of synapses—the connections between brain cells or neurons—followed by pruning as the brain matures. Synapses are the relays over which neurons communicate with each other and are the basis of the working circuitry of the brain. Already more numerous than an adult's at birth, synapses multiply rapidly in the first months of life. A 2-year-old has about half again as many synapses as an adult. (For an idea of the complexity of the brain: a cube of brain matter, 1 millimeter on each side, can contain between 35 and 70 million neurons and an estimated 500 billion synapses.)

Scientists believe that the loss of synapses as a child matures is part of the process by which the brain becomes more efficient. Although genes play a role in the decline in synapses, animal research has shown that experience also shapes the decline. Synapses "exercised" by experience survive and are strengthened, while others are pruned away. Scientists are working to determine to what extent the changes in gray matter on brain scans during the teen years reflect growth and pruning of synapses.

A Spectrum of Change

Research using many different approaches is showing that more than gray matter is changing:

- Connections between different parts of the brain increase throughout childhood and well into adulthood. As the brain develops, the fibers connecting nerve cells are wrapped in a protein that greatly increases the speed with which they can transmit impulses from cell to cell. The resulting increase in connectivity—a little like providing a growing city with a fast, integrated communication system—shapes how well different parts of the brain work in tandem. Research is finding that the extent of connectivity is related to growth in intellectual capacities such as memory and reading ability.

- Several lines of evidence suggest that the brain circuitry involved in emotional responses is changing during the teen years. Functional brain imaging studies, for example, suggest that the responses of teens to emotionally loaded images and situations are heightened relative to younger children and adults. The brain changes underlying these patterns involve brain centers and signaling molecules that are part of the reward system with which the brain motivates behavior. These age-related changes shape how much different parts of the brain are activated in response to experience, and in terms of behavior, the urgency and intensity of emotional reactions.

- Enormous hormonal changes take place during adolescence. Reproductive hormones shape not only sex-related growth and behavior, but overall social behavior. Hormone systems involved in the brain's response to stress are also changing during the teens. As with reproductive hormones, stress hormones can have complex effects on the brain, and as a result, behavior.

- In terms of sheer intellectual power, the brain of an adolescent is a match for an adult's. The capacity of a person to learn will never be greater than during adolescence. At the same time, behavioral tests, sometimes combined with functional brain imaging, suggest differences in how adolescents and adults carry out mental tasks. Adolescents and adults seem to engage different parts of the brain to different extents during tests requiring calculation and impulse control, or in reaction to emotional content.

- Research suggests that adolescence brings with it brain-based changes in the regulation of sleep that may contribute to teens' tendency to stay up late at night. Along with the obvious effects of sleep deprivation, such as fatigue and difficulty maintaining attention, inadequate sleep is a powerful contributor to irritability and depression. Studies of children and adolescents have found that sleep deprivation can increase impulsive behavior;

some researchers report finding that it is a factor in delinquency. Adequate sleep is central to physical and emotional health.

The Changing Brain and Behavior in Teens

One interpretation of all these findings is that in teens, the parts of the brain involved in emotional responses are fully online, or even more active than in adults, while the parts of the brain involved in keeping emotional, impulsive responses in check are still reaching maturity. Such a changing balance might provide clues to a youthful appetite for novelty, and a tendency to act on impulse—without regard for risk.

While much is being learned about the teen brain, it is not yet possible to know to what extent a particular behavior or ability is the result of a feature of brain structure—or a change in brain structure. Changes in the brain take place in the context of many other factors, among them, inborn traits, personal history, family, friends, community, and culture.

Alcohol and the Teen Brain

Adults drink more frequently than teens, but when teens drink they tend to drink larger quantities than adults. There is evidence to suggest that the adolescent brain responds to alcohol differently than the adult brain, perhaps helping to explain the elevated risk of binge drinking in youth. Drinking in youth, and intense drinking are both risk factors for later alcohol dependence. Findings on the developing brain should help clarify the role of the changing brain in youthful drinking, and the relationship between youth drinking and the risk of addiction later in life.

Teens and the Brain: More Questions for Research

- Scientists continue to investigate the development of the brain and the relationship between the changes taking place, behavior, and health. The following questions are among the important ones that are targets of research:

- How do experience and environment interact with genetic pre-programming to shape the maturing brain, and as a result, future abilities and behavior? In other words, to what extent does what a teen does and learns shape his or her brain over the rest of a lifetime?

- In what ways do features unique to the teen brain play a role in the high rates of illicit substance use and alcohol abuse in the late teen to young adult years? Does the adolescent capacity for learning make this a stage of particular vulnerability to addiction?

- Why is it so often the case that, for many mental disorders, symptoms first emerge during adolescence and young adulthood?

- This last question has been the central reason to study brain development from infancy to adulthood. Scientists increasingly view mental illnesses as developmental disorders that have their roots in the processes involved in how the brain matures. By studying how the circuitry of the brain develops, scientists hope to identify when and for what reasons development goes off track. Brain imaging studies have revealed distinctive variations in growth patterns of brain tissue in youth who show signs of conditions affecting mental health. Ongoing research is providing information on how genetic factors increase or reduce vulnerability to mental illness; and how experiences during infancy, childhood, and adolescence can increase the risk of mental illness or protect against it.

The Adolescent and Adult Brain

It is not surprising that the behavior of adolescents would be a study in change, since the brain itself is changing in such striking ways. Scientists emphasize that the fact that the teen brain is in transition doesn't mean it is somehow not up to par. It is different from both a child's and an adult's in ways that may equip youth to make the transition from dependence to independence. The capacity for learning at this age, an expanding social life, and a taste for exploration and limit testing may all, to some extent, be reflections of age-related biology.

Understanding the changes taking place in the brain at this age presents an opportunity to intervene early in mental illnesses that have their onset at this age. Research findings on the brain may also serve to help adults understand the importance of creating an environment in which teens can explore and experiment while helping them avoid behavior that is destructive to themselves and others.

Section 2.3

The Aging Brain

This section contains text excerpted from the following sources: Text in this section begins with excerpts from "How the Aging Brain Affects Thinking," National Institute on Aging (NIA), National Institutes of Health (NIH), May 17, 2017; Text beginning with the heading "Potential Threats to Brain Health" is excerpted from "Brain Health: You Can Make a Difference!" Administration for Community Living (ACL), September 2017.

The brain controls many aspects of thinking—remembering, planning, and organizing, making decisions, and much more. These cognitive abilities affect how well we do everyday tasks and whether we can live independently.

Some changes in thinking are common as people get older. For example, older adults may have:

- Increased difficulty finding words and recalling names

- More problems with multitasking

- Mild decreases in the ability to pay attention

Aging may also bring positive cognitive changes. People often have more knowledge and insight from a lifetime of experiences. Research shows that older adults can still:

- Learn new things

- Create new memories

- Improve vocabulary and language skills

The Older, Healthy Brain

As a person gets older, changes occur in all parts of the body, including the brain.

- Certain parts of the brain shrink, especially those important to learning and other complex mental activities.

- In certain brain regions, communication between neurons (nerve cells) can be reduced.

- Blood flow in the brain may also decrease.

- Inflammation, which occurs when the body responds to an injury or disease, may increase.

These changes in the brain can affect mental function, even in healthy older people. For example, some older adults find that they don't do as well as younger people on complex memory or learning tests. Given enough time, though, they can do as well. There is growing evidence that the brain remains "plastic"—able to adapt to new challenges and tasks—as people age.

It is not clear why some people think well as they get older while others do not. One possible reason is "cognitive reserve," the brain's ability to work well even when some part of it is disrupted. People with more education seem to have more cognitive reserve than others.

Some brain changes, like those associated with Alzheimer disease (AD), are NOT a normal part of aging. Talk with your healthcare provider if you are concerned.

Potential Threats to Brain Health

Health Conditions

Some health conditions can negatively affect your brain. Heart disease, high blood pressure, and diabetes can alter, or damage blood vessels throughout your body, including the brain. AD and other types of dementia also harm the brain. While no one knows how to prevent dementia, many approaches that are good for your health in other ways, including engaging in exercise and eating a healthy diet, are being tested.

Medicines

Some medications and certain combinations of drugs can affect your thinking and the way your brain works. Older adults taking medications should be particularly careful when consuming alcohol, as drugs may interact negatively with it.

Alcohol

Drinking alcohol can slow or impair communication among your brain cells. This can cause slurred speech, a fuzzy memory, drowsiness, and dizziness; it can also lead to long-term difficulties with your balance, memory, coordination, and body temperature.

Smoking

The risks associated with smoking are heart attacks, stroke, and lung disease.

Brain Injury

Older adults are at higher risk of falling and other accidents that can cause brain injury.

Actions You Can Take to Help Protect Your Brain

Take Charge

- Get recommended health screenings regularly.
- Manage health conditions, such as diabetes, high blood pressure, and high cholesterol.
- Be sure to talk with your doctor or pharmacist about the medications you take and any possible side effects on memory, sleep, and how your brain works.
- To learn more about how to move or exercise in a healthy way, ask your healthcare provider about your personal situation.

Eat Right

Try to maintain a balanced diet of fruits and vegetables, whole grains, lean meats (including fish and poultry), and low-fat or nonfat dairy products. Monitor your intake of solid fat, sugar, and salt, and eat proper portion sizes.

Get Moving

Being physically active may help reduce the risk of conditions that can harm brain health, such as diabetes, heart disease, depression, and stroke; it may also help improve connections among your brain cells. Older adults should get at least 150 minutes of exercise each week.

Drink Moderately, If at All

Staying away from alcohol can reverse some negative changes related to brain health.

Don't Smoke

Quitting smoking at any age will be beneficial to the health of your mind and body. Nonsmokers have a lower risk of heart attacks, stroke and lung diseases, as well as increased blood circulation.

Be Safe

To reduce the risk of falling, exercise to improve balance and coordination, take a falls prevention class, and make your home safer.

Think and Connect

Keep your mind active by doing mentally stimulating activities like reading, playing games, learning new things, teaching or taking a class and being social. Older adults who remain active and engaged with others by doing activities like volunteering report being happier and healthier overall.

Taking the First Step

You can start to support your brain health with some small, first steps, and build from there.

- Begin an exercise routine, such as a daily walk, with the goal of increasing the amount of time and speed.

- Add an extra serving of fruit and vegetables each day.

- Make an appointment for a health screening or a physical exam.

- Seek out volunteer opportunities that interest you.

- Sign up for a class or program at your community college or community center.

Chapter 3

How Toxins Affect the Brain

Chapter Contents

Section 3.1

Impact of Drug Abuse and Addiction on the Brain

This section includes text excerpted from "Understanding Drug Use and Addiction," National Institute on Drug Abuse (NIDA), August 2016.

Many people don't understand why or how other people become addicted to drugs. They may mistakenly think that those who use drugs lack moral principles or willpower and that they could stop their drug use simply by choosing to. In reality, drug addiction is a complex disease, and quitting usually takes more than good intentions or a strong will. Drugs change the brain in ways that make quitting hard, even for those who want to. Fortunately, researchers know more than ever about how drugs affect the brain and have found treatments that can help people recover from drug addiction and lead productive lives.

What Is Drug Addiction?

Addiction is a chronic disease characterized by drug seeking and use that is compulsive, or difficult to control, despite harmful consequences. The initial decision to take drugs is voluntary for most people, but repeated drug use can lead to brain changes that challenge an addicted person's self-control and interfere with their ability to resist intense urges to take drugs. These brain changes can be persistent, which is why drug addiction is considered a "relapsing" disease—people in recovery from drug use disorders are at increased risk for returning to drug use even after years of not taking the drug.

It's common for a person to relapse, but relapse doesn't mean that treatment doesn't work. As with other chronic health conditions, treatment should be ongoing and should be adjusted based on how the patient responds. Treatment plans need to be reviewed often and modified to fit the patient's changing needs.

28

What Happens to the Brain When a Person Takes Drugs?

Most drugs affect the brain's "reward circuit" by flooding it with the chemical messenger dopamine. This reward system controls the body's ability to feel pleasure and motivates a person to repeat behaviors needed to thrive, such as eating and spending time with loved ones. This overstimulation of the reward circuit causes the intensely pleasurable "high" that can lead people to take a drug again and again.

As a person continues to use drugs, the brain adjusts to the excess dopamine by making less of it and/or reducing the ability of cells in the reward circuit to respond to it. This reduces the high that the person feels compared to the high they felt when first taking the drug—an effect known as tolerance. They might take more of the drug, trying to achieve the same dopamine high. It can also cause them to get less pleasure from other things they once enjoyed, like food or social activities.

Long-term use also causes changes in other brain chemical systems and circuits as well, affecting functions that include:

- learning
- judgment
- decision-making
- stress
- memory
- behavior

Despite being aware of these harmful outcomes, many people who use drugs continue to take them, which is the nature of addiction.

Why Do Some People Become Addicted to Drugs While Others Don't?

No one factor can predict if a person will become addicted to drugs. A combination of factors influences risk for addiction. The more risk factors a person has, the greater the chance that taking drugs can lead to addiction. For example:

- **Biology.** The genes that people are born with account for about half of a person's risk for addiction. Gender, ethnicity, and the presence of other mental disorders may also influence risk for drug use and addiction.

- **Environment.** A person's environment includes many different influences, from family and friends to economic status and general quality of life. Factors such as peer pressure, physical and sexual abuse, early exposure to drugs, stress, and parental guidance can greatly affect a person's likelihood of drug use and addiction.

- **Development.** Genetic and environmental factors interact with critical developmental stages in a person's life to affect addiction risk. Although taking drugs at any age can lead to addiction, the earlier that drug use begins, the more likely it will progress to addiction. This is particularly problematic for teens. Because areas in their brains that control decision-making, judgment, and self-control are still developing, teens may be especially prone to risky behaviors, including trying drugs.

Can Drug Addiction Be Cured or Prevented?

As with most other chronic diseases, such as diabetes, asthma, or heart disease, treatment for drug addiction generally isn't a cure. However, addiction is treatable and can be successfully managed. People who are recovering from an addiction will be at risk for relapse for years and possibly for their whole lives. Research shows that combining addiction treatment medicines with behavioral therapy ensures the best chance of success for most patients. Treatment approaches tailored to each patient's drug use patterns and any co-occurring medical, mental, and social problems can lead to continued recovery.

More good news is that drug use and addiction are preventable. Results from National Institute on Drug Abuse (NIDA)-funded research have shown that prevention programs involving families, schools, communities, and the media are effective for preventing or reducing drug use and addiction. Although personal events and cultural factors affect drug use trends, when young people view drug use as harmful, they tend to decrease their drug taking. Therefore, education and outreach are key in helping people understand the possible risks of drug use. Teachers, parents, and healthcare providers have crucial roles in educating young people and preventing drug use and addiction.

Section 3.2

Mercury and Neurodevelopment

This section contains text excerpted from the following sources: Text
in this section begins with excerpts from "ToxFAQsTM—Mercury,"
Agency for Toxic Substances and Disease Registry (ATSDR),
Centers for Disease Control and Prevention (CDC), February 12,
2013. Reviewed February 2018; Text under the heading "Studies
on Neurodevelopmental Effects of Prenatal Mercury Exposure" is
excerpted from "Neurodevelopmental Disorders," U.S. Environmental
Protection Agency (EPA), October 2015; Text under the heading
"Brain Benefits of Aerobic Exercise Lost to Mercury Exposure" is
excerpted from "Brain Benefits of Aerobic Exercise Lost to
Mercury Exposure," National Institute of Environmental
Health Sciences (NIEHS), January 3, 2017.

Mercury is a naturally occurring metal which has several forms. The metallic mercury is a shiny, silver-white, odorless liquid. If heated, it is a colorless, odorless gas.

Mercury combines with other elements, such as chlorine, sulfur, or oxygen, to form inorganic mercury compounds or "salts," which are usually white powders or crystals. Mercury also combines with carbon to make organic mercury compounds. The most common one, methylmercury, is produced mainly by microscopic organisms in the water and soil. More mercury in the environment can increase the amounts of methylmercury that these small organisms make.

Metallic mercury is used to produce chlorine gas and caustic soda, and is also used in thermometers, dental fillings, and batteries. Mercury salts are sometimes used in skin lightening creams and as antiseptic creams and ointments.

What Happens to Mercury When It Enters the Environment?

- Inorganic mercury (metallic mercury and inorganic mercury compounds) enters the air from mining ore deposits, burning coal and waste, and from manufacturing plants.

31

• It enters the water or soil from natural deposits, disposal of wastes, and volcanic activity.

• Methylmercury may be formed in water and soil by small organisms called bacteria.

• Methylmercury builds up in the tissues of fish. Larger and older fish tend to have the highest levels of mercury.

How Might I Be Exposed to Mercury?

• Eating fish or shellfish contaminated with methylmercury.

• Breathing vapors in air from spills, incinerators, and industries that burn mercury-containing fuels.

• Release of mercury from dental work and medical treatments.

• Breathing contaminated workplace air or skin contact during use in the workplace.

• Practicing rituals that include mercury.

How Can Mercury Affect My Health?

The nervous system is very sensitive to all forms of mercury. Methylmercury and metallic mercury vapors are more harmful than other forms, because more mercury in these forms reaches the brain. Exposure to high levels of metallic, inorganic, or organic mercury can permanently damage the brain, kidneys, and developing fetus. Effects on brain functioning may result in irritability, shyness, tremors, changes in vision or hearing, and memory problems.

How Does Mercury Affect Children?

Very young children are more sensitive to mercury than adults. Mercury in the mother's body passes to the fetus and may accumulate there. It can also pass to a nursing infant through breast milk. However, the benefits of breastfeeding may be greater than the possible adverse effects of mercury in breast milk.

Mercury's harmful effects that may be passed from the mother to the fetus include brain damage, mental retardation, incoordination, blindness, seizures, and inability to speak.

How Can Families Reduce the Risk of Exposure to Mercury?

Carefully handle and dispose of products that contain mercury, such as thermometers or fluorescent light bulbs. Do not vacuum up spilled mercury, because it will vaporize and increase exposure. If a large amount of mercury has been spilled, contact your health department. Teach children not to play with shiny, silver liquids.

Properly dispose of older medicines that contain mercury. Keep all mercury-containing medicines away from children.

Pregnant women and children should keep away from rooms where liquid mercury has been used.

Learn about wildlife and fish advisories in your area from your public health or natural resources department.

Is There a Medical Test to Show Whether I've Been Exposed to Mercury?

Tests are available to measure mercury levels in the body. Blood or urine samples are used to test for exposure to metallic mercury and to inorganic forms of mercury. Mercury in whole blood or in scalp hair is measured to determine exposure to methylmercury. Your doctor can take samples and send them to a testing laboratory.

Studies on Neurodevelopmental Effects of Prenatal Mercury Exposure

U.S. Environmental Protection Agency (EPA) has determined that methylmercury is known to have neurotoxic and developmental effects in humans. Extreme cases of such effects were seen in people prenatally exposed during two high-dose mercury poisoning events in Japan and Iraq, who experienced severe adverse health effects such as cerebral palsy, mental retardation, deafness, and blindness. Prospective cohort studies have been conducted in island populations where frequent fish consumption leads to methylmercury exposure in pregnant women at levels much lower than in the poisoning incidents but much greater than those typically observed in the United States. Results from such studies in New Zealand and the Faroe Islands suggest that increased prenatal mercury exposure due to maternal fish consumption was associated with adverse effects on intelligence and decreased functioning in the areas of language, attention, and memory. More recent studies conducted in the United States have found associations between neurodevelopmental effects and blood mercury levels within the range typical for U.S. women, after accounting for the beneficial effects of fish consumption during pregnancy.

Brain Benefits of Aerobic Exercise Lost to Mercury Exposure

Cognitive function improves with aerobic exercise, but not in people exposed to high levels of mercury before birth, according to research funded in part by National Institute of Environmental Health Sciences (NIEHS).

Methylmercury is known to have toxic effects on the developing brain and nervous system. In vitro studies show that mercury is particularly toxic to neuronal stem cells. A team of scientists, led by Philippe Grandjean, M.D., of the Harvard T.H. Chan School of Public Health, suspected that prenatal exposure could limit the ability of nervous system tissues to grow and develop in response to increased aerobic fitness.

"If prenatal exposure to methylmercury causes a decrease in stem cells in the brain, this could represent an effect that may be silent at first, but could be unmasked later in life when stem cells are required to maintain or expand brain functions," Grandjean said.

Section 3.3

Dangers of Lead Exposure

This section contains text excerpted from the following sources: Text in this section begins with excerpts from "Learn about Lead," U.S. Environmental Protection Agency (EPA), May 26, 2017; Text beginning with the heading "Pathway of Lead Exposure in Children" is excerpted from "Lead Toxicity," Agency for Toxic Substances and Disease Registry (ATSDR), Centers for Disease Control and Prevention (CDC) June 12, 2017.

Lead is a naturally occurring element found in small amounts in the earth's crust. While it has some beneficial uses, it can be toxic to humans and animals causing health effects.

Where Is Lead Found?

Lead can be found in all parts of our environment—the air, the soil, the water, and even inside our homes. Much of our exposure comes from human activities including the use of fossil fuels including past use of leaded gasoline, some types of industrial facilities, and past use of lead-based paint in homes. Lead and lead compounds have been used in a wide variety of products found in and around our homes, including paint, ceramics, pipes and plumbing materials, solders, gasoline, batteries, ammunition, and cosmetics.

Lead may enter the environment from these past and current uses. Lead can also be emitted into the environment from industrial sources and contaminated sites, such as former lead smelters. While natural levels of lead in soil range between 50 and 400 parts per million (ppm), mining, smelting, and refining activities have resulted in substantial increases in lead levels in the environment, especially near mining and smelting sites.

When lead is released to the air from industrial sources or vehicles, it may travel long distances before settling to the ground, where it usually sticks to soil particles. Lead may move from soil into ground-water depending on the type of lead compound and the characteristics of the soil.

Federal and state regulatory standards have helped to reduce the amount of lead in air, drinking water, soil, consumer products, food, and occupational settings.

Lead Exposure in Pregnant Women

Lead can accumulate in our bodies over time, where it is stored in bones along with calcium. During pregnancy, lead is released from bones as maternal calcium and is used to help form the bones of the fetus. This is particularly true if a woman does not have enough dietary calcium. Lead can also cross the placental barrier exposing the fetus the lead. This can result in serious effects to the mother and her developing fetus, including:

- Reduced growth of the fetus
- Premature birth

Pathway of Lead Exposure in Children

- The nervous system is the most sensitive organ system for lead exposure in children

- Lead toxicity can affect every organ system.

- On a molecular level, proposed mechanisms for toxicity involve fundamental biochemical processes. These include lead's ability to inhibit or mimic the actions of calcium (which can affect calcium-dependent or related processes) and to interact with proteins (including those with sulfhydryl, amine, phosphate, and carboxyl groups)

- Lead's high affinity for sulfhydryl groups makes it particularly toxic to multiple enzyme systems including heme biosynthesis.

- The National Toxicology Program (NTP), and the American Academy of Pediatrics (AAP) have concluded that there is sufficient evidence for adverse health effects in children and adults at blood lead levels (BLLs) <5 micrograms per deciliter (μg/dL).

- "There is no identified threshold or safe level of lead in blood"

- It is important to control or eliminate all sources of lead in children's environments to prevent exposure.

Specific Neurological Effects for Population Groups

In children, there is no identified threshold or "safe" blood lead level below which no risk of poor developmental or intellectual function is expected. Data from the NTP showed that the effect of concurrent BLLs on IQ may be greater than currently believed.

Lead inhibits the bodies of growing children from absorbing iron, zinc and calcium, minerals essential to proper brain and nerve development.

- Children often show no signs of lead toxicity until they are in school, even as late as middle school, as expectations for academic achievement increase.

- The practicing healthcare provider can distinguish overt clinical symptoms and health effects that come with high exposure levels on an individual basis.

- However, lack of overt symptoms does not mean "no adverse impact."

- Lower levels of exposure have been shown to have many subtle adverse health effects.

- Medical research has established a connection between early childhood lead exposure and future criminal activity, especially of a violent nature. Numerous studies link elevated bone or blood lead levels with aggression, destructive and delinquent behavior, attention deficit hyperactivity disorder and criminal behavior.

- Acute exposure to very high levels of lead may produce encephalopathy in children.

While the immediate health effect of concern in children is typically neurological, it is important to remember that childhood lead poisoning can lead to health effects later in life, including

- attention deficit hyperactivity disorder (ADHD), delayed learning, and lower IQ (which will impact school performance),

- Developmental problems with their offspring,

- Hypertension,

- Renal effects, and

- Reproductive problems.

The neurological effects in an adult exposed to lead as an adult can be neuropathy, and may be different from those of an adult exposed to lead as a child when the brain was developing.

- Childhood neurological effects, including ADHD, may persist into adulthood.

- Lead-exposed adults may also experience many of the neurological symptoms experienced by children, but shown at higher blood lead levels

Section 3.4

Manganese and Brain Damage

This section includes text excerpted from "Public Health Statement—Manganese," Agency for Toxic Substances and Disease Registry (ATSDR), Centers for Disease Control and Prevention (CDC), January 21, 2015.

The U.S. Environmental Protection Agency (EPA) identifies the most serious hazardous waste sites in the nation. These sites are then placed on the National Priorities List (NPL) and are targeted for long-term federal clean-up activities. Manganese has been found in at least 869 of the 1,699 current or former NPL sites. Although the total number of NPL sites evaluated for this substance is not known, the possibility exists that the number of sites at which manganese is found may increase in the future as more sites are evaluated. This information is important because these sites may be sources of exposure, and exposure to this substance may harm you.

When a substance is released either from a large area, such as an industrial plant, or from a container, such as a drum or bottle, it enters the environment. Such a release does not always lead to exposure. You can be exposed to a substance only when you come in contact with it. You may be exposed by breathing, eating, or drinking the substance, or by skin contact.

If you are exposed to manganese, many factors will determine whether you will be harmed. These factors include the dose (how much), the duration (how long), and how you come in contact with it. You must also consider any other chemicals you are exposed to and your age, sex, diet, family traits, lifestyle, and state of health.

What Is Manganese?

Manganese is a naturally occurring substance found in many types of rocks and soil. Pure manganese is a silver-colored metal; however, it does not occur in the environment as a pure metal. Rather, it occurs combined with other substances such as oxygen, sulfur, and chlorine. Manganese is a trace element and is necessary for good health.

Uses

- **Manufacturing.** Manganese is used principally in steel production to improve hardness, stiffness, and strength. It is used in carbon steel, stainless steel, high-temperature steel, and tool steel, along with cast iron and superalloys.

- **Consumer products.** Manganese occurs naturally in most foods and may be added to food or made available in nutritional supplements. Manganese is also used in a wide variety of other products, including:

  - fireworks
  - dry-cell batteries
  - fertilizer
  - paints
  - a medical imaging agent
  - cosmetics

- It may also be used as an additive in gasoline to improve the octane rating of the gas.

Small amounts of manganese are used in a pharmaceutical product called mangafodipir trisodium (Mn DPDP) to improve lesion detection in magnetic resonance imaging of body organs.

What Happens to Manganese When It Enters the Environment?

Sources

Manganese is a normal constituent of air, soil, water, and food. Additional manganese can be found in air, soil, and water after release from the manufacture, use, and disposal of manganese-based products.

Breakdown

As with other elements, manganese cannot break down in the environment. It can only change its form or become attached or separated from particles. The chemical state of manganese and the type of soil determine how fast it moves through the soil and how much is retained in the soil. In water, most of the manganese tends to attach to particles in the water or settle into the sediment. The manganese-containing gasoline additive may degrade in the environment quickly when exposed to sunlight, releasing manganese.

How Might I Be Exposed to Manganese?

Food—Primary Source of Exposure

The primary way you can be exposed to manganese is by eating food or manganese-containing nutritional supplements. Vegetarians who consume foods rich in manganese such as grains, beans and nuts, as well as heavy tea drinkers, may have a higher intake of manganese than the average person.

Workplace Air

Certain occupations like welding or working in a factory where steel is made may increase your chances of being exposed to high levels of manganese.

Water and Soil

Because manganese is a natural component of the environment, you are always exposed to low levels of it in water, air, soil, and food. Manganese is routinely contained in groundwater, drinking water and soil at low levels. Drinking water containing manganese or swimming or bathing in water containing manganese may expose you to low levels of this chemical.

Air

Air also contains low levels of manganese, and breathing air may expose you to it. Releases of manganese into the air occur from:

- industries using or manufacturing products containing manganese,

- mining activities, and

- automobile exhaust.

Lifestyle traits may also lead to exposure to manganese. People who smoke tobacco or inhale second-hand smoke are typically exposed to manganese at levels higher than those not exposed to tobacco smoke.

How Can Manganese Enter and Leave My Body?

Enter Your Body

- **Inhalation.** When you breathe air containing manganese, a small amount of the manganese will enter your body through your lungs and the remainder can become trapped in your lungs. Some of the manganese in your lungs can also be trapped in mucus which you may cough up and swallow into your stomach.

- **Ingestion.** Manganese in food or water may enter your body through the digestive tract to meet your body's needs for normal functioning.

- **Dermal contact.** Only very small amounts of manganese can enter your skin when you come into contact with liquids containing manganese.

Leave Your Body

Once in your body, manganese-containing chemicals can break down into other chemicals. However, manganese is an element that cannot be broken down. Most manganese will leave your body in feces within a few days.

How Can Manganese Affect My Health?

General Population

Manganese is an essential nutrient, and eating a small amount of it each day is important to stay healthy.

Workers

Inhalation. The most common health problems in workers exposed to high levels of manganese involve the nervous system. These health effects include behavioral changes and other nervous system effects, which include movements that may become slow and clumsy. This combination of symptoms when sufficiently severe is referred to as "manganism." Other less severe nervous system effects such as slowed hand movements have been observed in some workers exposed to lower concentrations in the workplace.

The inhalation of a large quantity of dust or fumes containing manganese may cause irritation of the lungs which could lead to pneumonia.

Loss of sex drive and sperm damage has also been observed in men exposed to high levels of manganese in workplace air.

The manganese concentrations that cause effects such as slowed hand movements in some workers are approximately twenty thousand times higher than the concentrations normally found in the environment. Manganism has been found in some workers exposed to manganese concentrations about a million times higher than normal air concentrations of manganese.

Laboratory Animals

Inhalation. Respiratory effects, similar to those observed in workers, have been observed in laboratory monkeys exposed to high levels of manganese.

Laboratory Animals

Oral. Manganese has been shown to cross the blood-brain barrier and a limited amount of manganese is also able to cross the placenta during pregnancy, enabling it to reach a developing fetus.

Nervous system disturbances have been observed in animals after very high oral doses of manganese, including changes in behavior.

Sperm damage and adverse changes in male reproductive performance were observed in laboratory animals fed high levels of manganese. Impairments in fertility were observed in female rodents provided with oral manganese before they became pregnant.

Illnesses involving the kidneys and urinary tract have been observed in laboratory rats fed very high levels of manganese. These illnesses included inflammation of the kidneys and kidney stone formation.

Cancer

The EPA concluded that existing scientific information cannot determine whether or not excess manganese can cause cancer.

How Can Manganese Affect Children?

The potential health effects in humans from exposures during the period from conception to maturity at 18 years of age is discussed below.

Effects in Children

Studies in children have suggested that extremely high levels of manganese exposure may produce undesirable effects on brain development, including changes in behavior and decreases in the ability to learn and remember. In some cases, these same manganese exposure levels have been suspected of causing severe symptoms of manganism disease (including difficulty with speech and walking). We do not know for certain that these changes were caused by manganese alone. We do not know if these changes are temporary or permanent. We do not know whether children are more sensitive than adults to the effects of manganese, but there is some indication from experiments in laboratory animals that they may be.

Birth Defects

Studies of manganese workers have not found increases in birth defects or low birth weight in their children.

No birth defects were observed in animals exposed to manganese

In one human study where people were exposed to very high levels of manganese from drinking water, infants less than 1 year of age died at an unusually high rate. It is not clear, however, whether these deaths were attributable to the manganese level of the drinking water. The manganese toxicity may have involved exposures to the infant that occurred both before (through the mother) and after they were born.

How Can Families Reduce the Risk of Exposure to Manganese?

Avoid Inhalation of Manganese at Work

High levels of airborne manganese are observed in certain occupational settings such as steel factories or welding areas. You should take precautions to prevent inhalation of manganese by wearing an appropriate mask to limit the amount of manganese you breathe.

Avoid Wearing Manganese Dust-Contaminated Work Clothing in Your Home or Car

Workers exposed to high levels of airborne manganese in certain occupational settings may accumulate manganese dust on their work clothes. Manganese-contaminated work clothing should be removed before getting into your car or entering your home to help reduce the exposure hazard for yourself and your family.

Avoid Inhalation of Welding Fumes at Home

If you weld objects around your home, do so in a well-ventilated area and use an appropriate mask to decrease your risk of inhaling manganese-containing fumes. Children should be kept away from welding fumes.

Diet

Children are not likely to be exposed to harmful amounts of manganese in the diet. However, higher-than-usual amounts of manganese may be absorbed if their diet is low in iron. It is important to provide your child with a well-balanced diet.

Water

While tap and bottled water generally contain safe levels of manganese, well water may sometimes be contaminated with sufficiently high levels of manganese to create a potential health hazard. If drinking water is obtained from a well water source, it may be wise to have the water checked for manganese to ensure the level is below the current guideline level established by the EPA.

Smoking

Manganese is a minor constituent of tobacco smoke. Avoiding tobacco smoke may reduce your family's exposure to manganese.

If your doctor finds that you have been exposed to significant amounts of manganese, ask whether your children might also be exposed. Your doctor might need to ask your state health department to investigate.

Is There a Medical Test to Determine Whether I Have Been Exposed to Manganese?

Detecting Exposure

Several tests are available to measure manganese in blood, urine, hair, or feces. Because manganese is normally present in our body, some is always found in tissues or fluids.

Normal ranges of manganese levels are about 4–15 μg/L in blood, 1–8 μg/L in urine, and 0.4–0.85 μg/L in serum (the fluid portion of the blood).

Measuring Exposure

Because excess manganese is usually removed from the body within a few days, past exposures are difficult to measure with common laboratory tests.

A medical test known as magnetic resonance imaging, or MRI, can detect the presence of increased amounts of manganese in the brain. However, this type of test is qualitative, and has not been shown to reliably reflect or predict toxicologically meaningful exposures.

What Recommendations Has the Federal Government Made to Protect Human Health?

The federal government develops regulations and recommendations to protect public health. Regulations can be enforced by law. The EPA, the Occupational Safety and Health Administration (OSHA), and the U.S. Food and Drug Administration (FDA) are some federal agencies that develop regulations for toxic substances. Recommendations provide valuable guidelines to protect public health, but cannot be enforced by law. The Agency for Toxic Substances and Disease Registry (ATSDR) and the National Institute for Occupational Safety and Health (NIOSH) are two federal organizations that develop recommendations for toxic substances.

Regulations and recommendations can be expressed as "not-to-exceed" levels, that is, levels of a toxic substance in air, water, soil, or food that do not exceed a critical value that is usually based on levels that affect animals; they are then adjusted to levels that will help protect humans. Sometimes these not-to-exceed levels differ among federal organizations because they used different exposure times (an 8-hour workday or a 24-hour day), different animal studies, or other factors.

Recommendations and regulations are also updated periodically as more information becomes available. For the most current information, check with the federal agency or organization that provides it. Some regulations and recommendations for manganese include the following:

Drinking Water

The EPA has established that exposure to manganese in drinking water at concentrations of 1 mg/L for 1 or 10 days is not expected to cause any adverse effects in a child.

The EPA has established that lifetime exposure to 0.3 mg/L manganese is not expected to cause any adverse effects.

Bottled Water

The FDA has established that the manganese concentration in bottled drinking water should not exceed 0.05 mg/L.

Workplace Air

OSHA set a legal limit of 5 mg/m^3 manganese in air averaged over an 8-hour work day.

Chapter 4

Signs and Symptoms of Brain Disorders

Chapter Contents

Section 4.1

Symptom Overview

"Symptom Overview," © 2018 Omnigraphics.
Reviewed February 2018.

The nervous system includes the brain, spinal cord, and a large network of nerves and neurons. The brain is the control center of the body, and it manages everything from senses to thought to muscles. Damage to the brain can lead to serious medical conditions that can affect such functions as sensation, memory, and even the personality of an individual. Brain disorders include many different conditions and diseases that affect the brain and its processes. These disorders can be caused by illness, genetics, or traumatic injury.

A recent study reported that more than 600 neurological disorders have been identified, and these can disturb the functioning of the brain, nerves, and spinal cord. Brain disorders are a very broad category, and they differ significantly in signs and symptoms and severity. Some of the common types of disorders are discussed below.

Types of Physical Brain Disorders and Their Symptoms

Stroke

Strokes occur when the blood flow to an area of the brain is cut off, resulting in damage to brain cells. There are two kinds of stroke attacks: hemorrhagic (rupture of a blood vessel) and ischemic (blockage or clot in a blood vessel).

Some of the symptoms of stroke include:

- trouble in speaking and understanding
- difficulty walking
- loss of coordination and balance
- dizziness
- sudden numbness in leg, arm, or face
- weakness
- severe headache

Multiple Sclerosis

Multiple sclerosis is a disabling disease that affects the brain and spinal cord nerve cells that are responsible for the proper functioning of the nervous system. In multiple sclerosis, the protective sheath (myelin) that covers the nerve fibers is attacked by the body's immune system, causing an interruption of communication between the brain and other parts of the body.

The following are the most common symptoms of multiple sclerosis:

- weakness or numbness in one or more limbs or muscles
- fatigue, dizziness, or slurred speech
- double vision or vision loss
- trouble with thinking and memory
- lack of coordination

Brain Tumors

A collection of abnormal cells in the brain is known as a brain tumor. They can occur at any age and can be malignant (cancerous) or benign (noncancerous). When the tumors grow they can cause increase in intracranial pressure, which can be life-threatening. Tumors are divided into two types. Primary tumors originate in the brain and can be benign or cancerous in nature, while secondary tumors develop when cancer from another part of the body spreads to the brain.

Some of the symptoms of brain tumors include:

- headaches, usually severe in the morning and worsened by coughing, sneezing, or exercise
- vomiting
- nausea
- blurred or double vision
- seizures
- personality changes
- imbalance
- confusion and clumsiness
- memory loss
- eye problems
- difficulty swallowing
- vertigo or dizziness

- difficulty reading and writing
- muscle weakness
- loss of bowel and bladder control
- hand tremors
- loss of balance

Neurodegenerative Diseases

Neurodegenerative diseases can affect the neurons and nerves in the brain and cause them to deteriorate over time. They also damage brain tissues and nerves, frequently causing a change in the individual's personality. Common neurodegenerative diseases include Alzheimer disease (AD), amyotrophic lateral sclerosis (ALS, or Lou Gehrig disease), Huntington disease, Parkinson disease, and various forms of dementia.

Some of the symptoms of neurodegenerative diseases include:

- anxiety
- mood changes
- agitation
- apathy
- memory loss

Mental and Emotional Brain Disorders and Their Symptoms

Mental Disorders

Mental disorders are a group of conditions that can affect an individual's behavior patterns. Some mental disorders include depression, anxiety, posttraumatic stress disorder (PTSD), and schizophrenia. The kind of treatment administered to the patients for mental disorders depends on the type and severity of the condition.

Symptoms can vary depending on the particular condition but may include:

- withdrawal from social life
- inability to cope with stress and daily problems
- changes in sex drive
- changes in eating habits
- trouble understanding and relating to people and situations

- excessive anger or violence
- drug abuse or alcoholism
- confused thinking
- extreme mood swings
- extreme fear or worry
- hallucinations
- detachment from reality
- sleep issues
- tiredness and low energy

Emotional Disorders

An individual suffering from any kind of brain disorder may also experience a variety of emotional issues. And the symptoms of these issues can sometimes help identify underlying neurological problems.
Some of these emotional symptoms include:

- depression
- delusion
- mood swings
- sudden emotional outbursts

The appropriate medication is administered to patients experiencing neurological problems based on the symptoms and diagnosis of the disorder.

References

1. "5 Most Common Types of Neurological Disorders & Their Symptoms," Apollo Hospitals, September 23, 2016.
2. Lights, Verneda. "Brain Tumor," Healthline, April 21, 2017.
3. "Mental Illness," Mayo Clinic, October 13, 2015.
4. "Multiple Sclerosis," Mayo Clinic, August 4, 2017.
5. "Neurological Problem Symptoms, Causes, and Effects," PsychGuides.com, August 31, 2013.
6. Reed-Guy, Lauren. "Brain Disorders," Healthline, September 18, 2017.

Section 4.2

Headache

This section includes text excerpted from "Headache: Hope
through Research," National Institute of Neurological
Disorders and Stroke (NINDS), April 2016.

Anyone can experience a headache. Nearly 2 out of 3 children will
have a headache by age 15. More than 9 in 10 adults will experience a
headache sometime in their life. Headache is our most common form
of pain and a major reason cited for days missed at work or school as
well as visits to the doctor. Without proper treatment, headaches can
be severe and interfere with daily activities.

Certain types of headache run in families. Episodes of headache
may ease or even disappear for a time and recur later in life. It's possible to have more than one type of headache at the same time.

- **Primary headaches** occur independently and are not caused
  by another medical condition. It's uncertain what sets the process of a primary headache in motion. A cascade of events that
  affect blood vessels and nerves inside and outside the head
  causes pain signals to be sent to the brain. Brain chemicals
  called neurotransmitters are involved in creating head pain,
  as are changes in nerve cell activity (called cortical spreading
  depression). Migraine, cluster, and tension-type headache are
  the more familiar types of primary headache.

- **Secondary headaches** are symptoms of another health disorder that causes pain-sensitive nerve endings to be pressed on or
  pulled or pushed out of place. They may result from underlying
  conditions including fever, infection, medication overuse, stress
  or emotional conflict, high blood pressure, psychiatric disorders,
  head injury or trauma, stroke, tumors, and nerve disorders (particularly trigeminal neuralgia, a chronic pain condition that typically affects a major nerve on one side of the jaw or cheek).

Headaches can range in frequency and severity of pain. Some individuals may experience headaches once or twice a year, while others

may experience headaches more than 15 days a month. Some head-aches may recur or last for weeks at a time. Pain can range from mild to disabling and may be accompanied by symptoms such as nausea or increased sensitivity to noise or light, depending on the type of headache.

Why Headaches Hurt

Information about touch, pain, temperature, and vibration in the head and neck is sent to the brain by the *trigeminal* nerve, one of 12 pairs of cranial nerves that start at the base of the brain. The nerve has three branches that conduct sensations from the scalp, the blood vessels inside and outside of the skull, the lining around the brain (the *meninges*), and the face, mouth, neck, ears, eyes, and throat.

Brain tissue itself lacks pain-sensitive nerves and does not feel pain. Headaches occur when pain-sensitive nerve endings called *nociceptors* react to headache triggers (such as stress, certain foods or odors, or use of medicines) and send messages through the *trigeminal* nerve to the thalamus, the brain's "relay station" for pain sensation from all over the body. The thalamus controls the body's sensitivity to light and noise and sends messages to parts of the brain that manage awareness of pain and emotional response to it. Other parts of the brain may also be part of the process, causing nausea, vomiting, diarrhea, trouble concentrating, and other neurological symptoms.

When to See a Doctor

Not all headaches require a physician's attention. But headaches can signal a more serious disorder that requires prompt medical care. Immediately call or see a physician if you or someone you're with experience any of these symptoms:

- Sudden, severe headache that may be accompanied by a stiff neck.

- Severe headache accompanied by fever, nausea, or vomiting that is not related to another illness.

- "First" or "worst" headache, often accompanied by confusion, weakness, double vision, or loss of consciousness.

- Headache that worsens over days or weeks or has changed in pattern or behavior.

- Recurring headache in children.

- Headache following a head injury.

- Headache and a loss of sensation or weakness in any part of the body, which could be a sign of a stroke.

- Headache associated with convulsions.

- Headache associated with shortness of breath.

- Two or more headaches a week.

- Persistent headache in someone who has been previously headache-free, particularly in someone over age 50.

- New headaches in someone with a history of cancer or human immunodeficiency virus (HIV)/acquired immunodeficiency syndrome (AIDS).

Diagnosing Your Headache

How and under what circumstances a person experiences a headache can be key to diagnosing its cause. Keeping a headache journal can help a physician better diagnose your type of headache and determine the best treatment. After each headache, note the time of day when it occurred; its intensity and duration; any sensitivity to light, odors, or sound; activity immediately prior to the headache; use of prescription and nonprescription medicines; amount of sleep the previous night; any stressful or emotional conditions; any influence from weather or daily activity; foods and fluids consumed in the past 24 hours; and any known health conditions at that time. Women should record the days of their menstrual cycles. Include notes about other family members who have a history of headache or other disorder. A pattern may emerge that can be helpful to reducing or preventing headaches.

Once your doctor has reviewed your medical and headache history and conducted a physical and neurological exam, lab screening and diagnostic tests may be ordered to either rule out or identify conditions that might be the cause of your headaches. Blood tests and urinalysis can help diagnose brain or spinal cord infections, blood vessel damage, and toxins that affect the nervous system. Testing a sample of the fluid that surrounds the brain and spinal cord can detect infections, bleeding in the brain (called a brain hemorrhage), and measure any buildup of pressure within the skull. Diagnostic imaging, such as with computed tomography (CT) and magnetic resonance imaging (MRI), can detect irregularities in blood vessels and bones, certain brain tumors and cysts, brain damage from head injury, brain hemorrhage, inflammation, infection, and other disorders. Neuroimaging also gives doctors a way to see what's happening in the brain during headache attacks. An electroencephalogram (EEG) measures brainwave activity and can help diagnose brain tumors, seizures, head injury, and inflammation that may lead to headaches.

Secondary Headache Disorders

Secondary headache disorders are caused by an underlying illness or condition that affects the brain. Secondary headaches are usually diagnosed based on other symptoms that occur concurrently and the characteristics of the headaches. Some of the more serious causes of secondary headache include:

Brain tumor. A tumor that is growing in the brain can press against nerve tissue and pain-sensitive blood vessel walls, disrupting communication between the brain and the nerves or restricting the supply of blood to the brain. Headaches may develop, worsen, become more frequent, or come and go, often at irregular periods. Headache pain may worsen when coughing, changing posture, or straining, and may be severe upon waking. Treatment options include surgery, radiation therapy, and chemotherapy. However, the vast majority of individuals with headache do not have brain tumors.

Disorders of blood vessels in the brain, including stroke. Several disorders associated with blood vessel formation and activity can cause headache. Most notable among these conditions is stroke. Headache itself can cause stroke or accompany a series of blood vessel disorders that can cause a stroke.

There are two forms of stroke. A hemorrhagic stroke occurs when an artery in the brain bursts, spilling blood into the surrounding tissue. An ischemic stroke occurs when an artery supplying the brain with blood becomes blocked, suddenly decreasing or stopping blood flow and causing brain cells to die.

Hemorrhagic stroke. A hemorrhagic stroke is usually associated with disturbed brain function and an extremely painful headache that develops suddenly and may worsen with physical activity, coughing, or straining. Headache conditions associated with hemorrhagic stroke include:

- A **subarachnoid hemorrhage (SCH)** is the rupture of a blood vessel located within the subarachnoid space-a fluid-filled space between layers of connective tissue (meninges) that surround the brain. The first sign of a subarachnoid hemorrhage is typically a severe headache with a split-second onset and no known cause. Neurologists call this a thunderclap headache. Pain may also be felt in the neck and lower back. This sudden flood of blood can contaminate the cerebrospinal fluid that flows within the spaces of the brain and cause extensive damage throughout the brain.

• **Intracerebral hemorrhage (ICH)** is usually associated with severe headache. Several conditions can render blood vessels in the brain prone to rupture and hemorrhaging. Chronic hypertension can weaken the blood vessel wall. Poor blood clotting ability due to blood disorders or blood-thinning medications like warfarin further increase the risk of bleeding. And some venous strokes (caused by clots in the brain's veins) often cause bleeding into the brain. At risk are mothers in the postpartum period and persons with dehydration, cancer, or infections.

• An **aneurysm** is the abnormal ballooning of an artery that causes the artery wall to weaken. A ruptured cerebral aneurysm can cause hemorrhagic stroke and a sudden, incredibly painful headache that is generally different in severity and intensity from other headaches individuals may have experienced. Individuals usually describe the thunderclap-like headache as "the worst headache of my life." There may be loss of consciousness and other neurological features. "Sentinel" or sudden warning headaches sometimes occur from an aneurysm that leaks prior to rupture. Cerebral aneurysms that have leaked or ruptured are life-threatening and require emergency medical attention. Not all aneurysms burst, and people with very small aneurysms may be monitored to detect any growth or onset of symptoms. Treatment options include blocking the flow of blood to the aneurysm surgically (intra-arterial) and catheter techniques to fill the aneurysm with coils or balloons.

• **Arteriovenous malformation (AVM)**, an abnormal tangle of arteries and veins in the brain, causes headaches that vary in frequency, duration, and intensity as vascular malformations press on and displace normal tissue or leak blood into surrounding tissue. A headache consistently affecting one side of the head may be closely linked to the site of an AVM (although most one-sided headaches are caused by primary headache disorders).

Symptoms may include seizures and hearing pulsating noises. Treatment options include decreasing blood flow to and from the malformation by injecting particles or glue, or through focused radiotherapy or surgery.

Ischemic stroke. Headache that accompanies ischemic stroke can be caused by several problems with the brain's vascular system. Headache is prominent in individuals with clots in the brain's veins. Head pain occurs on the side of the brain in which the clot blocks blood flow and is often felt in the eyes or on the side of the head. Conditions of ischemic stroke that can cause headache include:

- **Arterial dissection** is a tear within an artery that supplies the brain with blood flow. The most common dissection occurs in the carotid artery in the neck, with head pain on the same side of the body where the tear occurs. Vertebral artery dissection causes pain in the rear upper part of the neck. Cervical artery dissection can lead to stroke or transient ischemic attacks (strokes that last only a few minutes but signal a subsequent, more severe stroke). They are usually caused by neck strain, i.e., trauma, chiropractic manipulation, sports injuries, or even pronounced bending of the head backward over a sink for hair washing ("beauty parlor stroke"). Immediate medical attention can be lifesaving.

- **Vascular inflammation** can cause the buildup of plaque, which can lead to ischemic stroke. Cerebral vasculitis, an inflammation of the brain's blood vessel system, may cause headache, stroke, and/or progressive cognitive decline. Severe headache attributed to a chronic inflammatory disease of blood vessels on the outside of the head, called giant cell arteritis (previously known as temporal arteritis), usually affects people older than age 60. It also causes muscle pain and tenderness in the temple area. Individuals also may experience temporary, followed by permanent, loss of vision on one or both eyes, pain with chewing, a tender scalp, muscle aches, depression, and fatigue. Corticosteroids are typically used to treat vascular inflammation and can prevent blindness.

Exposure to a substance or its withdrawal. Headaches may result from toxic states such as drinking alcohol, following carbon monoxide poisoning, or from exposure to toxic chemicals and metals, cleaning products or solvents, and pesticides. In the most severe cases, rising toxin levels can cause a pulsing, throbbing headache that, if left untreated, can lead to systemic poisoning, organ failure, and permanent neurological damage. These headaches are usually treated by identifying and removing the cause of the toxic buildup. The withdrawal from certain medicines or caffeine after frequent or excessive use can also cause headaches.

Head injury. Headaches are often a symptom of a concussion or other head injury. The headache may develop either immediately or months after a blow to the head, with pain felt at the injury site or throughout the head. Emotional disturbances may worsen headache pain. In most cases, the cause of posttraumatic headache is unknown. Sometimes the cause is ruptured blood vessels, which result in an accumulation of blood called a hematoma. This mass of blood can displace brain tissue and cause headaches as well as weakness, confusion, memory loss, and seizures. Hematomas can be drained surgically to produce rapid relief of symptoms. Bleeding between the dura (the outermost layer of the protective covering of the brain) and the skull, called epidural hematoma, usually occurs minutes to hours after a skull fracture and is especially dangerous. Bleeding between the brain and the dura, called subdural hematoma, is frequently associated with a dull, persistent ache on one side of the head. Nausea, vomiting, and mild disturbance of brain function also occur. Subdural hematoma may occur after head trauma but also occurs spontaneously in elderly persons or in individuals taking anticoagulant medications.

Increased intracranial pressure (ICP). A growing tumor, infection, or hydrocephalus (an extensive buildup of cerebrospinal fluid in the brain) can raise pressure in the brain and compress nerves and blood vessels, causing headaches. Hydrocephalus is most often treated with the surgical placement of a shunt system that diverts the fluid to a site elsewhere in the body, where it can be absorbed as part of the circulatory process. Headache attributed to idiopathic intracranial hypertension, previously known as pseudotumor cerebri (meaning "false brain tumor"), is associated with severe headache. It can be caused by clotting in the major cerebral veins or certain medications (some antibiotics, withdrawal of corticosteroids, human growth hormone replacement, and vitamin A and related compounds). It is most commonly seen in young, overweight females. Diagnosis usually requires a spinal fluid examination to document the high pressure and the rapid resolution of headache after the spinal fluid is removed.

Although called benign, the condition may lead to visual loss if left untreated. Weight loss, ending the use of the drug suspected of causing the problem, and diuretic treatment can help relieve the pressure.

Inflammation from meningitis, encephalitis, and other infections. Inflammation from infections can harm or destroy nerve cells and cause dull to severe headache pain, brain damage, or stroke, among other conditions. Inflammation of the brain and spinal cord (meningitis and encephalitis) requires urgent medical attention. Diagnosis and identification of the infection usually requires examination and culture of a sample of the cerebrospinal fluid. Treatment options include antibiotics, antiviral or antifungal drugs, corticosteroids, pain medications and sedatives, and anticonvulsants. Headaches may also occur with a fever or a flu-like infection. A headache may accompany a bacterial infection of the upper respiratory tract that spreads to and inflames the lining of the sinus cavities. When one or more of the cavities fills with fluid from the inflammation, the result is constant but dull facial pain and tenderness that worsens with straining or head movements. Treatment includes antibiotics, analgesics, and decongestants. Sinus infections do not generally cause chronic headaches.

Seizures. Migraine-like headache pain may occur during or after a seizure. Moderate to severe headache pain may last for several hours and worsen with sudden movements of the head or when sneezing, coughing, or bending. Other symptoms may include nausea, vomiting, fatigue, increased sensitivity to light or sound, and vision problems.

Spinal fluid leak. About one-fourth of people who undergo a lumbar puncture (which involves a small sampling of the spinal fluid being removed for testing) develop a headache due to a leak of cerebrospinal fluid following the procedure. Since the headache occurs only when the individual stands up, the "cure" is to lie down until the headache runs its course-anywhere from a few hours to several days. Severe postdural headaches may be treated by injecting a small amount of the individual's own blood into the low back to stop the leak (called an epidural blood patch). Occasionally spinal fluid leaks spontaneously, causing this "low-pressure headache."

Structural abnormalities of the head, neck, and spine. Headache pain and loss of function may be triggered by structural abnormalities in the head or spine, restricted blood flow through the neck, irritation to nerves anywhere along the path from the spinal cord to the brain, or stressful or awkward positions of the head and neck. Surgery is the only treatment available to correct the condition or halt the progression of damage to the central nervous system. Medications may ease the pain. Cervicogenic headaches are caused by structural irregularities in either the head or neck. In a Chiari malformation, the back of the skull is too small for the brain. This forces a part of the brain to block the normal flow of spinal fluid and press on the brainstem. Chiari malformations are present at birth but may not cause symptoms until later in life. Common symptoms include dizziness, muscle weakness, vision problems, and headache that worsen with coughing or straining. Syringomyelia, a fluid-filled cyst within the spinal cord, can cause pain, numbness, weakness, and headaches.

Trigeminal neuralgia (TN). The trigeminal nerve conducts sensations to the brain from the upper, middle, and lower portions of the face, as well as inside the mouth. The presumed cause of trigeminal neuralgia is a blood vessel pressing on the nerve as it exits the brainstem, but other causes have been described. Symptoms include headache and intense shock-like or stabbing pain that comes on suddenly and is typically felt on one side of the jaw or cheek. Muscle spasms may occur on the affected side of the face. The pain may occur spontaneously or be triggered by touching the cheek, as happens when shaving, washing, or applying makeup. The pain also may occur when eating, drinking, talking, smoking, or brushing teeth, or when the face is exposed to wind. Treatment options include anticonvulsants, antidepressants, and surgery to block pain signaling to the brain.

Section 4.3

Memory Loss (Amnesia)

This section includes text excerpted from "Coping with Memory Loss,"
U.S. Food and Drug Administration (FDA), December 13, 2017.

Everyone has mild memory lapses from time to time. You can't find your car keys one day, and your reading glasses go missing the next. These are usually just signs of a normal brain that's constantly prioritizing, sorting, storing, and retrieving all types of information. But how do you know when memory loss is abnormal—and should be evaluated by a healthcare professional? Here are some questions to consider:

- **Does the memory loss disrupt daily living**, such as driving, balancing a checkbook, and maintaining personal hygiene?

- **How often do memory lapses occur?** It's one thing to forget where you parked your car once in a while, but it's not normal to regularly forget your assigned parking spot or to miss appointments over and over. Frequent memory lapses are likely to be noticeable because they tend to interfere with daily living.

- **What's being forgotten?** Most people have trouble remembering some details of a conversation, but forgetting whole conversations could signal a problem. Other red flags: forgetting the name of a close friend or relative, frequently repeating yourself or asking the same questions in the same conversation.

- **Are there signs of confusion?** Serious memory lapses may cause individuals to get lost in a familiar place or put something in an inappropriate place because they can't remember where it goes (think car keys in the refrigerator).

- **Is the memory loss getting worse?** If you feel you're forgetting more and more over time, you should be evaluated by a health professional.

What Causes Memory Loss?

Anything that affects cognition—the process of thinking, learning, and remembering—can affect memory. Doctors use a combination of strategies to gain better insight into what's going on, says Ranjit Mani, M.D., a neurologist in U.S. Food and Drug Administration's (FDA), Division of Neurology Products (DNP).

Doctors evaluate memory loss by taking a medical history, asking questions to test mental ability, conducting a physical and neurological examination, and performing blood and urine tests. Brain imaging—either using computerized axial tomography (CAT) scans or magnetic resonance imaging (MRI)—can help to identify strokes and tumors, which can sometimes cause memory loss.

"The goal is to rule out factors that are potentially reversible and determine if the memory loss is due to a more serious brain disease," Mani says.

Some causes of memory loss can occur together or individually:

- **Medications** that can interfere with memory include over-the-counter (OTC) and prescription sleeping pills, OTC antihistamines, antianxiety medications, antidepressants, some drugs used to treat schizophrenia, and pain medicines used after surgery.

- **Heavy alcohol use** can cause deficiencies in vitamin B1 (thiamine), which can harm memory. Alcohol and illicit drugs can change chemicals in the brain and affect memory.

- **Stress**, particularly because of emotional trauma, can cause memory loss. In rare, extreme cases, a condition called psychogenic amnesia can result. "This can cause someone to wander around lost, unable to remember their name or date of birth or other basic information," Mani says. "It usually resolves on its own."

- **Depression**, which is common with aging, causes a lack of attention and focus that can affect memory. "Usually treating the depression will improve mood, and the memory problems may then also improve," Mani says.

- A **blow to the head** can cause a loss of consciousness and memory loss. "Memory loss from a single episode of head trauma typically stays the same or gradually gets better, but not worse," Mani says. However, repeated head trauma, as in boxers and footballers can result in progressive loss of memory and other effects.

- People with **human immunodeficiency virus (HIV), tuberculosis (TB), syphilis, herpes,** and other infections of the lining or substance of the brain may experience memory problems.

- **An underactive or overactive thyroid** can interfere with remembering recent events.

- **Lack of quality sleep** can affect memory.

- **Deficiencies of vitamins B_1 and B_{12} can affect memory**, and can be treated with a pill or an injection.

As part of the normal aging process, it can be harder for some people to recall some types of information, such as the names of individuals. Mild cognitive impairment (MCI), however, is a condition characterized by a memory deficit beyond that expected for age, but is not sufficient to impair day-to-day activities. The most serious form of memory loss is dementia. With dementia, there is increasing impairment of memory and other aspects of thinking that are sufficiently severe to impair daily activities. While this has many causes, the most common by far is Alzheimer disease (AD), in which there is a progressive loss of brain cells accompanied by other abnormalities of the brain.

Can Memory Loss Be Prevented?

Clinical trials are underway to test specific interventions for memory loss. Research has shown that the combination of shifting estrogen and progestin levels increased the risk of dementia in women older than 65. There is no evidence that the herb ginkgo biloba prevents memory loss.

But still, there are some things you can do that might help reduce the risk of developing memory problems:

- Lower your cholesterol and blood pressure. Several studies in recent years have suggested that vascular diseases (heart disease and stroke) that result from elevated cholesterol and blood pressure may contribute to the development of AD, its severity, or the development of multi-infarct dementia (also called vascular dementia).

- Don't smoke or abuse alcohol.

- Get regular exercise. Physical activity may help maintain blood flow to the brain and reduce risk factors associated with dementia.

- Maintain healthy eating habits. Eating more green leafy vegetables and less saturated fats has been shown to help slow cognitive decline. Also, eating fish with beneficial omega-3 fatty acids, such as salmon and tuna, may benefit brain health.

- Maintain social interactions, which can help reduce stress.

- Keep your brain active. Some experts suggest that challenging the brain with such activities as reading, writing, learning a new skill, playing games, and gardening stimulates brain cells and the connections between the cells, and may be associated with a lower risk of dementia.

Section 4.4

Seizures

This section contains text excerpted from the following sources:
Text in this section begins with excerpts from "Seizures,"
MedlinePlus, National Institutes of Health (NIH), June 29, 2017;
Text beginning with the heading "What Causes the Epilepsies?"
is excerpted from "The Epilepsies and Seizures: Hope through
Research," National Institute of Neurological Disorders and
Stroke (NINDS), April 2015.

Seizures are symptoms of a brain problem. They happen because of sudden, abnormal electrical activity in the brain. When people think of seizures, they often think of convulsions in which a person's body shakes rapidly and uncontrollably. Not all seizures cause convulsions. There are many types of seizures and some have mild symptoms. Seizures fall into two main groups. Focal seizures, also called partial seizures, happen in just one part of the brain. Generalized seizures are a result of abnormal activity on both sides of the brain.

Most seizures last from 30 seconds to 2 minutes and do not cause lasting harm. However, it is a medical emergency if seizures last longer than 5 minutes or if a person has many seizures and does not wake up between them. Seizures can have many causes, including medicines, high fevers, head injuries, and certain diseases. People who have recurring seizures due to a brain disorder have epilepsy.

What Causes the Epilepsies?

The epilepsies have many possible causes, but for up to half of people with epilepsy a cause is not known. In other cases, the epilepsies are clearly linked to genetic factors, developmental brain abnormalities, infection, traumatic brain injury, stroke, brain tumors, or other identifiable problems. Anything that disturbs the normal pattern of neuronal activity—from illness to brain damage to abnormal brain development—can lead to seizures.

The epilepsies may develop because of an abnormality in brain wiring, an imbalance of nerve signaling in the brain (in which some cells either over-excite or over-inhibit other brain cells from sending messages), or some combination of these factors. In some pediatric conditions abnormal brain wiring causes other problems such as intellectual impairment.

In other persons, the brain's attempts to repair itself after a head injury, stroke, or other problem may inadvertently generate abnormal nerve connections that lead to epilepsy. Brain malformations and abnormalities in brain wiring that occur during brain development also may disturb neuronal activity and lead to epilepsy.

Genetics

Genetic mutations may play a key role in the development of certain epilepsies. Many types of epilepsy affect multiple blood-related family members, pointing to a strong inherited genetic component. In other cases, gene mutations may occur spontaneously and contribute to development of epilepsy in people with no family history of the disorder (called "de novo" mutations). Overall, researchers estimate that hundreds of genes could play a role in the disorders.

Several types of epilepsy have been linked to mutations in genes that provide instructions for ion channels, the "gates" that control the flow of ions in and out of cells to help regulate neuronal signaling. For example, most infants with Dravet syndrome, a type of epilepsy associated with seizures that begin before the age of one year, carry a mutation in the *SCN1A* gene that causes seizures by affecting sodium ion channels.

Genetic mutations also have been linked to disorders known as the progressive myoclonic epilepsies, which are characterized by ultra-quick muscle contractions (myoclonus) and seizures over time. For example, Lafora disease, a severe, progressive form of myoclonic epilepsy that begins in childhood, has been linked to a gene that helps to break down carbohydrates in brain cells.

Mutations in genes that control neuronal migration—a critical step in brain development—can lead to areas of misplaced or abnormally formed neurons, called cortical dysplasia, in the brain that can cause these mis-wired neurons to misfire and lead to epilepsy.

Other genetic mutations may not cause epilepsy, but may influence the disorder in other ways. For example, one study showed that many people with certain forms of epilepsy have an abnormally active version of a gene that results in resistance to antiseizure drugs. Genes also may control a person's susceptibility to seizures, or seizure threshold, by affecting brain development.

Other Disorders

Epilepsies may develop as a result of brain damage associated with many types of conditions that disrupt normal brain activity. Seizures may stop once these conditions are treated and resolved. However, the chances of becoming seizure-free after the primary disorder is treated are uncertain and vary depending on the type of disorder, the brain region that is affected, and how much brain damage occurred prior to treatment. Examples of conditions that can lead to epilepsy include:

- Brain tumors, including those associated with neurofibromatosis or tuberous sclerosis complex, two inherited conditions that cause benign tumors called hamartomas to grow in the brain

- Head trauma

- Alcoholism or alcohol withdrawal

- Alzheimer disease

- Strokes, heart attacks, and other conditions that deprive the brain of oxygen (a significant portion of new-onset epilepsy in elderly people is due to stroke or other cerebrovascular disease)

- Abnormal blood vessel formation (arteriovenous malformations) or bleeding in the brain (hemorrhage)

- Inflammation of the brain

- Infections such as meningitis, human immunodeficiency virus (HIV), and viral encephalitis

Cerebral palsy (CP) or other developmental neurological abnormalities may also be associated with epilepsy. About 20 percent of seizures in children can be attributed to developmental neurological conditions. Epilepsies often co-occur in people with abnormalities of brain development or other neurodevelopmental disorders. Seizures are more common, for example, among individuals with autism spectrum disorder or intellectual impairment. In one study, fully a third of children with autism spectrum disorder had treatment-resistant epilepsy.

Seizure Triggers

Seizure triggers do not cause epilepsy but can provoke first seizures in those who are susceptible or can cause seizures in people with epilepsy who otherwise experience good seizure control with their medication. Seizure triggers include alcohol consumption or alcohol withdrawal, dehydration or missing meals, stress, and hormonal changes associated with the menstrual cycle. In surveys of people with epilepsy, stress is the most commonly reported seizure trigger. Exposure to toxins or poisons such as lead or carbon monoxide, street drugs, or even excessively large doses of antidepressants or other prescribed medications also can trigger seizures.

Sleep deprivation is a powerful trigger of seizures. Sleep disorders are common among people with the epilepsies and appropriate treatment of coexisting sleep disorders can often lead to improved control of seizures. Certain types of seizures tend to occur during sleep, while others are more common during times of wakefulness, suggesting to physicians how to best adjust a person's medication.

For some people, visual stimulation can trigger seizures in a condition known as photosensitive epilepsy. Stimulation can include such things as flashing lights or moving patterns.

How Are the Epilepsies Diagnosed?

A number of tests are used to determine whether a person has a form of epilepsy and, if so, what kind of seizures the person has.

Imaging and Monitoring

An electroencephalogram, or EEG, can assess whether there are any detectable abnormalities in the person's brainwaves and may help to determine if antiseizure drugs would be of benefit. This most common diagnostic test for epilepsy records electrical activity detected by electrodes placed on the scalp. Some people who are diagnosed with a specific syndrome may have abnormalities in brain activity, even when they are not experiencing a seizure. However, some people continue to show normal electrical activity patterns even after they have experienced a seizure. These occur if the abnormal activity is generated deep in the brain where the EEG is unable to detect it. Many people who do not have epilepsy also show some unusual brain activity on an EEG. Whenever possible, an EEG should be performed within 24 hours of an individual's first seizure. Ideally, EEGs should be performed while the person is drowsy as well as when he or she is awake because brain activity during sleep and drowsiness is often more revealing of activity resembling epilepsy. Video monitoring may be used in conjunction with EEG to determine the nature of a person's seizures and to rule out other disorders such as psychogenic nonepileptic seizures, cardiac arrhythmia, or narcolepsy that may look like epilepsy.

A magnetoencephalogram (MEG) detects the magnetic signals generated by neurons to help detect surface abnormalities in brain activity. MEG can be used in planning a surgical strategy to remove focal areas involved in seizures while minimizing interference with brain function.

The most commonly used brain scans include computed tomography (CT), positron emission tomography (PET), and magnetic resonance imaging (MRI). CT and MRI scans reveal structural abnormalities of the brain such as tumors and cysts, which may cause seizures. A type of MRI called functional MRI (fMRI) can be used to localize normal brain activity and detect abnormalities in functioning. Single photon emission computed tomography (SPECT) is sometimes used to locate seizure foci in the brain. A modification of SPECT, called ictal SPECT, can be very helpful in localizing the brain area generating seizures. In a person admitted to the hospital for epilepsy monitoring, the SPECT blood flow tracer is injected within 30 seconds of a seizure, then the images of brain blood flow at the time of the seizure are compared with blood flow images taken in between seizures. The seizure onset area shows a high blood flow region on the scan. PET scans can be used to identify brain regions with lower than normal metabolism, a feature of the epileptic focus after the seizure has stopped.

Medical History

Taking a detailed medical history, including symptoms and duration of the seizures, is still one of the best methods available to determine what kind of seizures a person has had and to determine any form of epilepsy. The medical history should include details about any past illnesses or other symptoms a person may have had, as well as any family history of seizures. Since people who have suffered a seizure often do not remember what happened, caregiver or other accounts of seizures are vital to this evaluation. The person who experienced the seizure is asked about any warning experiences. The observers will be asked to provide a detailed description of events in the timeline they occurred.

Blood Tests

Blood samples may be taken to screen for metabolic or genetic disorders that may be associated with the seizures. They also may be used to check for underlying health conditions such as infections, lead poisoning, anemia, and diabetes that may be causing or triggering the seizures. In the emergency department it is standard procedure to screen for exposure to recreational drugs in anyone with a first seizure.

Developmental, Neurological, and Behavioral Tests

Tests devised to measure motor abilities, behavior, and intellectual ability are often used as a way to determine how epilepsy is affecting an individual. These tests also can provide clues about what kind of epilepsy the person has.

Can the Epilepsies Be Prevented?

At this time there are no medications or other therapies that have been shown to prevent epilepsy. In some cases, the risk factors that lead to epilepsy can be modified. Good prenatal care, including treatment of high blood pressure and infections during pregnancy, may prevent brain injury in the developing fetus that may lead to epilepsy and other neurological problems later. Treating cardiovascular disease, high blood pressure, and other disorders that can affect the brain during adulthood and aging also may prevent some cases of epilepsy. Prevention or early treatment of infections such as meningitis in high-risk populations may also prevent cases of epilepsy. Also, the wearing of seatbelts and bicycle helmets, and correctly securing children in car seats, may avert some cases of epilepsy associated with head trauma.

How Can Epilepsy Be Treated?

Accurate diagnosis of the type of epilepsy a person has is crucial for finding an effective treatment. There are many different ways to successfully control seizures. Doctors who treat the epilepsies come from many different fields of medicine and include neurologists, pediatricians, pediatric neurologists, internists, and family physicians, as well as neurosurgeons. An epileptologist is someone who has completed advanced training and specializes in treating the epilepsies.

Once epilepsy is diagnosed, it is important to begin treatment as soon as possible. Research suggests that medication and other treatments may be less successful once seizures and their consequences become established. There are several treatment approaches that can be used depending on the individual and the type of epilepsy. If seizures are not controlled quickly, referral to an epileptologist at a specialized epilepsy center should be considered, so that careful consideration of treatment options, including dietary approaches, medication, devices, and surgery, can be performed in order to gain optimal seizure treatment.

Medications

The most common approach to treating the epilepsies is to prescribe antiseizure drugs. More than 20 different antiseizure medications are available, all with different benefits and side effects. Most seizures can be controlled with one drug (called monotherapy). Deciding on which drug to prescribe, and at what dosage, depends on many different factors, including seizure type, lifestyle and age, seizure frequency, drug side effects, medicines for other conditions, and, for a woman, whether she is pregnant or will become pregnant. It may take several months to determine the best drug and dosage. If one treatment is unsuccessful, another may work better.

For many people with epilepsy, seizures can be controlled with monotherapy at the optimal dosage. Combining medications may amplify side effects such as fatigue and dizziness, so doctors usually prescribe just one drug whenever possible. Combinations of drugs, however, are still sometimes necessary for some forms of epilepsy that do not respond to monotherapy.

When starting any new antiseizure medication, a low dosage will usually be prescribed initially followed by incrementally higher dosages, sometimes with blood-level monitoring, to determine when the optimal dosage has been reached. It may take time for the dosage to achieve optimal seizure control while minimizing side effects. The latter are usually worse when first starting a new medicine.

Most side effects of antiseizure drugs are relatively minor, such as fatigue, dizziness, or weight gain. Antiseizure medications have differing effects on mood: some may worsen depression, where others may improve depression or stabilize mood. However, severe and life-threatening reactions such as allergic reactions or damage to the liver or bone marrow can occur. Antiseizure medications can interact with many other drugs in potentially harmful ways. Some antiseizure drugs can cause the liver to speed the metabolism of other drugs and make the other drugs less effective, as may be the case with oral contraceptives. Since people can become more sensitive to medications as they age, blood levels of medication may need to be checked occasionally to see if dosage adjustments are necessary. The effectiveness of a medication can diminish over time, which can increase the risk of seizures. Some citrus fruit and products, in particular grapefruit juice, may interfere with the breakdown of many drugs, including antiseizure medications—causing them to build-up in the body, which can worsen side effects.

Some people with epilepsy may be advised to discontinue their anti-seizure drugs after 2–3 years have passed without a seizure. Others may be advised to wait for 4–5 years. Discontinuing medication should always be done with supervision of a healthcare professional. It is very important to continue taking antiseizure medication for as long as it is prescribed. Discontinuing medication too early is one of the major reasons people who have been seizure-free start having new seizures and can lead to status epilepticus. Some evidence also suggests that uncontrolled seizures may trigger changes in the brain that will make it more difficult to treat the seizures in the future.

The chance that a person will eventually be able to discontinue medication varies depending on the person's age and his or her type of epilepsy. More than half of children who go into remission with medication can eventually stop their medication without having new seizures. One study showed that 68 percent of adults who had been seizure-free for 2 years before stopping medication were able to do so without having more seizures and 75 percent could successfully discontinue medication if they had been seizure-free for 3 years. However, the odds of successfully stopping medication are not as good for people with a family history of epilepsy, those who need multiple medications, those with focal seizures, and those who continue to have abnormal EEG results while on medication.

There are specific syndromes in which certain antiseizure medications should not be used because they may make the seizures worse. For example, carbamazepine can worsen epilepsy in children diagnosed with Dravet syndrome.

Diet

Dietary approaches and other treatments may be more appropriate depending on the age of the individual and the type of epilepsy. A high-fat, very low carbohydrate ketogenic diet is often used to treat medication-resistant epilepsies. The diet induces a state known as ketosis, which means that the body shifts to breaking down fats instead of carbohydrates to survive. A ketogenic diet effectively reduces seizures for some people, especially children with certain forms of epilepsy. Studies have shown that more than 50 percent of people who try the ketogenic diet have a greater than 50 percent improvement in seizure control and 10 percent experience seizure freedom. Some children are able to discontinue the ketogenic diet after several years and remain seizure-free, but this is done with strict supervision and monitoring by a physician.

The ketogenic diet is not easy to maintain, as it requires strict adherence to a limited range of foods. Possible side effects include impaired growth due to nutritional deficiency and a buildup of uric acid in the blood, which can lead to kidney stones.

Researchers are looking at modified versions of and alternatives to the ketogenic diet. For example, studies show promising results for a modified Atkins diet and for a low-glycemic-index treatment, both of which are less restrictive and easier to follow than the ketogenic diet, but well-controlled randomized controlled trials have yet to assess these approaches.

Surgery

Evaluation of persons for surgery is generally recommended only after focal seizures persist despite the person having tried at least two appropriately chosen and well-tolerated medications, or if there is an identifiable brain lesion (a dysfunctional part of the brain) believed to cause the seizures. When someone is considered to be a good candidate for surgery experts generally agree that it should be performed as early as possible.

Surgical evaluation takes into account the seizure type, the brain region involved, and the importance of the area of the brain where seizures originate (called the focus) for everyday behavior. Prior to surgery, individuals with epilepsy are monitored intensively in order to pinpoint the exact location in the brain where seizures begin. Implanted electrodes may be used to record activity from the surface of the brain, which yields more detailed information than an external scalp EEG. Surgeons usually avoid operating in areas of the brain that are necessary for speech, movement, sensation, memory and thinking, or other important abilities. fMRI can be used to locate such "eloquent" brain areas involved in an individual.

While surgery can significantly reduce or even halt seizures for many people, any kind of surgery involves some level of risk. Surgery for epilepsy does not always successfully reduce seizures and it can result in cognitive or personality changes as well as physical disability, even in people who are excellent candidates for it. Nonetheless, when medications fail, several studies have shown that surgery is much more likely to make someone seizure-free compared to attempts to use other medications. Anyone thinking about surgery for epilepsy should be assessed at an epilepsy center experienced in surgical techniques and should discuss with the epilepsy specialists the balance between the risks of surgery and desire to become seizure-free.

Even when surgery completely ends a person's seizures, it is important to continue taking antiseizure medication for some time. Doctors generally recommend continuing medication for at least two years after a successful operation to avoid recurrence of seizures.

Surgical procedures for treating epilepsy disorders include:

- Surgery to remove a seizure focus involves removing the defined area of the brain where seizures originate. It is the most common type of surgery for epilepsy, which doctors may refer to as a lobectomy or lesionectomy, and is appropriate only for focal seizures that originate in just one area of the brain. In general, people have a better chance of becoming seizure-free after surgery if they have a small, well-defined seizure focus. The most common type of lobectomy is a temporal lobe resection, which is performed for people with medial temporal lobe epilepsy. In such individuals one hippocampus (there are two, one on each side of the brain) is seen to be shrunken and scarred on an MRI scan.

- Multiple subpial transection may be performed when seizures originate in part of the brain that cannot be removed. It involves making a series of cuts that are designed to prevent seizures from spreading into other parts of the brain while leaving the person's normal abilities intact.

- Corpus callosotomy, or severing the network of neural connections between the right and left halves (hemispheres) of the brain, is done primarily in children with severe seizures that start in one half of the brain and spread to the other side. Corpus callosotomy can end drop attacks and other generalized seizures. However, the procedure does not stop seizures in the side of the brain where they originate, and these focal seizures may even worsen after surgery.

- Hemispherectomy and hemispherotomy involve removing half of the brain's cortex, or outer layer. These procedures are used predominantly in children who have seizures that do not respond to medication because of damage that involves only half the brain, as occurs with conditions such as Rasmussen encephalitis. While this type of surgery is very excessive and is performed only when other therapies have failed, with intense rehabilitation, children can recover many abilities.

Devices

Electrical stimulation of the brain remains a therapeutic strategy of interest for people with medication-resistant forms of epilepsy who are not candidates for surgery.

The vagus nerve stimulation device for the treatment of epilepsy was approved by the U.S. Food and Drug Administration (FDA) in 1997. The vagus nerve stimulator is surgically implanted under the skin of the chest and is attached to the vagus nerve in the lower neck. The device delivers short bursts of electrical energy to the brain via the vagus nerve. On average, this stimulation reduces seizures by about 20–40 percent. Individuals usually cannot stop taking epilepsy medication because of the stimulator, but they often experience fewer seizures and they may be able to reduce the dosage of their medication.

Responsive stimulation involves the use of an implanted device that analyzes brain activity patterns to detect a forthcoming seizure. Once detected, the device administers an intervention, such as electrical stimulation or a fast-acting drug to prevent the seizure from occurring. These devices also are known as closed-loop systems. NeuroPace, one of the first responsive stimulation, closed-loop devices, received pre-market approval by the FDA in late 2013 and is available for adults with refractory epilepsy (hard to treat epilepsy that does not respond well to trials of at least two medicines).

Experimental devices: Not approved by the FDA for use in the United States (as of March 2015)

- Deep brain stimulation (DBS) using mild electrical impulses has been tried as a treatment for epilepsy in several different brain regions. It involves surgically implanting an electrode connected to an implanted pulse generator—similar to a heart pacemaker—to deliver electrical stimulation to specific areas in the brain to regulate electrical signals in neural circuits. Stimulation of an area called the anterior thalamic nucleus has been particularly helpful in providing at least partial relief from seizures in people who had medication-resistant forms of the disorder.

- A report on trigeminal nerve stimulation (using electrical signals to stimulate parts of the trigeminal nerve and affected brain regions) showed efficacy rates similar to those for vagal nerve stimulation, with responder rates hovering around 50 percent. (A responder is defined as someone having greater than a 50 percent reduction in seizure frequency.) Freedom from seizures, although reported, remains rare for both methods. At the time of this writing, a trigeminal nerve stimulation device was available for use in Europe, but it had not yet been approved in the United States.

- Transcutaneous magnetic stimulation involves a device being placed outside the head to produce a magnetic field to induce an electrical current in nearby areas of the brain. It has been shown to reduce cortical activity associated with specific epilepsy syndromes.

Chapter 5

Neurological Emergencies

Chapter Contents

Section 5.1

Brain Attack: Know the Signs, Act in Time

This section contains text excerpted from the following sources:
Text beginning with the heading "Stroke Basics" is excerpted from
"Stroke: Challenges, Progress, and Promise," National Institutes
of Health (NIH), February 2009. Reviewed February 2018; Text
beginning with the heading "Signs of Stroke in Men and Women" is
excerpted from "Stroke—Stroke Signs and Symptoms," Centers for
Disease Control and Prevention (CDC), January 17, 2017.

Stroke Basics

The effects of stroke manifest themselves rapidly. The five most
common symptoms of stroke are:

- Sudden weakness or numbness of the face or limbs, especially on
  one side of the body.

- Sudden confusion or difficulty speaking or understanding
  speech.

- Sudden trouble seeing in one or both eyes.

- Sudden trouble walking, dizziness, or loss of balance or
  coordination.

- Sudden severe headache with no known cause.

The exact symptoms depend on where in the brain's vascular system the blockage or rupture has occurred. Strokes that predominantly affect one hemisphere of the brain are common. Since each hemisphere controls the opposite side of the body, a stroke in the left hemisphere will cause motor and sensory deficits on the right side of the body, and vice versa.

The long-term outcomes after a stroke vary considerably and depend partly on the type of stroke and the age of the affected person. Although most stroke survivors regain their functional independence, 15–30 percent will have a permanent physical disability. Some will experience a permanent decline in cognitive function known as post-stroke or vascular dementia. Unfortunately, many stroke survivors face a danger of recurrent stroke in the future. About 20 percent of people who experience a first-ever stroke between ages 40 and 69 will have another stroke within five years. Finding treatments to help prevent stroke in this high-risk group is a major focus of National Institute of Neurological Disorders and Stroke (NINDS)-supported research.

Ischemic Stroke and Transient Ischemic Attack

Ischemic strokes make up about 80 percent of all strokes. Just as a heart attack occurs when there is insufficient blood flow to the heart, an ischemic stroke (sometimes called a "brain attack") occurs when there is a sudden interruption in blood flow to one or more regions of the brain. Like all cells in the body, neurons and other brain cells require oxygen and glucose delivered through the blood in order to function and survive. A few minutes of oxygen deprivation-called ischemia-is enough to kill millions of neurons. Moreover, ischemia can provoke inflammation, swelling (edema), and other processes that can continue to cause damage for hours to days after the initial insult.

Obstructive blood clots are the most common cause of ischemic stroke. Clotting (or coagulation) is a vital function that helps prevent bleeding when a blood vessel is damaged, but clots can also obstruct normal blood flow. When a clot forms in association with the wall of a blood vessel and grows large enough to impair blood flow, it is called a thrombus; a clot that breaks off the vessel wall and travels through the blood is an embolus. A cardioembolic stroke is caused by a clot that originates in the heart. Cardiac emboli are most likely to form in people with heart conditions such as atrial fibrillation (AF, an irregular heartbeat), heart failure, stenosis, or infections within the valves of the heart. They may also occur post-heart attack.

Another contributor to ischemic stroke is chronic atherosclerosis, which is a buildup of fatty deposits and cellular debris (plaque) on the inside of the blood vessel wall. As atherosclerotic plaques grow, they cause narrowing of the blood vessel (a condition called stenosis). Atherosclerosis can also activate cells involved in clotting.

Immediately after an ischemic stroke, the brain usually contains an irreversibly damaged core of tissue and an area of viable but at-risk tissue called the ischemic penumbra. Restoring normal blood flow-a process known as reperfusion-is essential to rescuing the penumbra. The longer reperfusion is delayed, the more cells in the penumbra will die. The region of brain tissue that is finally damaged is called an infarct.

If a stroke were a storm, a transient ischemic attack (TIA), or "ministroke," would be an ominous thunderclap. Symptoms of a TIA are similar to those of a full-blown stroke but resolve within 24 hours, typically in less than one hour. Still, the short-lived nature of TIAs does not mean that they leave the brain unharmed. In about 40–50 percent of people who have experienced a TIA, a tiny dot of infarct can be seen by brain imaging.

Even when there is no sign of brain infarction, a TIA is both a warning and an opportunity for intervention. While someone who has experienced a full-blown stroke has a two to seven percent risk of having another stroke within the next 90 days; the 90-day risk of stroke following a TIA is 10–20 percent. In many cases, TIAs may be caused by an unstable clot that could create a more permanent blockage within the brain's blood supply at any moment. Fortunately, there are a variety of treatments that can reduce the risk of stroke following a TIA, including medications to lower blood pressure and inhibit blood clotting. If necessary, surgical procedures can clear away plaque in the arteries that supply the brain, or a procedure called stenting can be used to widen the arteries. Severe strokes could be avoided if more people sought medical attention after a TIA.

Signs of Stroke in Men and Women

- Sudden numbness or weakness in the face, arm, or leg, especially on one side of the body.

- Sudden confusion, trouble speaking, or difficulty understanding speech.

- Sudden trouble seeing in one or both eyes.

- Sudden trouble walking, dizziness, loss of balance, or lack of coordination.

- Sudden severe headache with no known cause.

Acting F.A.S.T. Is Key for Stroke

Acting face, arms, speech, and time (F.A.S.T.) can help stroke patients get the treatments they desperately need. The stroke treatments that work best are available only if the stroke is recognized and diagnosed within 3 hours of the first symptoms. Stroke patients may not be eligible for these if they don't arrive at the hospital in time.

If you think someone may be having a stroke, act F.A.S.T. and do the following simple test:

F—Face: Ask the person to smile. Does one side of the face droop?

A—Arms: Ask the person to raise both arms. Does one arm drift downward?

S—Speech: Ask the person to repeat a simple phrase. Is the speech slurred or strange?

T—Time: If you see any of these signs, call 9-1-1 right away.

Note the time when any symptoms first appear. This information helps healthcare providers determine the best treatment for each person. Do not drive to the hospital or let someone else drive you. Call an ambulance so that medical personnel can begin life-saving treatment on the way to the emergency room.

Section 5.2

Brain Herniation

"Brain Herniation," © 2018 Omnigraphics.
Reviewed February 2018.

What Is Brain Herniation?

Brain herniation is a neurological emergency that occurs when there is a shift of brain tissue, cerebrospinal fluid, and blood from their normal positions to an adjacent space inside the skull. This emergency can occur because of increased pressure in the cranial cavity caused by stroke, head injury, bleeding, or brain tumor. The condition can be fatal if not treated immediately.

Types of Brain Herniation

Three types of brain herniation can occur depending on where the brain tissue has shifted:

1. **Subfalcine herniation.** This is the most common type of brain herniation. It occurs when the brain tissue is displaced

underneath the free edge of a membrane known as falx cerebri because of intracranial pressure.

2. **Transtentorial herniation.** This type of herniation is divided into two subtypes.

    - **Descending transtentorial or uncal:** This subtype usually takes place when the part of the temporal lobe known as uncus descends into an area called the posterior fossa.

    - **Ascending transtentorial herniation:** This subtype of herniation occurs when the brainstem and the cerebellum ascend through the tentorial notch.

3. **Cerebellar tonsillar herniation.** A condition in which the cerebellar tonsils descend through the foramen magnum, an opening at the base of the skull where the spinal cord passes, causing compression of the lower brainstem and upper cervical spinal cord.

Causes and Risk Factors

Any kind of swelling inside the brain increases pressure, which can cause brain tissue to move from its normal position resulting in brain herniation. Some of the major causes of swelling include:

- side effects of tumors in the brain

- brain hemorrhage (bleeding in the brain)

- stroke

- head injury that leads to subdural hematoma (when blood collects beneath the skull under the surface of the brain) or swelling (cerebral edema)

Some other reasons for an increase in intracranial pressure include:

- brain abscess (pus collection) from a fungal or bacterial infection or collection of other material in the brain

- brain surgery

- hydrocephalus (fluid collection in the brain)

- Chiari malformation (defect in brain structure)

People who are at higher risk for brain herniation include those with blood vessel problems (aneurysm) or brain tumors. Lifestyle or any physical activity that can increases the risk of head injury are also risk factors for brain herniation.

Brain herniation can occur in the following areas:

- the areas inside the skull separated by a rigid membrane, like the cerebral falx or the tentorium

- openings created during brain surgery

- the natural opening at the base of the skull

Symptoms

The signs and symptoms of brain herniation may include:

- headache

- drowsiness

- irregular or slow pulse

- weakness

- respiratory arrest

- difficulty concentrating

- dilated pupils

- coma

- loss of consciousness

- loss of reflexes

- seizures

- cardiac arrest

- abnormal body positions

Diagnosis

People affected with brain herniation tend to have persistent high blood pressure, irregular breathing patterns, and irregular or slow pulse. Diagnosis is based on exams that observe these symptoms, as well as tests that may include:

- computed tomography (CT) scan of the head

- magnetic resonance imaging (MRI) scan of the head

- X-rays of skull and neck

- blood tests to determine if an abscess is present

Treatment

Brain herniation is a potentially fatal medical emergency that requires immediate treatment. The focus is on relieving the swelling and pressure that causes the brain tissue to herniate. Some treatments that will help reverse or prevent brain herniation may involve:

- Removing cerebrospinal fluid (CSF) by placing a drain into the brain through a procedure called a ventriculostomy.

- Using corticosteroids to reduce swelling.

- Surgery to remove a tumor, a blood clot (hematoma), or abscess.

- Diuretics to help remove excess fluid from the body and reduce pressure inside the skull.

- Removing a section of the skull to make more space (craniectomy).

- Placing a tube in the airway to increase breathing rate and reduce carbon dioxide in the blood (endotracheal intubation).

During treatment for brain herniation, the patient may also receive:

- oxygen

- sedation

- breathing support through a tube placed in the airway

- medications for seizure control

- antibiotics to prevent infection or treat abscess

Prognosis

The prognosis for a person with brain herniation depends on its location, the severity of the injury, and how quickly treatment begins. Since herniation can affect the parts of the brain that control such functions as blood flow and respiration, the condition can be fatal. For this reason, it is essential to call a local emergency number if a person with a head injury or brain tumor experiences symptoms like decreased alertness, lethargy, or loss of consciousness.

Complications

Even with proper treatment, brain herniation can cause damage to vital structures in the body with results that can include:

* cardiac arrest

* coma

* permanent brain damage

* brain death

* death

References

1. "Brain Herniation," Milton S. Hershey Medical Center, Penn State Hershey, July 4, 2016.

2. Cafasso, Jacquelyn. "Brain Herniation," Healthline, October 20, 2017.

3. Kerkar, Pramod. "What Is Brain Herniation and How Is It Treated?" ePainAssist, March 8, 2017.

4. Skalski, Matt, MD, Laughlin Dawes, MD, et al. "Cerebral Herniation," Radiopaedia, September 20, 2016.

Section 5.3

Cerebral Hypoxia

This section includes text excerpted from "Cerebral Hypoxia Information Page," National Institute of Neurological Disorders and Stroke (NINDS), May 23, 2017.

Cerebral hypoxia refers to a condition in which there is a decrease of oxygen supply to the brain even though there is adequate blood flow. Drowning, strangling, choking, suffocation, cardiac arrest, head trauma, carbon monoxide poisoning, and complications of general anesthesia can create conditions that can lead to cerebral hypoxia. Symptoms of mild cerebral hypoxia include inattentiveness, poor judgment, memory loss, and a decrease in motor coordination. Brain cells are extremely sensitive to oxygen deprivation and can begin to die within five minutes after oxygen supply has been cut off. When hypoxia lasts for longer periods of time, it can cause coma, seizures, and even brain death. In brain death, there is no measurable activity in the brain, although cardiovascular function is preserved. Life support is required for respiration.

Prognosis

Recovery depends on how long the brain has been deprived of oxygen and how much brain damage has occurred, although carbon monoxide poisoning can cause brain damage days to weeks after the event. Most people who make a full recovery have only been briefly unconscious. The longer someone is unconscious, the higher the chances of death or brain death and the lower the chances of a meaningful recovery. During recovery, psychological and neurological abnormalities such as amnesia, personality regression, hallucinations, memory loss, and muscle spasms and twitches may appear, persist, and then resolve.

Treatment

Treatment depends on the underlying cause of the hypoxia, but basic life-support systems have to be put in place: mechanical ventilation to secure the airway; fluids, blood products, or medications to support blood pressure and heart rate; and medications to suppress seizures.

Section 5.4

Subarachnoid Hemorrhage

"Subarachnoid Hemorrhage," © 2018 Omnigraphics.
Reviewed February 2018.

A subarachnoid hemorrhage (SAH) is a type of stroke caused by the bleeding of a blood vessel into the arachnoid space, the space between the arachnoid and the pia mater, two of the three membranes that envelop the brain. Abnormalities in the blood vessels, particularly in an artery supplying blood to the brain, are the major causes of a subarachnoid hemorrhage. These abnormalities, known as aneurysms, result from a balloon-like swelling in the artery arising from weakened arterial walls. While small, unruptured aneurysms may be asymptomatic and harmless, large aneurysms can cause a rupture in the arterial wall leading to pooling of blood in the arachnoid space. An intracranial hemorrhage in the arachnoid space can also result from trauma or, less commonly, from a brain tumor, a brain infection (encephalitis), or an arteriovenous malformation (AVM), a prenatal condition that disrupts the normal circulation of blood. Whatever the cause, a subarachnoid hemorrhage is a serious, and possibly fatal, condition that requires immediate medical attention.

Risk Factors

Although cases of SAH in families have been reported, it's unclear if there is a certain genetic factor associated with them. Studies have shown that cerebral aneurysm, one of the leading causes of SAH, is associated with modifiable risk factors, including hypertension, excessive alcohol intake, and smoking. Some studies also indicate that SAH disproportionately affects women, particularly older women. While this may be attributed in part to female hormone levels, further studies are needed to draw definite conclusions on sex differences relating to the incidence, presentation, and outcome of SAH.

Signs and Symptoms

The classic symptoms of subarachnoid hemorrhage include photophobia (sensitivity to light), nuchal rigidity (resistance to neck flexion), and an excruciating headache, often termed a thunderclap headache due to its sudden onset and severity, followed by loss of consciousness. Other symptoms associated with SAH include blurred vision, seizures, nausea, and vomiting. SAH can also cause abnormal heart or respiratory rate, as well as loss or impairment of consciousness and other neurological problems, some of which may be debilitating and irreversible. Other signs are cranial nerve lesions, hemiparesis, and aphasia.

Diagnosis

If the characteristic symptoms are present, diagnosis for SAH proceeds immediately to prevent irreversible neurological damage and possible organ dysfunction. Diagnostic protocol for SAH typically includes:

- **Noncontrast computed tomography (CT).** This scan is one of the first to be performed to diagnose SAH, ideally within six hours of the presentation of symptoms. A CT angiogram using a contrast dye may also be performed to view the hemorrhaging blood vessel in greater detail.

- **Magnetic resonance imaging (MRI)** An MRI is typically used within the first 12 hours for a more accurate assessment and better visualization of the hemorrhaging blood vessel. More recently, MR angiogram using contrast dye has evolved as one of the most effective diagnostic procedures to detect the aneurysm and highlight blood flow, but this diagnostic tool comes with some limitations, including longer scan duration and difficulty in moving unstable, intubated patients.

- **Cerebral angiography.** Cerebral angiography, also called digital subtraction catheter angiography, is often considered the gold standard for the diagnosis of vascular abnormalities. It is performed even if the magnetic resonance angiography (MRA) or computed tomography angiography (CTA) has identified the causative lesion. This is carried out by inserting a catheter into an artery in the patient's leg and navigating it under X-ray guidance to the area under examination in the brain. Cerebral angiography is an important tool for helping plan surgery, if required.

Studies show that one-fifth of SAH cases caused by aneurysms do not show up on initial imaging tests. In such cases, when clinical presentation strongly points toward SAH a lumbar puncture (spinal tap) is usually indicated. This involves inserting a needle into the lower back to obtain a sample of the cerebrospinal fluid (CSF), the fluid surrounding the brain and spinal cord. The CSF is then analyzed to detect the presence of blood arising from a hemorrhaging vessel. The spinal tap is usually followed by imaging tests.

Treatment

The basic principles of treatment depend largely on the underlying cause of the hemorrhage and the potential complications associated with SAH. Treatment may include:

- **Early critical care management.** A diagnosis of SAH is followed immediately by close monitoring of the patient to stabilize vital functions, arrest the hemorrhage, and prevent re-bleed. This is usually carried out in a comprehensive stroke center, although some cases might require admission to a critical care unit (CCU). Patients with impaired consciousness might need to be intubated and mechanically ventilated for assisted breathing.

- **Pharmaceutical management.** Treatment for SAH may include medications to prevent delayed complications associated with the condition. Nimodipine, a calcium channel blocker, is the most common medication prescribed as part of the acute management protocol and is usually continued for 21 days to dilate blood vessels in the brain and prevent blockages. Other medications include anticonvulsants (for seizures), antiemetics (for nausea and vomiting), painkillers, and osmotic agents to decrease intracranial pressure. Corticosteroids may also be prescribed for their anti-inflammatory effects and potential to counteract infection and cerebral edema (hydrocephalus).

- **Surgery.** If diagnosis reveals aneurysm as the cause of SAH, surgery is performed to repair the ruptured blood vessel and prevent re-bleed. A portion of the skull is removed to expose the brain in a procedure called a craniotomy. The surgeon then places a permanent clip across the aneurysm to prevent blood flow to it.

Endovascular coiling. A minimally invasive technique, this procedure involves inserting a catheter into an artery in the leg or groin and guiding it to the site of the aneurysm. Platinum microcoils are then passed through the catheter into the aneurysm to induce clotting and prevent blood flow to it. In some cases, a stent (flexible mesh tube) may be permanently placed in the artery to provide a scaffold to keep the platinum coils in place. Termed stent-assisted coiling, this procedure is being increasingly used for wide-necked, large aneurysms and has been shown by studies to have better outcomes than surgery.

Complications

Subarachnoid hemorrhage can cause a number of short- and long-term complications, many of which are serious and potentially fatal. These can include:

- **Cerebral vasospasm.** One of the most important causes of mortality and permanent morbidity in the aftermath of SAH, cerebral vasospasm (CV) is characterized by intense constriction of the blood vessels around the aneurysm. CV generally develops about four days after aneurysmal rupture, and if untreated it could lead to delayed cerebral ischemia, a condition caused by insufficient blood flow to the brain. This in turn causes necrosis (death) of the brain tissue leading to increased risk of stroke. Because the cause of CV is not well understood, managing the condition can be challenging. Recent treatment includes increasing blood pressure (hypertension), increasing blood volume with IV fluids (hypervolemia), and reducing blood viscosity to increase flow through narrowed arteries (hemodilution).

- **Hydrocephalus.** A common complication of SAH is hydrocephalus, a buildup of clotted blood and fluid in the subarachnoid space. A potentially devastating condition, hydrocephalus may develop soon after SAH and is associated with elevated intracranial pressure. It requires immediate lowering of blood pressure to reduce further bleeding and prevent neurological deterioration. Treatment of hydrocephalus most often involves fluid drainage using a lumbar puncture. An external ventricular drain (EVD) may also be temporarily used to drain excess cerebrospinal fluid and blood. The drain is inserted into the ventricles (a communicating network of cavities filled with CSF) within the brain and allowed to remain in place for a specific period during which the risk of vasospasm is high. After this period, the EVD is clamped and removed, or it may be replaced by a permanent ventriculoperitoneal (VP) shunt if hydrocephalus has worsened.

- **Other complications.** SAH can also result in a number of other complications. For example, re-bleeding can take place at the site of the initial aneurysm within 6–8 weeks, requiring immediate repair in order to avoid permanent damage or even death. Other potential complications include hospital-acquired infections, deep-vein thrombosis (blood clots), and hyponatremia (fluid build-up).

Prognosis

The volume of hemorrhage has a direct bearing on the extent of neurological problems associated with SAH. Patients with smaller hemorrhages have relatively shorter recoveries and better outcomes than those who suffer large hemorrhages and become comatose or semi-comatose. Studies show that one-third of patients have good outcomes, while an equal number of them suffer from a series of neurological deficits from the hemorrhage, or the treatment, and may require long-term rehabilitation therapy to cope with the functional limitations associated with SAH. Some of the common problems involving physical and mental functions include:

- **Seizures.** Seizures can occur after SAH and are characterized by spasms that may last from a few seconds to a few minutes. Recurring seizures are called epilepsy and require treatment with antiepileptic drugs.

- **Cognitive problems.** These are a common result of SAH and include the inability to focus and organize even simple tasks, such as cleaning house or cooking a meal. Cognitive deficits also cause a change in perception. People, things, and places might begin to be perceived differently following SAH, and this may result in irritability, mood swings, and depression.

- **Speech and language issues.** Following SAH, speech and language problems can be caused by injury to the brain. This usually takes the form of aphasia that results in a total or partial loss of the ability to use words. While some people can experience a total recovery from aphasia, others may have permanent speech and language impairment, which can also make learning, reading, or writing difficult.

- **Motor function deficits.** These could include weakness or paralysis of the arms and legs. This typically affects either the right or the left side of the body and may either improve with time and rehabilitation or leave varying degrees of disability.

- **Fatigue.** This is one of the most common short-term results of SAH, characterized by an overwhelming lack of energy that usually persists for a few weeks and tends to decrease with time. Fatigue may also result from disturbances in the sleep-wake cycle, a common problem reported after SAH that can significantly affect the quality of life.

Rehabilitation for SAH survivors is supervised by an integrated team designed to help the patient reach maximum physical, cognitive, social, and vocational potential. This team may include a rehabilitation physician, a neuropsychologist, physical therapists, speech and language specialists, occupational therapists, social workers, and an orthotist. The principles of rehabilitation for SAH are similar to that for any type of acquired brain injury and are based on neuroplasticity, the ability of the brain to change and adapt. Studies have shown that over time new areas of the brain can be trained with the help of sensory inputs, learning, and experience. It's important that rehabilitation be initiated as soon as possible following SAH. In the majority of cases, early in-patient rehabilitation results in significant functional gains over the first 18 months following SAH, but some patients may continue to benefit from rehabilitation for as long as five years.

References

1. Diringer, Michael N., MD. "Management of Aneurysmal Subarachnoid Hemorrhage," National Center for Biotechnology Information (NCBI), February 10, 2010.

2. "Subarachnoid Haemorrhage," National Health Service (NHS), January 14, 2016.

3. "Subarachnoid Hemorrhage," The Internet Stroke Center, n.d.

4. "Subarachnoid Hemorrhage," Mayo Clinic, October 13, 2017.

Section 5.5

Delirium
(Acute Onset Cognitive Changes)

This section contains text excerpted from the following sources: Text in this section begins with excerpts from "Delirium," MedlinePlus, National Institutes of Health (NIH), May 13, 2016; Text beginning with the heading "Symptoms" is excerpted from "The Impact of Delirium," MedlinePlus, National Institutes of Health (NIH), 2015.

Delirium is a condition that features rapidly changing mental states. It causes confusion and changes in behavior. Besides falling in and out of consciousness, there may be problems with

- Attention and awareness
- Thinking and memory
- Emotion
- Muscle control
- Sleeping and waking

Causes of delirium include medications, poisoning, serious illnesses, or infections, and severe pain. It can also be part of some mental illnesses or dementia.

Delirium and dementia have similar symptoms, so it can be hard to tell them apart. They can also occur together. Delirium starts suddenly and can cause hallucinations. The symptoms may get better or worse, and can last for hours or weeks. On the other hand, dementia develops slowly and does not cause hallucinations. The symptoms are stable, and may last for months or years.

Delirium tremens is a serious type of alcohol withdrawal syndrome. It usually happens to people who stop drinking after years of alcohol abuse.

People with delirium often, though not always, make a full recovery after their underlying illness is treated.

Symptoms

Delirium often involves a quick change between mental states (for example, from lethargy to agitation and back to lethargy) Symptoms may include:

- Fluctuating alertness (usually more alert in the morning, less at night)
- Hallucinations and delusions
- Variable levels of consciousness or awareness
- Disrupted sleep patterns, drowsiness
- Confusion (disorientation) about time or place
- Declines in short-term memory and recall
- Disorganized thinking, talking in a way that doesn't make sense
- Emotional changes: anger, agitation, depression, irritability, overexcitement
- Incontinence
- Problem concentrating

Contributing Factors

A number of medical and physical conditions may play a role in the onset of delirium, especially in older people:

- Use of pain medication or sedatives, or sedative drug withdrawal

- Drug or alcohol abuse

- Dehydration

- Electrolyte or other body chemical disturbances

- Infections such as urinary tract infections or pneumonia

- Poisons

- Recent surgery

- Disrupted and/or insufficient sleep

Treatment

Treatment depends on the condition of the patient, the level of pain, the medical history, and a variety of other considerations. The goal of treatment is to manage the symptoms. The person may need to stay in the hospital for a short time. Some examples of ways to manage symptoms include:

- Allowing older people to sleep undisturbed between 10 p.m. and 6 a.m. so that their normal sleep cycle is less disrupted.

- Stopping or changing medications that may contribute to delirium to try to improve mental function. After asking about your medical history to establish a "baseline," for example, your doctor may discuss medicines and substances that can worsen confusion, such as alcohol.

- Using low doses of medicines that control aggression or agitation, and adjusting the dose. These are usually started as needed.

- Behavior modification to control unacceptable or dangerous behaviors.

- Reality orientation to reduce disorientation. Reality orientation can include calendars, clocks, and anything that stimulates the senses to the present surroundings.

- Ensuring the patient has a hearing aid, glasses, or other devices necessary to aid communication.

Disorders that contribute to delirium should be treated. These may include:

- Anemia

- Decreased oxygen (hypoxia)

- Heart failure
- High carbon dioxide levels (hypercapnia)
- Infections
- Kidney failure
- Liver failure
- Nutritional disorders
- Psychiatric conditions (such as depression)
- Thyroid disorders

Prognosis

Cognitive dysfunction due to delirium in the setting of dementia may be reversible by treating the underlying acute illness. Full recovery is common, but depends on the underlying cause of the delirium. It may take several weeks for cognitive function to return to normal. However, more and more clinical data suggests that delirium may persist for weeks and even months.

Possible Complications

- Loss of ability to function or care for self
- Loss of ability to interact
- Increased likelihood of hospital acquired infections, longer hospital stays, and nursing home placements
- Side effects of medications used to treat the disorder

When to Contact a Medical Professional

Call your healthcare provider if there is a rapid change in mental status.

Prevention

Treating the conditions that may produce delirium can reduce its risk. In hospitalized patients, avoiding sedatives, prompt treatment of metabolic disorders and infections, and using reality orientation programs may reduce the risk of delirium in those at high risk.

Chapter 6

Coma

What Is Coma?

A coma, sometimes also called persistent vegetative state (PVS), is a profound or deep state of unconsciousness. PVS is not brain death. An individual in a state of coma is alive but unable to move or respond to his or her environment. Coma may occur as a complication of an underlying illness, or as a result of injuries, such as head trauma. Individuals in such a state have lost their thinking abilities and awareness of their surroundings, but retain noncognitive function and normal sleep patterns. Even though those in a PVS lose their higher brain functions, other key functions such as breathing and circulation remain relatively intact. Spontaneous movements may occur, and the eyes may open in response to external stimuli. Individuals may even occasionally grimace, cry, or laugh. Although individuals in a PVS may appear somewhat normal, they do not speak and they are unable to respond to commands.

Treatment

Once an individual is out of immediate danger, the medical care team focuses on preventing infections and maintaining a healthy

This chapter includes text excerpted from "Coma Information Page," National Institute of Neurological Disorders and Stroke (NINDS), May 24, 2017.

physical state. This will often include preventing pneumonia and bed-sores and providing balanced nutrition. Physical therapy may also be used to prevent contractures (permanent muscular contractions) and deformities of the bones, joints, and muscles that would limit recovery for those who emerge from coma.

Prognosis

The outcome for coma and PVS depends on the cause, severity, and site of neurological damage. Individuals may emerge from coma with a combination of physical, intellectual, and psychological difficulties that need special attention. Recovery usually occurs gradually, with some acquiring more and more ability to respond. Some individuals never progress beyond very basic responses, but many recover full awareness. Individuals recovering from coma require close medical supervision. A coma rarely lasts more than 2–4 weeks. Some patients may regain a degree of awareness after persistent vegetative state. Others may remain in that state for years or even decades. The most common cause of death for someone in a PVS is infection, such as pneumonia.

Part Two

Diagnosing and Treating Brain Disorders

Chapter 7

Neurological Tests and Procedures

Chapter Contents

Section 7.1

Common Screening and Diagnostic Tests for Neurological Disorders

This section includes text excerpted from "Neurological Diagnostic Tests and Procedures Fact Sheet," National Institute of Neurological Disorders and Stroke (NINDS), May 9, 2017.

Diagnostic tests and procedures are vital tools that help physicians confirm or rule out the presence of a neurological disorder or other medical condition. A century ago, the only way to make a positive diagnosis for many neurological disorders was by performing an autopsy after a patient had died. But decades of basic research into the characteristics of disease, and the development of techniques that allow scientists to see inside the living brain and monitor nervous system activity as it occurs, have given doctors powerful and accurate tools to diagnose disease and to test how well a particular therapy may be working.

Perhaps the most significant changes in diagnostic imaging over the past 20 years are improvements in spatial resolution (size, intensity, and clarity) of anatomical images and reductions in the time needed to send signals to and receive data from the area being imaged. These advances allow physicians to simultaneously see the structure of the brain and the changes in brain activity as they occur. Scientists continue to improve methods that will provide sharper anatomical images and more detailed functional information.

Researchers and physicians use a variety of diagnostic imaging techniques (DIT) and chemical and metabolic analyses to detect, manage, and treat neurological disease. Some procedures are performed in specialized settings, conducted to determine the presence of a particular disorder or abnormality. Many tests that were previously conducted in a hospital are now performed in a physician's office or at an outpatient testing facility, with little if any risk to the patient. Depending on the type of procedure, results are either immediate or may take several hours to process.

What Are Some of the More Common Screening Tests?

Laboratory screening tests of blood, urine, or other substances are used to help diagnose disease, better understand the disease process, and monitor levels of therapeutic drugs. Certain tests, ordered by the physician as part of a regular check-up, provide general information, while others are used to identify specific health concerns. For example, blood and blood product tests can detect brain and/or spinal cord infection, bone marrow disease, hemorrhage, blood vessel damage, toxins that affect the nervous system, and the presence of antibodies that signal the presence of an autoimmune disease. Blood tests are also used to monitor levels of therapeutic drugs used to treat epilepsy and other neurological disorders. Genetic testing of deoxyribonucleic acid (DNA) extracted from white cells in the blood can help diagnose Huntington disease (HD) and other congenital diseases. Analysis of the fluid that surrounds the brain and spinal cord can detect meningitis, acute and chronic inflammation, rare infections, and some cases of multiple sclerosis (MS). Chemical and metabolic testing of the blood can indicate protein disorders, some forms of muscular dystrophy (MD) and other muscle disorders, and diabetes. Urinalysis can reveal abnormal substances in the urine or the presence or absence of certain proteins that cause diseases including the mucopolysaccharidoses.

Genetic testing or counseling can help parents who have a family history of a neurological disease determine if they are carrying one of the known genes that cause the disorder or find out if their child is affected. Genetic testing can identify many neurological disorders, including spina bifida, in utero (while the child is inside the mother's womb). Genetic tests include the following:

- Amniocentesis, usually done at 14–16 weeks of pregnancy, tests a sample of the amniotic fluid in the womb for genetic defects (the fluid and the fetus have the same DNA). Under local anesthesia, a thin needle is inserted through the woman's abdomen and into the womb. About 20 milliliters of fluid (roughly 4 teaspoons) is withdrawn and sent to a lab for evaluation. Test results often take 1–2 weeks.

- Chorionic villus sampling, or CVS, is performed by removing and testing a very small sample of the placenta during early pregnancy. The sample, which contains the same DNA as the fetus, is removed by catheter or fine needle inserted through the cervix or by a fine needle inserted through the abdomen. It is tested for genetic abnormalities and results are usually available within 2 weeks. CVS should not be performed after the tenth week of pregnancy.

- Uterine ultrasound is performed using a surface probe with gel. This noninvasive test can suggest the diagnosis of conditions such as chromosomal disorders.

What Is a Neurological Examination?

- A neurological examination assesses motor and sensory skills, the functioning of one or more cranial nerves, hearing and speech, vision, coordination, and balance, mental status, and changes in mood or behavior, among other abilities. Items including a tuning fork, flashlight, reflex hammer, ophthalmoscope, and needles are used to help diagnose brain tumors, infections such as encephalitis and meningitis, and diseases such as Parkinson disease (PD), HD, amyotrophic lateral sclerosis (ALS), and epilepsy. Some tests require the services of a specialist to perform and analyze results.

- X-rays of the patient's chest and skull are often taken as part of a neurological workup. X-rays can be used to view any part of the body, such as a joint or major organ system. In a conventional X-ray, also called a radiograph, a technician passes a concentrated burst of low dose ionized radiation through the body and onto a photographic plate. Since calcium in bones absorbs X-rays more easily than soft tissue or muscle, the bony structure appears white on the film. Any vertebral misalignment or fractures can be seen within minutes. Tissue masses such as injured ligaments or a bulging disc are not visible on conventional X-rays. This fast, noninvasive, painless procedure is usually performed in a doctor's office or at a clinic.

- Fluoroscopy is a type of X-ray that uses a continuous or pulsed beam of low dose radiation to produce continuous images of a body part in motion. The fluoroscope (X-ray tube) is focused on the area of interest and pictures are either videotaped or sent to a monitor for viewing. A contrast medium may be used to highlight the images. Fluoroscopy can be used to evaluate the flow of blood through arteries.

What Are Some Diagnostic Tests Used to Diagnose Neurological Disorders?

Based on the result of a neurological exam, physical exam, patient history, X-rays of the patient's chest and skull, and any previous screening or testing, physicians may order one or more of the following diagnostic tests to determine the specific nature of a suspected neurological disorder or injury. These diagnostics generally involve either nuclear medicine imaging (NMI), in which very small amounts of radioactive materials are used to study organ function and structure, or diagnostic imaging, which uses magnets and electrical charges to study human anatomy.

The following list of available procedures—in alphabetical rather than sequential order—includes some of the more common tests used to help diagnose a neurological condition.

Angiography is a test used to detect blockages of the arteries or veins. A cerebral angiogram can detect the degree of narrowing or obstruction of an artery or blood vessel in the brain, head, or neck. It is used to diagnose stroke and to determine the location and size of a brain tumor, aneurysm, or vascular malformation. This test is usually performed in a hospital outpatient setting and takes up to 3 hours, followed by a 6- to 8-hour resting period. The patient, wearing a hospital or imaging gown, lies on a table that is wheeled into the imaging area. While the patient is awake, a physician anesthetizes a small area of the leg near the groin and then inserts a catheter into a major artery located there. The catheter is threaded through the body and into an artery in the neck. Once the catheter is in place, the needle is removed and a guide wire is inserted. A small capsule containing a radiopaque dye (one that is highlighted on X-rays) is passed over the guidewire to the site of release. The dye is released and travels through the bloodstream into the head and neck. A series of X-rays is taken and any obstruction is noted. Patients may feel a warm to hot sensation or slight discomfort as the dye is released.

Biopsy involves the removal and examination of a small piece of tissue from the body. Muscle or nerve biopsies are used to diagnose neuromuscular disorders and may also reveal if a person is a carrier of a defective gene that could be passed on to children. A small sample of muscle or nerve is removed under local anesthetic and studied under a microscope. The sample may be removed either surgically, through a slit made in the skin, or by needle biopsy, in which a thin hollow needle is inserted through the skin and into the muscle. A small piece of muscle or nerve remains in the hollow needle when it is removed from the body. The biopsy is usually performed at an outpatient testing facility. A brain biopsy, used to determine tumor type, requires surgery to remove a small piece of the brain or tumor. Performed in a

105

hospital, this operation is riskier than a muscle biopsy and involves a longer recovery period.

Brain scans are imaging techniques used to diagnose tumors, blood vessel malformations, or hemorrhage in the brain. These scans are used to study organ function or injury or disease to tissue or muscle. Types of brain scans include computed tomography (CT), magnetic resonance imaging (MRI), and positron emission tomography (PET).

Cerebrospinal fluid analysis involves the removal of a small amount of the fluid that protects the brain and spinal cord. The fluid is tested to detect any bleeding or brain hemorrhage, diagnose infection to the brain and/or spinal cord, identify some cases of multiple sclerosis and other neurological conditions, and measure intracranial pressure.

The procedure is usually done in a hospital. The sample of fluid is commonly removed by a procedure known as a lumbar puncture, or spinal tap. The patient is asked to either lie on one side, in a ball position with knees close to the chest, or lean forward while sitting on a table or bed. The doctor will locate a puncture site in the lower back, between two vertebrate, then clean the area and inject a local anesthetic. The patient may feel a slight stinging sensation from this injection. Once the anesthetic has taken effect, the doctor will insert a special needle into the spinal sac and remove a small amount of fluid (usually about three teaspoons) for testing. Most patients will feel a sensation of pressure only as the needle is inserted.

A common after-effect of a lumbar puncture is headache, which can be lessened by having the patient lie flat. Risk of nerve root injury or infection from the puncture can occur but it is rare. The entire procedure takes about 45 minutes.

Computed tomography, also known as a CT scan, is a noninvasive, painless process used to produce rapid, clear two-dimensional images of organs, bones, and tissues. Neurological CT scans are used to view the brain and spine. They can detect bone and vascular irregularities, certain brain tumors and cysts, herniated discs, epilepsy, encephalitis, spinal stenosis (narrowing of the spinal canal), a blood clot or intracranial bleeding in patients with stroke, brain damage from head injury, and other disorders. Many neurological disorders share certain characteristics and a CT scan can aid in proper diagnosis by differentiating the area of the brain affected by the disorder.

Scanning takes about 20 minutes (a CT of the brain or head may take slightly longer) and is usually done at an imaging center or hospital on an outpatient basis. The patient lies on a special table that slides into a narrow chamber. A sound system built into the chamber allows the patient to communicate with the physician or technician. As the patient lies still, X-rays are passed through the body at various angles and are detected by a computerized scanner. The data is processed and displayed as cross-sectional images, or "slices," of the internal structure of the body or organ. A light sedative may be given to patients who are unable to lie still and pillows may be used to support and stabilize the head and body. Persons who are claustrophobic may have difficulty taking this imaging test.

Occasionally a contrast dye is injected into the bloodstream to highlight the different tissues in the brain. Patients may feel a warm or cool sensation as the dye circulates through the bloodstream or they may experience a slight metallic taste.

Although very little radiation is used in CT, pregnant women should avoid the test because of potential harm to the fetus from ionizing radiation.

Discography is often suggested for patients who are considering lumbar surgery or whose lower back pain has not responded to conventional treatments. This outpatient procedure is usually performed at a testing facility or a hospital. The patient is asked to put on a metal free hospital gown and lie on an imaging table. The physician numbs the skin with anesthetic and inserts a thin needle, using X-ray guidance, into the spinal disc. Once the needle is in place, a small amount of contrast dye is injected and CT scans are taken. The contrast dye outlines any damaged areas. More than one disc may be imaged at the same time. Patient recovery usually takes about an hour. Pain medicine may be prescribed for any resulting discomfort.

An **intrathecal contrast enhanced CT scan** (also called cisternography) is used to detect problems with the spine and spinal nerve roots. This test is most often performed at an imaging center. The patient is asked to put on a hospital or imaging gown. Following application of a topical anesthetic, the physician removes a small sample of the spinal fluid via lumbar puncture. The sample is mixed with a contrast dye and injected into the spinal sac located at the base of the lower back. The patient is then asked to move to a position that will allow the contrast fluid to travel to the area to be studied. The dye allows the spinal canal and nerve roots to be seen more clearly on a CT scan. The scan may take up to an hour to complete. Following the test, patients may experience some discomfort and/or headache that may be caused by the removal of spinal fluid.

Electroencephalography, or EEG, monitors brain activity through the skull. EEG is used to help diagnose certain seizure disorders, brain tumors, brain damage from head injuries, inflammation of the brain and/or spinal cord, alcoholism, certain psychiatric disorders, and metabolic and degenerative disorders that affect the brain. EEGs are also used to evaluate sleep disorders, monitor brain activity when a patient has been fully anesthetized or loses consciousness, and confirm brain death.

This painless, risk-free test can be performed in a doctor's office or at a hospital or testing facility. Prior to taking an EEG, the person must avoid caffeine intake and prescription drugs that affect the nervous system. A series of cup-like electrodes are attached to the patient's scalp, either with a special conducting paste or with extremely fine needles. The electrodes (also called leads) are small devices that are attached to wires and carry the electrical energy of the brain to a machine for reading. A very low electrical current is sent through the electrodes and the baseline brain energy is recorded. Patients are then exposed to a variety of external stimuli—including bright or flashing light, noise or certain drugs—or are asked to open and close the eyes, or to change breathing patterns. The electrodes transmit the resulting changes in brainwave patterns. Since movement and nervousness can change brainwave patterns, patients usually recline in a chair or on a bed during the test, which takes up to an hour. Testing for certain disorders requires performing an EEG during sleep, which takes at least 3 hours.

Electromyography, or EMG, is used to diagnose nerve and muscle dysfunction and spinal cord disease. It records the electrical activity from the brain and/or spinal cord to a peripheral nerve root (found in the arms and legs) that controls muscles during contraction and at rest.

During an EMG, very fine wire electrodes are inserted into a muscle to assess changes in electrical voltage that occur during movement and when the muscle is at rest. The electrodes are attached through a series of wires to a recording instrument. Testing usually takes place at a testing facility and lasts about an hour but may take longer, depending on the number of muscles and nerves to be tested. Most patients find this test to be somewhat uncomfortable.

An EMG is usually done in conjunction with a nerve conduction velocity (NCV) test, which measures electrical energy by assessing the nerve's ability to send a signal. This two-part test is conducted most often in a hospital. A technician tapes two sets of flat electrodes on the skin over the muscles. The first set of electrodes is used to send small pulses of electricity (similar to the sensation of static electricity) to stimulate the nerve that directs a particular muscle. The second set of electrodes transmits the responding electrical signal to a recording machine. The physician then reviews the response to verify any nerve damage or muscle disease. Patients who are preparing to take an EMG or NCV test may be asked to avoid caffeine and not smoke for 2–3 hours prior to the test, as well as to avoid aspirin and nonsteroidal anti-inflammatory drugs for 24 hours before the EMG. There is no discomfort or risk associated with this test.

Electronystagmography (ENG) describes a group of tests used to diagnose involuntary eye movement, dizziness, and balance disorders, and to evaluate some brain functions. The test is performed at an imaging center. Small electrodes are taped around the eyes to record eye movements. If infrared photography is used in place of electrodes, the patient wears special goggles that help record the information. Both versions of the test are painless and risk-free.

Evoked potentials (also called evoked response) measure the electrical signals to the brain generated by hearing, touch, or sight. These tests are used to assess sensory nerve problems and confirm neurological conditions including multiple sclerosis, brain tumor, acoustic neuroma (small tumors of the inner ear), and spinal cord injury. Evoked potentials are also used to test sight and hearing (especially in infants and young children), monitor brain activity among coma patients, and confirm brain death.

Testing may take place in a doctor's office or hospital setting. It is painless and risk-free. Two sets of needle electrodes are used to test for nerve damage. One set of electrodes, which will be used to measure the electrophysiological response to stimuli, is attached to the patient's scalp using conducting paste. The second set of electrodes is attached to the part of the body to be tested. The physician then records the amount of time it takes for the impulse generated by stimuli to reach the brain. Under normal circumstances, the process of signal transmission is instantaneous.

Auditory evoked potentials (also called brainstem auditory evoked response) are used to assess high frequency hearing loss, diagnose any damage to the acoustic nerve, and auditory pathways in the brainstem, and detect acoustic neuromas. The patient sits in a soundproof room and wears headphones. Clicking sounds are delivered one at a time to one ear while a masking sound is sent to the other ear. Each ear is usually tested twice, and the entire procedure takes about 45 minutes.

Visual evoked potentials detect loss of vision from optic nerve damage (in particular, damage caused by multiple sclerosis). The patient sits close to a screen and is asked to focus on the center of a shifting checkerboard pattern. Only one eye is tested at a time; the other eye is either kept closed or covered with a patch. Each eye is usually tested twice. Testing takes 30–45 minutes.

Somatosensory evoked potentials measure response from stimuli to the peripheral nerves and can detect nerve or spinal cord damage or nerve degeneration from multiple sclerosis and other degenerating diseases. Tiny electrical shocks are delivered by electrode to a nerve in an arm or leg. Responses to the shocks, which may be delivered for more than a minute at a time, are recorded. This test usually lasts less than an hour.

Magnetic resonance imaging (MRI) uses computer generated radio waves and a powerful magnetic field to produce detailed images of body structures including tissues, organs, bones, and nerves. Neurological uses include the diagnosis of brain and spinal cord tumors, eye disease, inflammation, infection, and vascular irregularities that may lead to stroke. MRI can also detect and monitor degenerative disorders such as multiple sclerosis and can document brain injury from trauma.

The equipment houses a hollow tube that is surrounded by a very large cylindrical magnet. The patient, who must remain still during the test, lies on a special table that is slid into the tube. The patient will be asked to remove jewelry, eyeglasses, removable dental work, or other items that might interfere with the magnetic imaging. The patient should wear a sweatshirt and sweatpants or other clothing free of metal eyelets or buckles. MRI scanning equipment creates a magnetic field around the body strong enough to temporarily realign water molecules in the tissues. Radio waves are then passed through the body to detect the "relaxation" of the molecules back to a random alignment and trigger a resonance signal at different angles within the body. A computer processes this resonance into either a three-dimensional picture or a two-dimensional "slice" of the tissue being scanned, and differentiates between bone, soft tissues and fluid-filled spaces by their water content and structural properties. A contrast dye may be used to enhance visibility of certain areas or tissues. The patient may hear grating or knocking noises when the magnetic field is turned on and off. (Patients may wear special earphones to block out the sounds.) Unlike CT scanning, MRI does not use ionizing radiation to produce images. Depending on the part(s) of the body to be scanned, MRI can take up to an hour to complete. The test is painless and risk-free, although persons who are obese or claustrophobic may find it somewhat uncomfortable. (Some centers also use open MRI machines that do not completely surround the person being tested and are less confining. However, open MRI does not currently provide the same picture quality as standard MRI and some tests may not be available using this equipment). Due to the incredibly strong magnetic field generated by an MRI, patients with implanted medical devices such as a pacemaker should avoid the test.

Functional MRI (fMRI) uses the blood's magnetic properties to produce real time images of blood flow to particular areas of the brain. An fMRI can pinpoint areas of the brain that become active and note how long they stay active. It can also tell if brain activity within a region occurs simultaneously or sequentially. This imaging process is used to assess brain damage from head injury or degenerative disorders such as Alzheimer disease (AD) and to identify and monitor other neurological disorders, including MS, stroke, and brain tumors.

Myelography involves the injection of a water or oil-based contrast dye into the spinal canal to enhance X-ray imaging of the spine. Myelograms are used to diagnose spinal nerve injury, herniated discs, fractures, back or leg pain, and spinal tumors.

The procedure takes about 30 minutes and is usually performed in a hospital. Following an injection of anesthesia to a site between two vertebrae in the lower back, a small amount of the cerebrospinal fluid is removed by spinal tap and the contrast dye is injected into the spinal canal. After a series of X-rays is taken, most or all of the contrast dye is removed by aspiration. Patients may experience some pain during the spinal tap and when the dye is injected and removed. Patients may also experience headache following the spinal tap. The risk of fluid leakage or allergic reaction to the dye is slight.

Positron emission tomography (PET) scans provide two and three-dimensional pictures of brain activity by measuring radioactive isotopes that are injected into the bloodstream. PET scans of the brain are used to detect or highlight tumors and diseased tissue, measure cellular and/or tissue metabolism, show blood flow, evaluate patients who have seizure disorders that do not respond to medical therapy and patients with certain memory disorders, and determine brain changes following injury or drug abuse, among other uses. PET may be ordered as a follow-up to a CT or MRI scan to give the physician a greater understanding of specific areas of the brain that may be involved with certain problems. Scans are conducted in a hospital or at a testing facility, on an outpatient basis. A low level radioactive isotope, which binds to chemicals that flow to the brain, is injected into the bloodstream and can be traced as the brain performs different functions. The patient lies still while overhead sensors detect gamma rays in the body's tissues. A computer processes the information and displays it on a video monitor or on film. Using different compounds, more than one brain function can be traced simultaneously. PET is painless and relatively risk-free. Length of test time depends on the part of the body to be scanned. PET scans are performed by skilled technicians at highly sophisticated medical facilities.

A **polysomnogram** measures brain and body activity during sleep. It is performed over one or more nights at a sleep center. Electrodes are pasted or taped to the patient's scalp, eyelids, and/or chin. Throughout the night and during the various wake/sleep cycles, the electrodes record brainwaves, eye movement, breathing, leg, and skeletal muscle activity, blood pressure, and heart rate. The patient may be videotaped to note any movement during sleep. Results are then used to identify any characteristic patterns of sleep disorders, including restless legs syndrome (RLS), periodic limb movement disorder (PLMD), insomnia, and breathing disorders such as obstructive sleep apnea (OSA). Polysomnograms are noninvasive, painless, and risk-free.

Single photon emission computed tomography (SPECT), a nuclear imaging test involving blood flow to tissue, is used to evaluate certain brain functions. The test may be ordered as a follow-up to an MRI to diagnose tumors, infections, degenerative spinal disease, and stress fractures. As with a PET scan, a radioactive isotope, which binds to chemicals that flow to the brain, is injected intravenously into the body. Areas of increased blood flow will collect more of the isotope. As the patient lies on a table, a gamma camera rotates around the head and records where the radioisotope has traveled. That information is converted by computer into cross-sectional slices that are stacked to produce a detailed three-dimensional image of blood flow and activity within the brain. The test is performed at either an imaging center or a hospital.

Thermography uses infrared sensing devices to measure small temperature changes between the two sides of the body or within a specific organ. Also known as digital infrared thermal imaging, thermography may be used to detect vascular disease of the head and neck, soft tissue injury, various neuromusculoskeletal disorders, and the presence or absence of nerve root compression. It is performed at an imaging center, using infrared light recorders to take thousands of pictures of the body from a distance of 5–8 feet. The information is converted into electrical signals which results in a computer generated two-dimensional picture of abnormally cold or hot areas indicated by color or shades of black and white. Thermography does not use radiation and is safe, risk-free, and noninvasive.

Ultrasound imaging, also called ultrasound scanning or sonography, uses high frequency sound waves to obtain images inside the body. Neurosonography (ultrasound of the brain and spinal column) analyzes blood flow in the brain and can diagnose stroke, brain tumors, hydrocephalus (buildup of cerebrospinal fluid in the brain), and vascular problems. It can also identify or rule out inflammatory processes causing pain. It is more effective than an X-ray in displaying soft tissue masses and can show tears in ligaments, muscles, tendons, and other soft tissue masses in the back. Transcranial Doppler ultrasound is used to view arteries and blood vessels in the neck and determine blood flow and risk of stroke.

During ultrasound, the patient lies on an imaging table and removes clothing around the area of the body to be scanned. A jelly-like lubricant is applied and a transducer, which both sends and receives high frequency sound waves, is passed over the body. The sound wave echoes are recorded and displayed as a computer generated real-time visual image of the structure or tissue being examined. Ultrasound is painless, noninvasive, and risk-free. The test is performed on an outpatient basis and takes between 15 and 30 minutes to complete.

Section 7.2

Neurological Imaging

This section includes text excerpted from "Neurological Imaging," National Institutes of Health (NIH), March 29, 2013. Reviewed February 2018.

Neurological Imaging in the Past

- Neurologists and neurosurgeons made clinical decisions based on first generation computed tomography (CT) scans. This was a quantum advance over the insensitive plain film X-ray techniques of previous generations.

- Early positron emission tomography (PET) and single photon emission computed tomography (SPECT) techniques utilized first generation radiographic tracers (or tags) to map brain function.

- Functional magnetic resonance imaging (fMRI) allowed researchers to measure blood oxygen level dependent (BOLD) changes in the brain of humans for the first time. fMRI enabled the noninvasive study of everything from finger movements to thoughts and emotions.

Neurological Imaging in the Present Day

- Advanced magnetic resonance imaging (MRI) is revolutionizing the care of patients with neurologic disorders, as well as research in understanding the brain. Magnetic resonance spectroscopy (MRS) allows measurement of brain chemicals in living patients. PET imaging using compounds that bind to brain receptors now allows the study of molecular details not previously visualized.

- The resolution of brain and spinal cord imaging has increased tremendously. For example, modern techniques allow the neuroimaging of subtle abnormalities of neurological development that give rise to seizures and enable many more persons to benefit from a surgical treatment of epilepsy. MRI can now identify spinal vascular malformations that are amenable to treatment. Many of these went undiagnosed previously.

- Functional MRI BOLD imaging enables researchers not only to localize and measure important brain functions, but also to assess functional changes in the brain resulting from disease processes, injury, or response to treatment. fMRI is also being used to guide operative strategy in neurosurgery.

- Diffusion tensor imaging, a technique that allows for the visualization and characterization of white matter tracts in the human brain, is allowing researchers to assess changes in the brain's maturation from childhood to adulthood, as well as to detect differences in white matter integrity between healthy and diseased populations.

- Advanced diagnostics in many neurological diseases/disorders now are increasingly used as a means to monitor the progression of disease and response to treatment. For example, the

114

development of Pittsburgh compound B (PiB) now permits the molecular imaging of the amyloid beta-protein (ABP) in patients with Alzheimer disease (AD). In addition, MRI has become invaluable in the diagnosis of patients with multiple sclerosis (MS) and spinal cord disorders.

- Advanced image processing allows clinicians and researchers to measure the subtle shrinkage of brain regions over time (from chronic disease progression) and use this information to test new therapies. Furthermore, neuroimaging has made it possible to detect, characterize, and monitor objective brain changes after insults such as traumatic brain injury (TBI).

- Neuroimaging has played a crucial role in advancing under-standing and treatment of stroke, and is now recommended by national guidelines for acute assessment and treatment decisions and for secondary prevention. Studies are using different forms of imaging at different time points after stroke to help hospitals better identify patients who could benefit from treatment beyond the current window.

Neurological Imaging in Future

- Advanced neuroimaging techniques will allow researchers to understand all of the structural and functional pathways in the entire, living human brain. This groundbreaking advance could lead to more accurate diagnosis and treatment of a variety of neurological and mental disorders. The National Institutes of Health (NIH) has launched the Human Connectome Project (HCP) a $30 million multisite project that aims to understand genetic and environmental influences on brain connectivity, as well as how dysfunction in connectivity can contribute to neuro-logical and mental conditions.

- Scientists will be able to use imaging to understand cognitive impairment in neurodegenerative diseases such as Alzheimer. The ongoing AD Neuroimaging Initiative (ADNI) a multisite, longitu-dinal, prospective study of normal cognitive aging, mild cognitive impairment (MCI), and early AD, will enable researchers to define rates of impairment, design improved methods for clinical trials, and develop more effective techniques to treat and prevent AD.

- In the future, scientists will be able to use neuroimaging to determine consciousness states of individuals. A series of intriguing studies has improved the clinical assessment of states such as coma, vegetative state, minimally conscious state, and locked-in syndrome, providing information about evaluation of brain function, formation of diagnoses, and estimation of prognosis.

Section 7.3

Carotid Ultrasound

This section includes text excerpted from "Carotid Ultrasound," National Heart, Lung, and Blood Institute (NHLBI), June 11, 2014. Reviewed February 2018.

What Is Carotid Ultrasound?

Carotid ultrasound is a painless and harmless test that uses high frequency sound waves to create pictures of the insides of your carotid arteries.

You have two common carotid arteries, one on each side of your neck. They each divide into internal and external carotid arteries. The internal carotid arteries supply oxygen-rich blood to your brain. The external carotid arteries supply oxygen-rich blood to your face, scalp, and neck.

Carotid ultrasound shows whether a waxy substance called plaque has built up in your carotid arteries. The buildup of plaque in the carotid arteries is called carotid artery disease (CAD).

Over time, plaque can harden or rupture (break open). Hardened plaque narrows the carotid arteries and reduces the flow of oxygen-rich blood to the brain. If the plaque ruptures, a blood clot can form on its surface. A clot can mostly or completely block blood flow through a carotid artery, which can cause a stroke. A piece of plaque or a blood clot also can break away from the wall of the carotid artery. The plaque or clot can travel through the bloodstream and get stuck in one of the brain's smaller arteries. This can block blood flow in the artery and cause a stroke. A standard carotid ultrasound shows the structure of your carotid arteries. Your carotid ultrasound test might include a Doppler ultrasound. Doppler ultrasound is a special test that shows

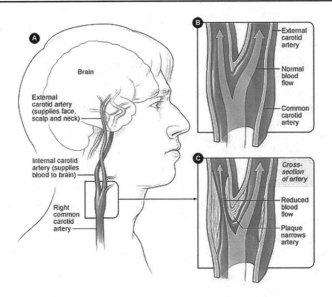

Figure 7.1. *Carotid Arteries*

Figure A shows the location of the right carotid artery in the head and neck. Figure B is a cross-section of a normal carotid artery that has normal blood flow. Figure C shows a carotid artery that has plaque buildup and reduced blood flow.

the movement of blood through your blood vessels. Your doctor might need results from both types of ultrasound to fully assess whether you have a blood flow problem in your carotid arteries.

Who Needs Carotid Ultrasound?

A carotid ultrasound shows whether you have plaque buildup in your carotid arteries. Over time, plaque can harden or rupture (break open). This can reduce or block the flow of oxygen-rich blood to your brain and cause a stroke.

Your doctor may recommend a carotid ultrasound if you:

- **Had a stroke or mini-stroke recently**. During a mini-stroke, you may have some or all of the symptoms of a stroke. However, the symptoms usually go away on their own within 24 hours.

- **Have an abnormal sound called a carotid bruit in one of your carotid arteries**. Your doctor can hear a carotid bruit using a stethoscope. A bruit might suggest a partial blockage in your carotid artery, which could lead to a stroke.

117

Your doctor also may recommend a carotid ultrasound if he or she thinks you have:

• Blood clots in one of your carotid arteries

• A split between the layers of your carotid artery wall. The split can weaken the wall or reduce blood flow to your brain.

A carotid ultrasound also might be done to see whether carotid artery surgery, also called carotid endarterectomy (CEA), has restored normal blood flow through a carotid artery. If you had a procedure called carotid stenting, your doctor might use carotid ultrasound afterward to check the position of the stent in your carotid artery. (The stent, a small mesh tube, supports the inner artery wall.). Carotid ultrasound sometimes is used as a preventive screening test in people at increased risk of stroke, such as those who have high blood pressure and diabetes.

What to Expect before Carotid Ultrasound

Carotid ultrasound is a painless test. Typically, there is little to do in advance of the test. Your doctor will tell you how to prepare for your carotid ultrasound.

What to Expect during Carotid Ultrasound

Carotid ultrasound usually is done in a doctor's office or hospital. The test is painless and often doesn't take more than 30 minutes. The ultrasound machine includes a computer, a screen, and a transducer. The transducer is a hand-held device that sends and receives ultrasound waves.

You will lie on your back on an exam table for the test. Your technician or doctor will put gel on your neck where your carotid arteries are located. The gel helps the ultrasound waves reach the arteries.

Your technician or doctor will put the transducer against different spots on your neck and move it back and forth. The transducer gives off ultrasound waves and detects their echoes as they bounce off the artery walls and blood cells. Ultrasound waves can't be heard by the human ear. The computer uses the echoes to create and record pictures of the insides of the carotid arteries. These pictures usually appear in black and white. The screen displays these live images for your doctor to review. Your carotid ultrasound test might include a Doppler ultrasound. Doppler ultrasound is a special test that shows the movement

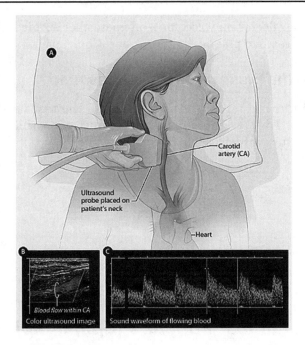

Figure 7.2. *Carotid Ultrasound*

Figure A shows how the ultrasound probe (transducer) is placed over the carotid artery. Figure B is a color ultrasound image showing blood flow (the red color in the image) in the carotid artery. Figure C is a waveform image showing the sound of flowing blood in the carotid artery.

of blood through your arteries. Blood flow through the arteries usually appears in color on the ultrasound pictures.

What to Expect after Carotid Ultrasound

You usually can return to your normal activities as soon as the carotid ultrasound is over. Your doctor will likely be able to tell you the results of the carotid ultrasound when it occurs or soon afterward.

What Does a Carotid Ultrasound Show?

A carotid ultrasound can show whether plaque buildup has narrowed one or both of your carotid arteries. If so, you might be at risk of having a stroke. The risk depends on the extent of the blockage and how much it has reduced blood flow to your brain. To lower your risk of stroke, your doctor may recommend medical or surgical treatments to reduce or remove plaque from your carotid arteries.

What Are the Risks of Carotid Ultrasound?

Carotid ultrasound has no risks because the test uses harmless sound waves. They are the same type of sound waves that doctors use to record pictures of fetuses in pregnant women.

Section 7.4

Lumbar Puncture (Spinal Tap)

This section includes text excerpted from "Lumbar Puncture Fact Sheet," National Institute on Aging (NIA), National Institutes of Health (NIH), June 11, 2010. Reviewed February 2018.

What Is Lumbar Puncture?

A lumbar puncture (spinal tap) test is a procedure to remove a small sample of cerebral spinal fluid from the lower spine. A needle is inserted between the vertebrae (backbones) in the lower back and into the space containing the spinal fluid which surrounds and cushions the brain and spinal cord.

How Long Does It Take?

About 20–30 minutes. There is an additional recovery period of about 30 minutes after the test, when you will remain at the clinic.

Why Is the Lumbar Puncture Test Performed?

To obtain a specimen of fluid for testing. Cerebrospinal fluid (CSF) bathes the brain and contains proteins that can provide clues about disorders such as Alzheimer disease (AD) or changes in the brain that accompany aging.

Does It Hurt?

You may experience pressure when the needle is inserted. You may also feel some very brief leg pain while the needle is positioned because it may briefly touch a floating nerve ending.

How Is It Performed?

- You will lie on your side with your knees drawn up toward your chin as far as possible or you will sit on the edge of an exam table, in a hunched forward position.
- The doctor will cleanse the skin over your spinal column with iodine.
- An injection of local anesthetic may be given at the puncture site.
- A needle is inserted into your spinal fluid space.
- Spinal fluid is collected into specimen tubes for laboratory testing.
- The needle is withdrawn, your back is cleaned, and a band-aid is placed over the spot.

After the Test

- You will be asked to lie down for about 30 minutes.
- You will be given something to eat and drink.
- While you are recovering, please report any of the following symptoms to the doctor or nurse:
  - Headache
  - Tingling
  - Numbness or pain in your lower back and legs
  - Problems with urination
- You will return home after the recovery period.

Instructions to follow at home:
- Drink at least 6 glasses of fluid (no alcohol) in the next 12 hours.
- Remain quiet for the next 24 hours.

- Avoid any strenuous physical activity for 48 hours–no exercising, heavy lifting, or repeated bending.

- A mild headache may follow a lumbar puncture. It is often relieved by caffeine, aspirin or tylenol, and drinking plenty of fluids.

- If you develop a headache that persists more than 24 hours, in particular one that is worse on sitting or standing, and better when lying down, then call the doctor or study coordinator at the clinic.

Section 7.5

Intracranial Pressure Monitoring

This section includes text excerpted from "Non-Invasive
Intracranial Pressure Measurement," National Aeronautics
and Space Administration (NASA), July 14, 2017.

An acknowledged objective of critical care medicine is a timely, accurate, readily deployable, cost-effective, and, importantly, safe means of assessing and/or monitoring critical aspects/parameters of patient condition such as intracranial pressure (ICP). However, ICP monitoring is complicated by a large set of variables related to the patients themselves—presented symptoms, circumstances, and related information indicating such measurement; and relevant accompanying issues. These conditions and the various combinations thereof present attending physicians with the choice of many alternatives regarding key parameters, including but not limited to urgency, availability, appropriability, and accuracy to a minimum standard. Cost, complexity, ease of use and other issues are also meaningful factors, but the bottom line for any of the various technical approaches, whether invasive or noninvasive, is performance. Key to this technology is its capability to correlate closely with established tympanic membrane displacement (TMD) ICP monitoring technology.

Benefits

- Based on known and well understood principles, yielding data that demonstrate close correlation with a known noninvasive ICP monitoring technology, tympanic membrane displacement.

- Implementation of the technology would be straightforward and of low impact to the patient in a clinical setting.

Applications

- Application of the technology to limited and narrowly defined settings, such as on board emergency vehicles responding to medical emergencies and other medical triage situations outside of medical facilities, may present opportunities such as specific application subsets of ICP monitoring, as in remote, nonmedical facilities and in emergency/triage facilities and/or equipment (e.g., battlefield settings, ambulances/emergency medical service (EMS) vehicles, etc.) in which the products likely low cost, small footprint and ease of use may constitute compelling advantages.

- Further refinement of the technology to yield ICP monitoring data more closely matching those of invasive procedures may be possible.

The Technology

This technology and a product based on it offer new analytical capabilities for assessment of intracranial dynamics. It offers the possibility for the monitoring of transcranial expansion and related physiological phenomena in humans resulting from variations in intracranial pressure (ICP) caused by injuries to the head and/or brain pathologies. The technology uses constant frequency pulse phase locked loop (CFPPLL) technology to measure skull expansion caused by pressure and its variations in time. This approach yields a more accurate, more robust measurement capability with improved bandwidth that allows new analytical approaches for assessing the physiology of skull expansion under pulsatile cerebral blood flow (pCBF). The dynamical quantities assessable with the CFPPLL include skull volume expansion and total fluid. Such an instrument can serve to measure intracranial dynamics with equation based algorithms, and offers a path to measure or determine quasi-static intracranial pressure, along with the pulsatile related intracranial pressure incre-ments. Supportive measurements, such as time dependence of arterial pressure waveforms together with time-dependent phase change of transcranial expansions can serve as the basis of noninvasive tech-niques to measure intracranial pressure.

Chapter 8

Chemotherapy and the Brain

Chapter Contents

Section 8.1

Chemobrain

This section includes text excerpted from "Understanding "Chemobrain" and Cognitive Impairment after Cancer Treatment," National Cancer Institute (NCI), March 28, 2017.

For decades, cancer survivors have described experiencing problems with memory, attention, and processing information months or even years after treatment. Because so many of these survivors had chemotherapy, this phenomenon has been called "chemobrain" or "chemofog," but researchers say those terms don't always fit the varied impairments experienced by these patients. Why cancer treatment related cognitive impairment occurs isn't fully understood. But research, including the largest study to date of breast cancer survivors to focus on this problem, aims to find the factors that might predict which patients will have cognitive impairment (CI) after treatment and to identify what can be done to lessen its impact.

A Frequent Problem

Although cognitive changes have been associated with treatment for many kinds of cancer, research has focused on cognitive changes in breast cancer survivors. In an update on the state of the science in 2012, Tim Ahles, Ph.D., of Memorial Sloan Kettering Cancer Center (MSKCC), and his colleagues reported that studies of breast cancer survivors found that 17–75 percent of these women experienced cognitive deficits—problems with attention, concentration, planning, and working memory—from 6 months to 20 years after receiving chemotherapy.

According to Julia Rowland, Ph.D., director of National Cancer Institute's (NCI) Office of Cancer Survivorship (OCS), for a long time many women who brought up these issues with their doctors found their concerns dismissed. But now, "people are finally taking it very seriously," she said. Doctors are realizing that "you have to understand what the consequences of therapy are and that very few if any of our treatments are entirely benign."

Early researchers assumed that cognitive problems were a result of chemotherapy alone. More research has suggested that the combination of chemotherapy and hormonal therapy, or even hormonal therapy alone, may cause cognitive change.

"From many sources of data, we now know patients experience impairments not just after chemo, but after surgery, radiation, hormonal therapy," and other treatments, said Patricia Ganz, M.D., an oncologist and director of Cancer Prevention and Control Research (CPCR) at The University of California, Los Angeles (UCLA's) Jonsson Comprehensive Cancer Center (JCCC).

In one study, Dr. Ganz and her colleagues gave 53 breast cancer survivors and 19 matched healthy women a comprehensive neurocognitive test and took measures of mood, energy level, and self-reported cognitive functioning. They found that the survivors who'd had adjuvant chemotherapy performed significantly worse than those who'd had surgery only, with the worst performance among those who'd received chemotherapy and the antiestrogen drug tamoxifen (Nolvadex®).

One challenge in studying these issues has been that many cancer survivors who report cognitive difficulties still perform within the normal range on neuropsychological tests. "You assess people's memory, and it tends to be fine," said Dr. Ahles. "But because of problems with attention and being able to sort out relevant information, it's harder for them to store information properly."

Imaging studies conducted by Dr. Ganz and others show that, despite performing within the normal range on these tests, women who report cognitive challenges are still struggling. For example, in one study, a set of identical twins—one who had received chemotherapy treatment for breast cancer and one who did not have cancer—was evaluated with self-reported measures, neuropsychological tests, and magnetic resonance imaging (MRI). The results showed small differences in the neuropsychological tests, but the twin who had cancer treatment had substantially more self-reported cognitive complaints. Imaging tests in this twin showed greater recruitment of brain areas during working memory processing. These patients "have to work harder," Dr. Ganz said. "Often they'll get the answer right on a neuropsychology test, but it takes much more effort for them to come up with that," than people who haven't been exposed to treatment.

Investigating Different Reactions to Treatment

But why do some cancer survivors experience cognitive decline after treatment while others don't? "Clearly there's a subset of people who aren't affected," said Dr. Rowland. "So the question is: Who are they? What are the factors there?"

And do these cognitive issues sometimes develop prior to cancer treatment? In a study, more than 20 percent of patients with breast cancer had lower cognitive performance at the pretreatment assessment than would be expected for their age and education, and other studies have had similar findings. This shows that "it's not just the treatment that you get but what you bring to the diagnosis that increases your risk," Dr. Ahles said.

To explore these and other factors, a team led by Michelle Janelsins, Ph.D., of the University of Rochester's Wilmot Cancer Institute, carried out a nationwide prospective longitudinal study in which they compared cognitive difficulties among 581 breast cancer patients treated at community clinical sites across the United States with 364 age-matched healthy women. Researchers used a tool called the Functional Assessment of Cancer Therapy-Cognitive Function (FACT-Cog), which allowed women to report their own cognitive function.

The study found that, from the time of diagnosis to after completing chemotherapy, 45.2 percent of patients self-reported a clinically significant decline in cognitive function, compared with 10.4 percent of healthy people over the same time period. And from before chemotherapy to 6 months after completing chemotherapy, 36.5 percent of patients reported a decline in cognitive function, compared with 13.6 percent of the healthy women.

In further analyses of pretreatment factors, the researchers found that both higher anxiety and higher levels of depressive symptoms before treatment were associated with lower FACT-Cog scores. This finding led the researchers to conclude that managing anxiety and depression after diagnosis and during treatment may lessen cognitive impairment and its impact on quality of life. The neuropsychological outcomes from the study have not yet been published.

Dr. Ahles, a coauthor, said this study is significant, not only because of its size, but also because it's one of the first studies of cognitive impairment in cancer patients to focus on patients seen in community-based settings. Dr. Rowland added that it's important because of the visibility it brings to the issue. "Once you start getting these reports published in journals that have a wide clinical readership, my sense is you have a greater willingness to say, 'this is a problem,'" she said.

Directions for Research and Treatment

The need to determine who is most at risk for developing cognitive problems after cancer treatment is driving research in several different ways. Dr. Ahles has been investigating the interplay between cancer and aging. "With regard to cognition, the question becomes, 'are the changes that we're seeing due to specific effects of chemotherapy on the brain, or are they a reflection of accelerating aging on some level?'" he said. "This is a new, interesting area of research to explore."

Dr. Ahles has also investigated potential genetic markers for increased vulnerability to cognitive impairment after cancer treatment, including a form (or allele) of the *APOE* gene called ε4, which is associated with Alzheimer disease (AD). Other studies have shown that breast cancer survivors who have a variant of the *COMT* gene, which influences how quickly the brain metabolizes dopamine, are at greater risk of cognitive impairment and that a variant of the *BDNF* gene can protect against chemotherapy associated cognitive impairment.

Dr. Ahles said that, although these are all small studies, together they point to imbalances or deficits in neurotransmitter activity as risk factors for cognitive impairment after cancer treatment, a conclusion that could have a variety of treatment implications. For example, research shows that in animal models, the antidepressant fluoxetine can prevent or improve memory problems associated with the chemotherapy treatment 5-fluorouracil (5-FU).

Dr. Ganz believes inflammation may be a factor in cognitive impairment after cancer treatment. In their research, she and her colleagues have found a strong association between fatigue and cognitive complaints after cancer treatment in patients with specific polymorphisms in the genes that regulate the cytokines that promote inflammation.

Finding biological risk factors like this, she noted, could be extremely helpful in devising ways to limit the cognitive effects of treatment. "If we could identify people who might be more susceptible biologically to this long-term treatment, we could test whether an intervention might be helpful," she said.

One randomized trial found that using a cognitive rehabilitation program (CRP) in which cancer survivors report cognitive symptoms after chemotherapy led to lower levels of anxiety, depression, fatigue, and stress. Dr. Ganz is also planning on testing a cognitive behavioral therapy intervention, and some research has already shown this kind of therapy can be effective for cognitive problems after cancer treatment. "I think for some of the patients, it's not so much that they're severely impaired, but they get distressed and they can't do things, so cognitive behavioral therapy might be helpful in that situation," she said.

Dr. Ganz said the latest studies are valuable because they highlight the need to listen to patients expressing these concerns. "I think the importance of research is that if patients say they have pain, they feel sad, they can't sleep, we don't send them for complicated testing—instead, we believe what they say," she said. "So if somebody says, 'I'm really forgetful. I can't find my words very easily. I can't concentrate,' when they're telling us those things and it hasn't gotten better 6 months or a year after their treatment, they've had some kind of injury."

Section 8.2

Questions about Chemotherapy Treatments

This section includes text excerpted from "Chemotherapy to Treat Cancer," National Cancer Institute (NCI), April 29, 2015.

What Is Chemotherapy?

Chemotherapy (also called chemo) is a type of cancer treatment that uses drugs to kill cancer cells.

How Chemotherapy Works against Cancer

Chemotherapy works by stopping or slowing the growth of cancer cells, which grow and divide quickly. Chemotherapy is used to:

Treat cancer. Chemotherapy can be used to cure cancer, lessen the chance it will return, or stop or slow its growth.

Ease cancer symptoms. Chemotherapy can be used to shrink tumors that are causing pain and other problems.

How Is Chemotherapy Used with Other Cancer Treatments?

When used with other treatments, chemotherapy can:

- Make a tumor smaller before surgery or radiation therapy. This is called neoadjuvant chemotherapy.
- Destroy cancer cells that may remain after treatment with surgery or radiation therapy. This is called adjuvant chemotherapy.
- Help other treatments work better.
- Kill cancer cells that have returned or spread to other parts of your body.

Are There Any Side Effects of Chemotherapy?

Chemotherapy not only kills fast-growing cancer cells, but also kills or slows the growth of healthy cells that grow and divide quickly. Examples are cells that line your mouth and intestines and those that cause your hair to grow. Damage to healthy cells may cause side effects, such as mouth sores, nausea, and hair loss. Side effects often get better or go away after you have finished chemotherapy.

The most common side effect is fatigue, which is feeling exhausted and worn out. You can prepare for fatigue by:

- Asking someone to drive you to and from chemotherapy
- Planning time to rest on the day of and day after chemotherapy
- Asking for help with meals and child care on the day of and at least one day after chemotherapy

There are many ways you can help manage chemotherapy side effects.

How Much Does Chemotherapy Cost?

The cost of chemotherapy depends on:

- The types and doses of chemotherapy used
- How long and how often chemotherapy is given
- Whether you get chemotherapy at home, in a clinic or office, or during a hospital stay
- The part of the country where you live

131

Talk with your health insurance company about what services it will pay for. Most insurance plans pay for chemotherapy. To learn more, talk with the business office where you go for treatment.

If you need financial assistance, there are organizations that may be able to help. To find such organizations, go to the National Cancer Institute (NCI) database, Organizations that Offer Support Services and search for "financial assistance." Or call toll-free 800-4-CANCER (800-422-6237) to ask for information on organizations that may help.

How Is Chemotherapy Given?

Chemotherapy may be given in many ways. Some common ways include:

- **Oral.** The chemotherapy comes in pills, capsules, or liquids that you swallow

- **Intravenous (IV).** The chemotherapy goes directly into a vein

- **Injection.** The chemotherapy is given by a shot in a muscle in your arm, thigh, or hip, or right under the skin in the fatty part of your arm, leg, or belly

- **Intrathecal.** The chemotherapy is injected into the space between the layers of tissue that cover the brain and spinal cord

- **Intraperitoneal (IP).** The chemotherapy goes directly into the peritoneal cavity, which is the area in your body that contains organs such as your intestines, stomach, and liver

- **Intra-arterial (IA).** The chemotherapy is injected directly into the artery that leads to the cancer

- **Topical.** The chemotherapy comes in a cream that you rub onto your skin

Chemotherapy is often given through a thin needle that is placed in a vein on your hand or lower arm. Your nurse will put the needle in at the start of each treatment and remove it when treatment is over. IV chemotherapy may also be given through catheters or ports, sometimes with the help of a pump.

- **Catheter.** A catheter is a thin, soft tube. A doctor or nurse places one end of the catheter in a large vein, often in your chest area. The other end of the catheter stays outside your body.

Most catheters stay in place until you have finished your chemotherapy treatments. Catheters can also be used to give you other drugs and to draw blood. Be sure to watch for signs of infection around your catheter. See the section about infection for more information.

- **Port.** A port is a small, round disc that is placed under your skin during minor surgery. A surgeon puts it in place before you begin your course of treatment, and it remains there until you have finished. A catheter connects the port to a large vein, most often in your chest. Your nurse can insert a needle into your port to give you chemotherapy or draw blood. This needle can be left in place for chemotherapy treatments that are given for longer than one day. Be sure to watch for signs of infection around your port. See the section about infection for more information.

- **Pump.** Pumps are often attached to catheters or ports. They control how much and how fast chemotherapy goes into a catheter or port, allowing you to receive your chemotherapy outside of the hospital. Pumps can be internal or external. External pumps remain outside your body. Internal pumps are placed under your skin during surgery.

How Does Your Doctor Decide Which Chemotherapy Drugs to Give You?

There are many different chemotherapy drugs. Which ones are included in your treatment plan depends mostly on:

- The type of cancer you have and how advanced it is
- Whether you have had chemotherapy before
- Whether you have other health problems, such as diabetes or heart disease

Where Will You Get Chemotherapy?

You may receive chemotherapy during a hospital stay, at home, or as an outpatient at a doctor's office, clinic, or hospital. Outpatient means you do not stay overnight. No matter where you go for chemotherapy, your doctor and nurse will watch for side effects and help you manage them.

How Often Will You Receive Chemotherapy?

Treatment schedules for chemotherapy vary widely. How often and how long you get chemotherapy depends on:

- Your type of cancer and how advanced it is
- Whether chemotherapy is used to:
  - Cure your cancer
  - Control its growth
  - Ease symptoms
- The type of chemotherapy you are getting
- How your body responds to the chemotherapy

You may receive chemotherapy in cycles. A cycle is a period of chemotherapy treatment followed by a period of rest. For instance, you might receive chemotherapy every day for 1 week followed by 3 weeks with no chemotherapy. These 4 weeks make up one cycle. The rest period gives your body a chance to recover and build new healthy cells.

What Happens If You Miss a Chemotherapy Treatment?

It is best not to skip a chemotherapy treatment. But, sometimes your doctor may change your chemotherapy schedule if you are having certain side effects. If this happens, your doctor or nurse will explain what to do and when to start treatment again.

How Chemotherapy Can Affect You?

Chemotherapy affects people in different ways. How you feel depends on:

- The type of chemotherapy you are getting
- The dose of chemotherapy you are getting
- Your type of cancer
- How advanced your cancer is
- How healthy you are before treatment

Since everyone is different and people respond to chemotherapy in different ways, your doctor and nurses cannot know for sure how you will feel during chemotherapy.

How Will I Know If My Chemotherapy Is Working?

You will see your doctor often. During these visits, she will ask you how you feel, do a physical exam, and order medical tests and scans. Tests might include blood tests. Scans might include magnetic resonance imaging (MRI), computerized tomography (CT), or positron emission tomography (PET) scans.

You cannot tell if chemotherapy is working based on its side effects. Some people think that severe side effects mean that chemotherapy is working well, or that no side effects mean that chemotherapy is not working. The truth is that side effects have nothing to do with how well chemotherapy is fighting your cancer.

Do You Require Any Special Diet While Receiving Chemotherapy?

Chemotherapy can damage the healthy cells that line your mouth and intestines and cause eating problems. Tell your doctor or nurse if you have trouble eating while you are receiving chemotherapy. You might also find it helpful to speak with a dietitian. For more information about coping with eating problems see the booklet Eating Hints or the section on side effects.

Can You Go to Work during Chemotherapy Sessions?

Many people can work during chemotherapy, as long as they match their work schedule to how they feel. Whether or not you can work may depend on what kind of job you have. If your job allows, you may want to see if you can work part-time or from home on days you do not feel well. Many employers are required by law to change your work schedule to meet your needs during cancer treatment. Talk with your employer about ways to adjust your work during chemotherapy. You can learn more about these laws by talking with a social worker.

Chapter 9

Brain Surgery

Surgery is the usual first treatment for most brain tumors. Before surgery begins, you may be given general anesthesia, and your scalp is shaved. You probably won't need your entire head shaved.

Surgery to open the skull is called a craniotomy. The surgeon makes an incision in your scalp and uses a special type of saw to remove a piece of bone from the skull.

You may be awake when the surgeon removes part or all of the brain tumor. The surgeon removes as much tumor as possible. You may be asked to move a leg, count, say the alphabet, or tell a story. Your ability to follow these commands helps the surgeon protect important parts of the brain.

After the tumor is removed, the surgeon covers the opening in the skull with the piece of bone or with a piece of metal or fabric. The surgeon then closes the incision in the scalp.

Sometimes surgery isn't possible. If the tumor is in the brainstem or certain other areas, the surgeon may not be able to remove the tumor without harming normal brain tissue. People who can't have surgery may receive radiation therapy or other treatment.

You may have a headache or be uncomfortable for the first few days after surgery. However, medicine can usually control pain. Before surgery, you should discuss the plan for pain relief with your healthcare team. After surgery, your team can adjust the plan if you need more relief.

This chapter includes text excerpted from "What You Need to Know about TM–Brain Tumors," National Cancer Institute (NCI), May 2009. Reviewed February 2018.

You may also feel tired or weak. The time it takes to heal after surgery is different for everyone. You will probably spend a few days in the hospital.

Other, less common problems may occur after surgery for a brain tumor. The brain may swell or fluid may build up within the skull. The healthcare team will monitor you for signs of swelling or fluid buildup.

You may receive steroids to help relieve swelling. A second surgery may be needed to drain the fluid. The surgeon may place a long, thin tube (shunt) in a ventricle of the brain. (For some people, the shunt is placed before performing surgery on the brain tumor.)

The tube is threaded under the skin to another part of the body, usually the abdomen. Excess fluid is carried from the brain and drained into the abdomen.

Sometimes the fluid is drained into the heart instead. Infection is another problem that may develop after surgery. If this happens, the healthcare team will give you an antibiotic.

Brain surgery may harm normal tissue. Brain damage can be a serious problem. It can cause problems with thinking, seeing, or speaking. It can also cause personality changes or seizures. Most of these problems lessen or disappear with time. But sometimes damage to the brain is permanent. You may need physical therapy, speech therapy, or occupational therapy.

Rehabilitation

Rehabilitation can be a very important part of the treatment plan. The goals of rehabilitation depend on your needs and how the tumor has affected your ability to carry out daily activities.

Some people may never regain all the abilities they had before the brain tumor and its treatment. But your healthcare team makes every effort to help you return to normal activities as soon as possible.

Several types of therapists can help:

- **Physical therapists**

  Brain tumors and their treatment may cause paralysis. They may also cause weakness and problems with balance. Physical therapists help people regain strength and balance.

- **Speech therapists**

  Speech therapists help people who have trouble speaking, expressing thoughts, or swallowing.

- **Occupational therapists**

  Occupational therapists help people learn to manage activities of daily living, such as eating, using the toilet, bathing, and dressing.

- **Physical medicine specialists**

  Medical doctors with special training help people with brain tumors stay as active as possible. They can help people recover lost abilities and return to daily activities.

Children with brain tumors may have special needs. Sometimes children have tutors in the hospital or at home. Children who have problems learning or remembering what they learn may need tutors or special classes when they return to school.

Chapter 10

Deep Brain Stimulation

Deep brain stimulation (DBS) was first developed as a treatment for Parkinson disease to reduce tremor, stiffness, walking problems and uncontrollable movements. In DBS, a pair of electrodes is implanted in the brain and controlled by a generator that is implanted in the chest. Stimulation is continuous and its frequency and level are customized to the individual.

DBS has been studied as a treatment for depression or obsessive-compulsive disorder (OCD). Currently, there is a Humanitarian Device Exemption for the use of DBS to treat OCD, but its use in depression remains only on an experimental basis. A review of all 22 published studies testing DBS for depression found that only three of them were of high quality because they not only had a treatment group but also a control group which did not receive DBS. The review found that across the studies,

40–50 percent of people showed receiving DBS greater than 50 percent improvement.

DBS: How It works

DBS requires brain surgery. The head is shaved and then attached with screws to a sturdy frame that prevents the head from moving during the surgery. Scans of the head and brain using magnetic

This chapter includes text excerpted from "Brain Stimulation Therapies," National Institute of Mental Health (NIMH), June 2016.

resonance imaging (MRI) are taken. The surgeon uses these images as guides during the surgery. Patients are awake during the procedure to provide the surgeon with feedback, but they feel no pain because the head is numbed with a local anesthetic and the brain itself does not register pain.

Once ready for surgery, two holes are drilled into the head. From there, the surgeon threads a slender tube down into the brain to place electrodes on each side of a specific area of the brain. In the case of depression, the first area of the brain targeted by DBS is called Area 25, or the subgenual cingulate cortex. This area has been found to be overactive in depression and other mood disorders. But later research targeted several other areas of the brain affected by depression. So DBS is now targeting several areas of the brain for treating depression. In the case of OCD, the electrodes are placed in an area of the brain (the ventral capsule/ventral striatum) believed to be associated with the disorder.

After the electrodes are implanted and the patient provides feedback about their placement, the patient is put under general anesthesia. The electrodes are then attached to wires that are run inside the body from the head down to the chest, where a pair of battery-operated generators are implanted. From here, electrical pulses are continuously delivered over the wires to the electrodes in the brain. Although it is unclear exactly how the device works to reduce depression or OCD, scientists believe that the pulses help to "reset" the area of the brain that is malfunctioning so that it works normally again.

DBS Side Effects

DBS carries risks associated with any type of brain surgery. For example, the procedure may lead to:

- Bleeding in the brain or stroke
- Infection
- Disorientation or confusion
- Unwanted mood changes
- Movement disorders
- Lightheadedness
- Trouble sleeping

Because the procedure is still being studied, other side effects not yet identified may be possible. Long-term benefits and side effects are unknown.

Chapter 11

Radiation Therapy

Chapter Contents

Section 11.1

Introduction to Radiotherapy

This section includes text excerpted from "Radiation Therapy for Cancer," National Cancer Institute (NCI), July 19, 2017.

Radiation therapy (also called radiotherapy) is a cancer treatment that uses high doses of radiation to kill cancer cells and shrink tumors. At low doses, radiation is used as an X-ray to see inside your body and take pictures, such as X-rays of your teeth or broken bones.

How Is Radiation Therapy Given?

Radiation therapy can be external beam or internal. External beam involves a machine outside your body that aims radiation at cancer cells. Internal radiation therapy involves placing radiation inside your body, in or near the cancer. Sometimes people get both forms of radiation therapy.

Who Gets Radiation Therapy?

Many people with cancer need treatment with radiation therapy. In fact, more than half (about 60%) of people with cancer have radiation therapy. Sometimes, radiation therapy is the only kind of cancer treatment people have.

What Does Radiation Therapy Do to Cancer Cells?

Given in high doses, radiation kills or slows the growth of cancer cells.

Radiation therapy is used to:

- Treat cancer. Radiation can be used to cure cancer, to prevent it from returning, or to stop or slow its growth.

- Reduce symptoms. When a cure is not possible, radiation may be used to treat pain and other problems caused by the cancer tumor. Or, it can prevent problems that may be caused by a growing tumor, such as blindness or loss of bowel and bladder control.

How Long Does Radiation Therapy Take to Work?

Radiation therapy does not kill cancer cells right away. It takes days or weeks of treatment before cancer cells start to die. Then, cancer cells keep dying for weeks or months after radiation therapy ends.

What Does Radiation Therapy Do to Healthy Cells?

Radiation not only kills or slows the growth of cancer cells, it can also affect nearby healthy cells. The healthy cells almost always recover after treatment is over. But sometimes people may have side effects that are severe or do not get better. Other side effects may show up months or years after radiation therapy is over. These are called late side effects.

Doctors try to protect healthy cells during treatment by:

- **Using as low a dose of radiation as possible.** The radiation dose is balanced between being high enough to kill cancer cells, yet low enough to limit damage to healthy cells.

- **Spreading out treatment over time.** You may get radiation therapy once a day, or in smaller doses twice a day for several weeks. Spreading out the radiation dose allows normal cells to recover while cancer cells die.

- **Aiming radiation at a precise part of your body.** Some types of radiation therapy allow your doctor to aim high doses of radiation at your cancer while reducing radiation to nearby healthy tissue. These techniques use a computer to deliver precise radiation doses to a cancer tumor or to specific areas within the tumor.

Does Radiation Therapy Hurt?

No, radiation therapy does not hurt while it is being given. But the side effects that people may get from radiation therapy can cause pain and discomfort.

Is Radiation Therapy Used with Other Types of Cancer Treatment?

Yes, radiation therapy is often used with other cancer treatments. Here are some examples:

- **Radiation therapy and surgery**

  Radiation may be given before, during, or after surgery. Doctors may use radiation to shrink the size of the cancer before surgery, or they may use radiation after surgery to kill any cancer cells that remain. Sometimes, radiation therapy is given during surgery, so that it goes straight to the cancer without passing through the skin. Radiation therapy given during surgery is called intraoperative radiation.

- **Radiation therapy and chemotherapy**

  Radiation may be given before, during, or after chemotherapy. Before or during chemotherapy, radiation therapy can shrink the cancer so that chemotherapy works better. After chemotherapy, radiation therapy can be used to kill any cancer cells that remain.

Is Radiation Therapy Expensive?

Yes, radiation therapy costs a lot of money. It uses complex machines and involves the services of many healthcare providers. The exact cost of your radiation therapy depends on the cost of healthcare where you live, what kind of radiation therapy you get, and how many treatments you need.

Talk with your health insurance company about what services it will pay for. Most insurance plans pay for radiation therapy. To learn more, talk with the business office of the clinic or hospital where you go for treatment. If you need financial assistance, there are organizations that may be able to help. To find such organizations, go to the National Cancer Institute database, Organizations that Offer Support Services at: supportorgs.cancer.gov and search "financial assistance." Or call toll-free 800-4-CANCER (800-422-6237) to ask for information on organizations that may help.

Should I Follow a Special Diet While I Am Getting Radiation Therapy?

Your body uses a lot of energy to heal during radiation therapy. It is important that you eat enough calories and protein to keep your weight the same during this time. Ask your doctor or nurse if you need a special diet while you are receiving radiation therapy. You might also find it helpful to speak with a dietitian.

Can I Continue to Work during Radiation Therapy?

Some people are able to work full time during radiation therapy. Others can work only part time or not at all. How much you are able to work depends on how you feel. Ask your doctor or nurse what you may expect from the treatment you will have.

You are likely to feel well enough to work when you first start your radiation treatments. As time goes on, do not be surprised if you are more tired, have less energy, or feel weak. Once you have finished treatment, it may take a few weeks or many months for you to feel better.

You may get to a point during your radiation therapy when you feel too sick to work. Talk with your employer to find out if you can go on medical leave. Make sure that your health insurance will pay for treatment while you are on medical leave.

How Do I Make the Most of Radiation Therapy?

You have an important role to play in your radiation therapy. To get the most from this treatment:

- Arrive on time for all radiation therapy sessions.

- Ask questions and talk about your concerns.

- Tell someone on your radiation therapy team when you have side effects and changes with eating or bowel habits.

- Tell your doctor or nurse if you are in pain.

Follow the advice of your doctors and nurses about how to care for yourself at home, such as:

- Taking care of your skin

- Drinking enough liquids

- Eating foods to help with side effects

- Maintaining your weight

What Happens When Radiation Therapy Is Over?

Once you have finished radiation therapy, you will need follow-up care for the rest of your life. Follow-up care refers to regular checkups once treatment is over. During these checkups, your doctor or nurse will see how well the radiation therapy worked, check for signs of cancer, talk with you about your treatment and care, and look for late side effects. Late side effects are those that occur six or more months after you have completed radiation therapy. During these checkups, your doctor or nurse will:

- Examine you and review how you have been feeling. Your doctor can prescribe medicine or suggest other ways to treat any side effects you may have.

- Order lab and imaging tests, which are tests that make pictures of areas inside the body. These tests may include blood tests, X-rays, or computed tomography (CT), magnetic resonance imaging (MRI), or positron emission tomography (PET) scans.

- Discuss treatment. Your doctor may suggest that you have more treatment, such as extra radiation treatments, chemotherapy, or other types of treatment.

- Answer your questions and respond to your concerns. It may be helpful to write down your questions ahead of time and bring them with you.

After I Have Finished Radiation Therapy, What Symptoms Should I Look For?

You have gone through a lot with cancer and radiation therapy. Now you may be even more aware of your body and how you feel each day. Pay attention to changes in your body. Tell your doctor or nurse if you have:

- A pain that does not go away
- New lumps, bumps, swellings, rashes, bruises, or bleeding
- Appetite changes, nausea, vomiting, diarrhea, or constipation
- Weight loss that you cannot explain
- A fever, cough, or hoarseness that does not go away
- Any other symptoms that worry you

Section 11.2

Types of Radiation Therapies

This section includes text excerpted from "Radiation Therapy for Cancer," National Cancer Institute (NCI), July 19, 2017.

External Beam Radiation Therapy

External beam radiation therapy (EBRT) comes from a machine that aims radiation at your cancer. The machine is large and may be noisy. It does not touch you, but can move around you, sending radiation to a part of your body from many directions.

EBRT is a local treatment, which means it treats a specific part of your body. For example, if you have cancer in your lung, you will have radiation only to your chest, not to your whole body.

Internal Radiation Therapy

Internal radiation therapy is a treatment in which a source of radiation is put inside your body. The radiation source can be solid or liquid.

Internal radiation therapy with a solid source is called brachytherapy. In this type of treatment, seeds, ribbons, or capsules that contain a radiation source are placed in your body in or near the tumor. Like external beam radiation therapy, brachytherapy is a local treatment and treats only a specific part of your body.

Internal radiation therapy with a liquid source is called systemic therapy. Systemic means that the treatment travels in the blood to tissues throughout your body, seeking out and killing cancer cells. You receive systemic radiation therapy by swallowing or through a vein, via an IV line.

The type of radiation therapy that you may have depends on many factors, including:

- The type of cancer

- The size of the tumor

- The tumor's location in the body

- How close the tumor is to normal tissues that are sensitive to radiation

- Your general health and medical history

- Whether you will have other types of cancer treatment

- Other factors, such as your age and other medical conditions

Why People with Cancer Receive Radiation Therapy

Radiation therapy (RT) is used to treat cancer and ease cancer symptoms.

When treatments are used to ease symptoms, they are known as palliative treatments. External beam radiation may shrink tumors to treat pain and other problems caused by the tumor, such as trouble breathing or loss of bowel and bladder control. Pain from cancer that has spread to the bone can be treated with systemic radiation therapy drugs called radiopharmaceuticals.

When used to treat cancer, radiation therapy can cure cancer, prevent it from returning, or stop or slow its growth.

Types of Cancer That Are Treated with Radiation Therapy

External beam radiation therapy is used to treat many types of cancer.

Brachytherapy is often used to treat cancers of the head and neck, breast, cervix, prostate, and eye.

Systemic radiation therapy is most often used to treat certain types of thyroid cancer. This treatment uses radioactive iodine, which is also known as I-131.

Lifetime Dose Limits

There is a limit to the amount of radiation an area of your body can safely receive over the course of your lifetime. Depending on how much radiation an area has already been treated with, you may not be able to have radiation therapy to that area a second time. But, if one area of the body has already received the safe lifetime dose of radiation, another area might still be treated if the distance between the two areas is large enough.

What to Expect When Having External Beam Radiation Therapy

How Often You Will Have External Beam Radiation Therapy

Most people have external beam radiation therapy once a day, five days a week, Monday through Friday. Radiation is given in a series of treatments to allow healthy cells to recover and to make radiation more effective. How many weeks you have treatment depends on the type of cancer you have, the goal of your treatment, the radiation dose, and the radiation schedule.

The span of time from your first radiation treatment to the last is called a course of treatment.

Researchers are looking at different ways to adjust the radiation dose or schedule in order to reach the total dose of radiation more quickly or to limit damage to healthy cells. Different ways of delivering the total radiation dose include:

- Accelerated fractionation, which is treatment given in larger daily or weekly doses to reduce the number of weeks of treatment.

- Hyperfractionation, which is a smaller dose than the usual daily dose of radiation given more than once a day.

- Hypofractionation, which is larger doses given once a day or less often to reduce the number of treatments.

Researchers hope these different schedules for delivering radiation may be more effective and cause fewer side effects than the usual way of doing it or be as effective but more convenient.

Where You Go for External Beam Radiation Therapy

Most of the time, you will get external beam radiation therapy as an outpatient. This means that you will have treatment at a clinic or radiation therapy center and will not stay the night in the hospital.

What Happens before Your First External Beam Radiation Therapy Treatment

You will have a 1- to 2-hour meeting with your doctor or nurse before you begin radiation therapy. At this time, you will have a physical exam, talk about your medical history, and maybe have imaging tests. Your doctor or nurse will discuss external beam radiation therapy, its benefits and side effects, and ways you can care for yourself during and after treatment. You can then choose whether to have external beam radiation therapy.

If you decide to have external beam radiation therapy, you will be scheduled for a treatment planning session called a simulation. At this time:

A radiation oncologist (a doctor who specializes in using radiation to treat cancer) and radiation therapist will figure out your treatment area. You may also hear the treatment area referred to as the treatment port or treatment field. These terms refer to the places in your body that will get radiation. You will be asked to lie very still while X-rays or scans are taken.

- The radiation therapist will tattoo or draw small dots of colored ink on your skin to mark the treatment area. These dots will be needed throughout your course of radiation therapy. The radiation therapist will use them to make sure you are in exactly the same position for every treatment. The dots are about the size of a freckle. If the dots are tattooed, they will remain on your skin for the rest of your life. Ink markings will fade over time. Be careful not to remove them and tell the radiation therapist if they have faded or lost color.

- A body mold may be made of the part of the body that is being treated. This is a plastic or plaster form that keeps you from moving during treatment. It also helps make sure that you are in exactly the same position for each treatment

- If you are getting radiation to the head and neck area you may be fitted for a mask. The mask has many air holes. It attaches to the table where you will lie for your treatments. The mask helps keep your head from moving so that you are in exactly the same position for each treatment.

What to Wear for Your Treatments

Wear clothes that are comfortable and made of soft fabric, such as fleece or cotton. Choose clothes that are easy to take off, since you may need to expose the treatment area or change into a hospital gown. Do not wear clothes that are tight, such as close-fitting collars or waistbands, near your treatment area. Also, do not wear jewelry, adhesive bandages, or powder in the treatment area.

What Happens during a Treatment Session

- You may be asked to change into a hospital gown or robe.

- You will go to the treatment room where you will receive radiation. The temperature in this room will be very cool.

- Depending on where your cancer is, you will either lie down on a treatment table or sit in a special chair. The radiation therapist will use the dots on your skin and body mold or face mask, if you have one, to help you get into the right position.

- You may see colored lights pointed at your skin marks. These lights are harmless and help the therapist position you for treatment.

- You will need to stay very still so the radiation goes to the exact same place each time. You will get radiation for 1–5 minutes. During this time, you can breathe normally.

The radiation therapist will leave the room just before your treatment begins. He or she will go to a nearby room to control the radiation machine. The therapist watches you on a TV screen or through a window and talks with you through a speaker in the treatment room. Make sure to tell the therapist if you feel sick or are uncomfortable. He or she can stop the radiation machine at any time. You will hear the radiation machine and see it moving around, but you won't be able to feel, hear, see, or smell the radiation.

Most visits last from 30 minutes to an hour, with most of that time spent helping you get into the correct position.

External Beam Radiation Therapy Will Not Make You Radioactive

People often wonder if they will be radioactive when they are having treatment with radiation. External beam radiation therapy will not make you radioactive. You may safely be around other people, even pregnant women, babies, and young children.

What to Expect When Having Internal Radiation Therapy

What Happens before Your First Internal Radiation Therapy Treatment

You will have a 1- to 2-hour meeting with your doctor or nurse to plan your treatment before you begin internal radiation therapy. At

153

this time, you will have a physical exam, talk about your medical history, and maybe have imaging tests. Your doctor will discuss the type of internal radiation therapy that is best for you, its benefits and side effects, and ways you can care for yourself during and after treatment. You can then decide whether to have internal radiation therapy.

How Brachytherapy Is Put in Place

Most brachytherapy is put in place through a catheter, which is a small, stretchy tube. Sometimes, brachytherapy is put in place through a larger device called an applicator. The way the brachytherapy is put in place depends on your type of cancer. Your doctor will place the catheter or applicator into your body before you begin treatment.

Techniques for placing brachytherapy include:

- Interstitial brachytherapy, in which the radiation source is placed within the tumor. This technique is used for prostate cancer, for instance.

- Intracavity brachytherapy, in which the radiation source is placed within a body cavity or a cavity created by surgery. For example, radiation can be placed in the vagina to treat cervical or endometrial cancer.

- Episcleral brachytherapy, in which the radiation source is attached to the eye. This technique is used to treat melanoma of the eye.

Once the catheter or applicator is in place, the radiation source is placed inside it. The radiation source may be kept in place for a few minutes, for many days, or for the rest of your life. How long it remains in place depends on the type of radiation source, your type of cancer, where the cancer is in your body, your health, and other cancer treatments you have had.

Types of Brachytherapy

There are three types of brachytherapy:

- **Low-dose rate (LDR) implants**

  In this type of brachytherapy, the radiation source stays in place for 1–7 days. You are likely to be in the hospital during this time. Once your treatment is finished, your doctor will remove the radiation source and the catheter or applicator.

- **High-dose rate (HDR) implants**

  In this type of brachytherapy, the radiation source is left in place for just 10–20 minutes at a time and then taken out. You may have treatment twice a day for 2–5 days or once a week for 2–5 weeks. The schedule depends on your type of cancer. During the course of treatment, your catheter or applicator may stay in place, or it may be put in place before each treatment. You may be in the hospital during this time, or you may make daily trips to the hospital to have the radiation source put in place. As with LDR implants, your doctor will remove the catheter or applicator once you have finished treatment.

- **Permanent implants**

  After the radiation source is put in place, the catheter is removed. The implants remain in your body for the rest of your life, but the radiation gets weaker each day. As time goes on, almost all the radiation will go away. When the radiation is first put in place, you may need to limit your time around other people and take other safety measures. Be extra careful not to spend time with children or pregnant women.

Internal Radiation Therapy Makes You Give Off Radiation

With systemic radiation, your body fluids (urine, sweat, and saliva) will give off radiation for a while. With brachytherapy, your body fluids will not give off radiation, but the radiation source in your body will. If the radiation you receive is a very high dose, you may need to follow some safety measures. These measures may include:

- Staying in a private hospital room to protect others from radiation coming from your body

- Being treated quickly by nurses and other hospital staff. They will provide all the care you need, but may stand at a distance, talk with you from the doorway of your room, and wear protective clothing.

Your visitors will also need to follow safety measures, which may include:

- Not being allowed to visit when the radiation is first put in

- Needing to check with the hospital staff before they go to your room

155

- Standing by the doorway rather than going into your hospital room.

- Keeping visits short (30 minutes or less each day). The length of visits depends on the type of radiation being used and the part of your body being treated.

- Not having visits from pregnant women and children younger than a year old

You may also need to follow safety measures once you leave the hospital, such as not spending much time with other people. Your doctor or nurse will talk with you about any safety measures you should follow when you go home.

What to Expect When the Catheter Is Removed

Once you finish treatment with LDR or HDR implants, the catheter will be removed. Here are some things to expect:

- You will get medicine for pain before the catheter or applicator is removed.

- The area where the catheter or applicator was might be tender for a few months.

- There is no radiation in your body after the catheter or applicator is removed. It is safe for people to be near you—even young children and pregnant women.

For a week or two, you may need to limit activities that take a lot of effort. Ask your doctor what kinds of activities are safe for you and which ones you should avoid.

Chapter 12

Brain Rehabilitation

Chapter Contents

Section 12.1

Rehabilitation Therapies

This section contains text excerpted from the following sources:
Text in this section begins with excerpts from "Spinal Cord Injury:
Hope through Research," National Institute of Neurological Disorders
and Stroke (NINDS), February 8, 2017; Text beginning with the
heading "What Is Post-Stroke Rehabilitation?" is excerpted from "Post-
Stroke Rehabilitation," National Institute of Neurological Disorders
and Stroke (NINDS), September 2014. Reviewed February 2018.

Rehabilitation programs combine physical therapies with skill-building activities and counseling to provide social and emotional support. The education and active involvement of the newly injured person and his or her family and friends is crucial.

A rehabilitation team is usually led by a doctor specializing in physical medicine and rehabilitation (called a physiatrist), and often includes social workers, physical and occupational therapists, recreational therapists, rehabilitation nurses, rehabilitation psychologists, vocational counselors, nutritionists, a case worker, and other specialists.

In the initial phase of rehabilitation, therapists emphasize regaining communication skills and leg and arm strength. For some individuals, mobility will only be possible with the assistance of devices such as a walker, leg braces, or a wheelchair. Communication skills such as writing, typing, and using the telephone may also require adaptive devices for some people with tetraplegia.

Physical therapy includes exercise programs geared toward muscle strengthening. Occupational therapy helps redevelop fine motor skills, particularly those needed to perform activities of daily living such as getting in and out of a bed, self-grooming, and eating. Bladder and bowel management programs teach basic toileting routines. People acquire coping strategies for recurring episodes of spasticity, autonomic dysreflexia, and neurogenic pain.

Vocational rehabilitation includes identifying the person's basic work skills and physical and cognitive capabilities to determine the likelihood for employment; identifying potential workplaces and any assistive equipment that will be needed; and arranging for a user-friendly workplace. If necessary, educational training is provided to develop skills for a new line of work that may be less dependent upon physical abilities and more dependent upon computer or communication skills. Individuals with disabilities that prevent them from returning to the workforce are encouraged to maintain productivity by participating in activities that provide a sense of satisfaction and self-esteem, such as educational classes, hobbies, memberships in special interest groups, and participation in family and community events.

Recreation therapy encourages people with central nervous system (CNS) injury to participate in recreational sports or activities at their level of mobility, as well as achieve a more balanced and normal lifestyle that provides opportunities for socialization and self-expression.

Adaptive devices also may help people with CNS injury to regain independence and improve mobility and quality of life. Such devices may include a wheelchair, electronic stimulators, assisted gait training, neural prostheses, computer adaptations, and other computer-assisted technology.

What Is Post-Stroke Rehabilitation?

Rehabilitation helps stroke survivors relearn skills that are lost when part of the brain is damaged. For example, these skills can include coordinating leg movements in order to walk or carrying out the steps involved in any complex activity. Rehabilitation also teaches survivors new ways of performing tasks to circumvent or compensate for any residual disabilities. Individuals may need to learn how to bathe and dress using only one hand, or how to communicate effectively when their ability to use language has been compromised. There is a strong consensus among rehabilitation experts that the most important element in any rehabilitation program is carefully directed, well-focused, repetitive practice—the same kind of practice used by all people when they learn a new skill, such as playing the piano or pitching a baseball.

Rehabilitative therapy begins in the acute-care hospital after the person's overall condition has been stabilized, often within 24–48 hours after the stroke. The first steps involve promoting independent movement because many individuals are paralyzed or seriously weakened. Patients are prompted to change positions frequently while lying in bed and to engage in passive or active range of motion exercises to strengthen their stroke-impaired limbs. ("Passive" range-of-motion exercises are those in which the therapist actively helps the patient move a limb repeatedly, whereas "active" exercises are performed by the patient with no physical assistance from the therapist.) Depending on many factors—including the extent of the initial injury—patients may progress from sitting up and being moved between the bed and a chair to standing, bearing their own weight, and walking, with or without assistance. Rehabilitation nurses and therapists help patients who are able to perform progressively more complex and demanding tasks, such as bathing, dressing, and using a toilet, and they encourage patients to begin using their stroke-impaired limbs while engaging in those tasks. Beginning to reacquire the ability to carry out these basic activities of daily living represents the first stage in a stroke survivor's return to independence.

For some stroke survivors, rehabilitation will be an ongoing process to maintain and refine skills and could involve working with specialists for months or years after the stroke.

What Medical Professionals Specialize in Post-Stroke Rehabilitation?

Physicians

Physicians have the primary responsibility for managing and coordinating the long-term care of stroke survivors, including recommending which rehabilitation programs will best address individual needs. Physicians also are responsible for caring for the stroke survivor's general health and providing guidance aimed at preventing a second stroke, such as controlling high blood pressure or diabetes and eliminating risk factors such as cigarette smoking, excessive weight, a high-cholesterol diet, and high alcohol consumption.

Neurologists usually lead acute-care stroke teams and direct patient care during hospitalization. They sometimes participate on the long-term rehabilitation team. Other subspecialists often lead the rehabilitation stage of care, especially physiatrists, who specialize in physical medicine and rehabilitation.

Rehabilitation Nurses

Nurses specializing in rehabilitation help survivors relearn how to carry out the basic activities of daily living. They also educate survivors about routine healthcare, such as how to follow a medication schedule, how to care for the skin, how to move out of a bed and into a wheelchair, and special needs for people with diabetes. Rehabilitation nurses also work with survivors to reduce risk factors that may lead to a second stroke, and provide training for caregivers.

Nurses are closely involved in helping stroke survivors manage personal care issues, such as bathing and controlling incontinence. Most stroke survivors regain their ability to maintain continence, often with the help of strategies learned during rehabilitation. These strategies include strengthening pelvic muscles through special exercises and following a timed voiding schedule. If problems with incontinence continue, nurses can help caregivers learn to insert and manage catheters and to take special hygienic measures to prevent other incontinence-related health problems from developing.

Physical Therapists

Physical therapists specialize in treating disabilities related to motor and sensory impairments. They are trained in all aspects of anatomy and physiology related to normal function, with an emphasis on movement. They assess the stroke survivor's strength, endurance, range of motion, gait abnormalities, and sensory deficits to design individualized rehabilitation programs aimed at regaining control over motor functions.

Physical therapists help survivors regain the use of stroke-impaired limbs, teach compensatory strategies to reduce the effect of remaining deficits, and establish ongoing exercise programs to help people retain their newly learned skills. Disabled people tend to avoid using impaired limbs, a behavior called learned nonuse. However, the repetitive use of impaired limbs encourages brain plasticity and helps reduce disabilities.

Strategies used by physical therapists to encourage the use of impaired limbs include selective sensory stimulation such as tapping or stroking, active and passive range-of-motion exercises, and temporary restraint of healthy limbs while practicing motor tasks.

In general, physical therapy emphasizes practicing isolated movements, repeatedly changing from one kind of movement to another, and rehearsing complex movements that require a great deal of coordination and balance, such as walking up or down stairs or moving safely between obstacles. People too weak to bear their own weight can still practice repetitive movements during hydrotherapy (in which water provides sensory stimulation as well as weight support) or while being partially supported by a harness. A recent trend in physical therapy emphasizes the effectiveness of engaging in goal-directed activities, such as playing games, to promote coordination. Physical therapists frequently employ selective sensory stimulation to encourage use of impaired limbs and to help survivors with neglect regain awareness of stimuli on the neglected side of the body.

161

Occupational and Recreational Therapists

Like physical therapists, occupational therapists are concerned with improving motor and sensory abilities, and ensuring patient safety in the post-stroke period. They help survivors relearn skills needed for performing self-directed activities (also called occupations) such as personal grooming, preparing meals, and housecleaning. Therapists can teach some survivors how to adapt to driving and provide on-road training. They often teach people to divide a complex activity into its component parts, practice each part, and then perform the whole sequence of actions. This strategy can improve coordination and may help people with apraxia relearn how to carry out planned actions.

Occupational therapists also teach people how to develop compensatory strategies and change elements of their environment that limit activities of daily living. For example, people with the use of only one hand can substitute hook and loop fasteners (such as Velcro) for buttons on clothing. Occupational therapists also help people make changes in their homes to increase safety, remove barriers, and facilitate physical functioning, such as installing grab bars in bathrooms.

Recreational therapists help people with a variety of disabilities to develop and use their leisure time to enhance their health, independence, and quality of life.

Speech-Language Pathologists

Speech-language pathologists help stroke survivors with aphasia relearn how to use language or develop alternative means of communication. They also help people improve their ability to swallow, and they work with patients to develop problem-solving and social skills needed to cope with the after-effects of a stroke.

Many specialized therapeutic techniques have been developed to assist people with aphasia. Some forms of short-term therapy can improve comprehension rapidly. Intensive exercises such as repeating the therapist's words, practicing following directions, and doing reading or writing exercises form the cornerstone of language rehabilitation. Conversational coaching and rehearsal, as well as the development of prompts or cues to help people remember specific words, are sometimes beneficial. Speech-language pathologists also help stroke survivors develop strategies for circumventing language disabilities. These strategies can include the use of symbol boards or sign language. Recent advances in computer technology have spurred the development of new types of equipment to enhance communication.

Speech-language pathologists use special types of imaging techniques to study swallowing patterns of stroke survivors and identify the exact source of their impairment. Difficulties with swallowing have many possible causes, including a delayed swallowing reflex, an inability to manipulate food with the tongue, or an inability to detect food remaining lodged in the cheeks after swallowing. When the cause has been pinpointed, speech-language pathologists work with the individual to devise strategies to overcome or minimize the deficit. Sometimes, simply changing body position and improving posture during eating can bring about improvement. The texture of foods can be modified to make swallowing easier; for example, thin liquids, which often cause choking, can be thickened. Changing eating habits by taking small bites and chewing slowly can also help alleviate dysphagia.

Vocational Therapists

Approximately one-fourth of all strokes occur in people between the ages of 45 and 65. For most people in this age group, returning to work is a major concern. Vocational therapists perform many of the same functions that ordinary career counselors do. They can help people with residual disabilities identify vocational strengths and develop résumés that highlight those strengths. They also can help identify potential employers, assist in specific job searches, and provide referrals to stroke vocational rehabilitation agencies.

Most important, vocational therapists educate disabled individuals about their rights and protections as defined by the Americans with Disabilities Act (ADA) of 1990. This law requires employers to make "reasonable accommodations" for disabled employees. Vocational therapists frequently act as mediators between employers and employees to negotiate the provision of reasonable accommodations in the workplace.

When Can a Stroke Patient Begin Rehabilitation?

Rehabilitation should begin as soon as a stroke patient is stable, sometimes within 24–48 hours after a stroke. This first stage of rehabilitation can occur within an acute-care hospital; however, it is very dependent on the unique circumstances of the individual patient.

Recently, in the largest stroke rehabilitation study in the United States, researchers compared two common techniques to help stroke patients improve their walking. Both methods—training on a body-weight supported treadmill or working on strength and balance exercises at home with a physical therapist—resulted in equal improvements in the individual's ability to walk by the end of one year. Researchers found that functional improvements could be seen as late as one year after the stroke, which goes against the conventional wisdom that most recovery is complete by 6 months. The trial showed that 52 percent of the participants made significant improvements in walking, everyday function and quality of life, regardless of how severe their impairment was, or whether they started the training at 2 or 6 months after the stroke.

Where Can a Stroke Patient Get Rehabilitation?

At the time of discharge from the hospital, the stroke patient and family coordinate with hospital social workers to locate a suitable living arrangement. Many stroke survivors return home, but some move into some type of medical facility.

Inpatient Rehabilitation Units

Inpatient facilities may be freestanding or part of larger hospital complexes. Patients stay in the facility, usually for 2–3 weeks, and engage in a coordinated, intensive program of rehabilitation. Such programs often involve at least 3 hours of active therapy a day, 5 or 6 days a week. Inpatient facilities offer a comprehensive range of medical services, including full-time physician supervision and access to the full range of therapists specializing in post-stroke rehabilitation.

Outpatient Units

Outpatient facilities are often part of a larger hospital complex and provide access to physicians and the full range of therapists specializing in stroke rehabilitation. Patients typically spend several hours, often 3 days each week, at the facility taking part in coordinated therapy sessions and return home at night. Comprehensive outpatient facilities frequently offer treatment programs as intense as those of inpatient facilities, but they also can offer less demanding regimens, depending on the patient's physical capacity.

Nursing Facilities

Rehabilitative services available at nursing facilities are more variable than are those at inpatient and outpatient units. Skilled nursing facilities usually place a greater emphasis on rehabilitation, whereas traditional nursing homes emphasize residential care. In addition, fewer hours of therapy are offered compared to outpatient and inpatient rehabilitation units.

Home-Based Rehabilitation Programs

Home rehabilitation allows for great flexibility so that patients can tailor their program of rehabilitation and follow individual schedules. Stroke survivors may participate in an intensive level of therapy several hours per week or follow a less demanding regimen. These arrangements are often best suited for people who require treatment by only one type of rehabilitation therapist. Patients dependent on Medicare coverage for their rehabilitation must meet Medicare's "homebound" requirements to qualify for such services; at this time lack of transportation is not a valid reason for home therapy. The major disadvantage of home-based rehabilitation programs is the lack of specialized equipment. However, undergoing treatment at home gives people the advantage of practicing skills and developing compensatory strategies in the context of their own living environment. In the recent stroke rehabilitation trial, intensive balance and strength rehabilitation in the home was equivalent to treadmill training at a rehabilitation facility in improving walking.

Section 12.2

Cognitive Rehabilitation Therapy

This section includes text excerpted from "Cognitive Impairment in Adults with Non–Central Nervous System Cancers (PDQ®)–Health Professional Version," National Cancer Institute (NCI), November 2, 2017.

When people talk about cognitive rehabilitation therapy (CRT), they're actually not talking about one therapy—they're talking about a constellation of techniques that are used to try to improve an individual's ability to function after injury. In other words, CRT is not a single therapy, but a collection of individual treatment strategies designed to improve problems with memory, attention, perception, learning, planning and judgment brought about by brain injury, neurological disorders or other illnesses.

Examples of cognitive rehabilitation therapies include writing tasks and interaction with computer-assisted programs. The goal of many of these therapies is to improve functions of memory, attention processing, social communications, problem-solving and the regulation of emotions.

It should be noted that in cases of mild traumatic brain injury (mTBI), nearly 90 percent of patients recover with no residual problems and only those with persistent symptoms need to be evaluated and treated. Diagnostic tools for mTBI are not precise and neuropsychological assessments can be difficult to interpret. Therefore, medical evidence for effectiveness of cognitive rehabilitation therapies has been difficult to measure.

Frequently Asked Questions

Who May Benefit Most from CRT?

Patients who have experienced moderate to severe TBI and who suffer from recurring symptoms such as attention and memory deficits, problems with executive functioning and social pragmatics deficits are most likely to benefit from CRT. In cases of mild TBI, nearly 90 percent recover with no residual problems and only those with persistent symptoms need to be evaluated and treated.

Why Is It Difficult to Determine How Effective CRTs Can Be; There Seems to Be Great Disparity of Opinion on the Subject?

Limited data on the effectiveness of cognitive rehabilitation programs are available, and this is in part due to the heterogeneity of the subjects, interventions and outcomes studied. Lack of rigorous methodology (i.e., randomized controlled trials) in efficacy studies has also contributed to the disparity in opinion on the effectiveness of CRT.

Are There "Specialists" in CRTs, or Do Most Doctors Understand Their Uses?

Neuropsychologists specialize in neuropsychological cognitive testing that is used to determine if a patient will benefit from cognitive rehabilitation. They are also the primary providers who develop the individualized cognitive rehabilitation plan for patients. However, cognitive rehabilitation may be performed by an occupational therapist, physical therapist, speech/language pathologist, neuropsychologist, or a physician.

Approaches to Cognitive rehabilitation Interventions

CR has shown promise in reducing the impact of cognitive problems on cancer patients and survivors. CR originated to treat populations with brain injuries such as stroke or traumatic brain injury, and it has been adapted for the cancer setting. Several rehabilitation approaches have been blended to varying degrees in CR interventions:

- **Psychoeducation** provides useful information about brain functioning, cognitive deficits, and their consequences for daily life.

- **Compensatory training** focuses on the acquisition of new behaviors and strategies to compensate for chronic dysfunction. This intervention may include modifying or restructuring the environment by substituting external aids (such as calendars and electronic diaries) so that individuals rely less on their cognitive abilities; or learning new coping strategies (such as pacing cognitive activities and minimizing distractions).

- **Cognitive training** involves the use of repetitive, increasingly challenging tasks (often via computer) to improve, maintain, or restore cognitive function in the areas of attention, memory, and executive function.

The following table will discuss about the therapy types and procedures along with the specific examples.

Table 12.1. Types of Therapies

Therapy	Area of Cognitive Impairment	Specific Examples	Procedure/Treatment
Attention Process Training	Attention	Letter cancellation tasks with distracting Noise in background	Consists of sequential hierarchical interventions aimed at specific attentional processes including sustained attention, selective attention, and divided attention. Increasing levels of distraction are introduced to gradually make the task more challenging
Error Management Training	Attention Memory Executive functioning Social pragmatics	Individual and group self-awareness training	A group support program that includes components of cognitive rehabilitation, cognitive behavioral therapy, and social skills training and focuses on self-regulation and psychosocial functioning. The 16-week intervention is designed to improve self-awareness deficits that are common following TBI and targets error awareness and self-correction in real life settings at home and work.
Emotional Regulation Training	Attention Memory Executive functioning Social pragmatics	Anger Management Training	The goal is to increase the patient's awareness of their negative emotional states, particularly anger, through training in recognition of cognitive, physical and emotional reactions. Patients are provided with an outline of anger syndromes and handouts summarizing the sessions as well as practice in relaxation techniques, self-talk methods and time outs.

Table 12.1. Continued

Therapy	Area of Cognitive Impairment	Specific Examples	Procedure/Treatment
External Cuing	Attention Memory Executive functioning	Supervised living BlackBerry Cell phone PDA	Provides the patient with technology aids such as alarm watches, pagers, etc. Includes restructuring the environment using labels, signs and directions. Other aids for memory and executive functioning include voice organizers, mobile phone computer interactive systems, and devices such as PDAs and BlackBerry cell phones. External cueing strategies may require family as well as individual treatments to select and train the appropriate cues.
Integrated Use	Attention Memory Executive functioning Social pragmatics		Provide individual and group cognitive, psychological and functional interventions. These programs are multidisciplinary and employ multiple treatment modalities in a holistic program that is typically delivered to patients three to five times per week over several months. Treatment is individualized and uses psychosocial interventions to enhance effectiveness. These programs also address self-awareness, behavioral and affective regulation, and community reintegration. The group treatments focus on improving executive functioning and generalizing strategies learned in treatment to the naturalistic environment. The treatment team is usually comprised of a neuropsychologist, speech-language pathologist, occupational therapist, vocational therapist, recreation therapist, and physician and meets regularly to develop individualized treatment goals and monitor patient progress.

Table 12.1. Continued

Therapy	Area of Cognitive Impairment	Specific Examples	Procedure/Treatment
			Community re-entry is a goal of this treatment, so outings to community settings to practice new skills are an integral component of this treatment; vocational trials are also often included. Families are involved in psychoeducation and family therapy to support the patient's treatment progress.
Memory Notebook	Attention Memory Executive functioning	Prosthetics PDA	A memory compensation strategy in which the patient is taught how to use a diary and then how to use this diary to solve problems in daily activities. A memory notebook includes sections for autobiographical and injury related information, a memory log, a calendar to-do list, transportation information such as bus schedules, names and identifying information, and a feelings log to record emotions that occur in specific situations. Other sections can be added that are personally relevant to the patient. During the first phase of treatment, the patient is familiarized with the sections of the notebook and the overall purpose of the notebook. In the next phase of treatment, the patient learns to use the notebook with therapist guidance during simulated situations. During the final phase, the patient is coached about how to use the notebook at home or at work. A PDA is the electronic equivalent of a memory notebook. PDAs and memory notebooks serve as memory prosthetics for the traumatic brain injury patient with impaired prospective memory. An important component in this intervention is therapist facilitation of the patient's emotional

Table 12.1. Continued

Therapy	Area of Cognitive Impairment	Specific Examples	Procedure/Treatment
			acceptance of the necessity of using a memory notebook and the acceptability of the use of devices in the patient's social environment.
Problem Solving Training	Attention Memory Executive functioning Social pragmatics	Internal problem-solving Internal dialogue	Problem solving training interventions address issues in the ability to formulate goals, initiate behavior, anticipate the consequences of action; plan, organize, and monitor behavior; and to change behavior in accordance with feedback. Training provides patients with techniques for analyzing complex problems by breaking them into manageable steps. Steps taught include defining the problem, generating alternatives, making a decision, and verifying the solution. The patient is taught to use an internal dialogue or self-instructions to approach problems in everyday life; self-awareness and self-regulation are emphasized. Training methods include cue cards, feedback, modeling, and the keeping of a diary. Problem solving training can occur in individual or group treatments.
Social Communications Skills Training Groups	Executive functioning Social pragmatics	Group cognitive therapy	Social communication skills training is a group treatment approach that is jointly facilitated by mental health and rehabilitation professionals. These groups emphasize self-awareness to set individual goals. Group process is used to foster interaction, problem solving, a social support system, and awareness that one is not alone. A treatment protocol has been used which was comprised of 12 ninety minute sessions.

Table 12.1. Continued

Therapy	Area of Cognitive Impairment	Specific Examples	Procedure/Treatment
Various Mneumonic Techniques	Memory	Story method Acronyms Sentence/acrostics Method of loci Chunking Repetition	Mnemonic Strategies are memory-enhancing strategies that help patients develop techniques to enhance registration and encoding of information. Examples of mnemonic strategies include verbal organization strategies such as forming acronyms and making paired associations with target words and semantic elaboration which refers to linking target words or ideas in a story. Rehearsal or repetition is another strategy for improving retention of information. These techniques are typically taught in individual treatment sessions as they are difficult to learn, require assistance to identify applicable situations for use in the patient's life, and require repeated practice for generalization from the treatment session to the patient's own environment to occur. Additional efficiency can be achieved when a group format is used for practice after individual strategy training.
Visual Imagery Mneumonics	Memory	Imagery-based training	Visual imagery is a popular mnemonic strategic in which the patient is taught to make a movie or picture of what needs to be recalled. Application of this technique is useful for improving recall of everyday verbal material such as stories, names, and appointments. Treatment occurs three times weekly and is of 10 weeks duration.

Table 12.1. Continued

Therapy	Area of Cognitive Impairment	Specific Examples	Procedure/Treatment
Working Memory Training	Attention	Completing two cognitive tasks simultaneously	Working memory training refers to a treatment designed to improve and optimize the temporary maintenance and manipulation of mental representations of information. This cognitive process is particularly important when information is presented rapidly or there are multiple sources of information. Working memory training teaches patients strategies to improve their regulation and allocation of attentional resources. Tasks are administered in a hierarchical sequence with task complexity and additional components added as mastery is obtained. In the n-back procedure, for example, a sequence of stimuli is presented and the patient is asked to recall stimuli early in the sequence. Number strings or playing cards presented in random sequence have been used for the training task. The therapist modifies the conditions of the task such as changing from self-paced to externally based presentation. The working memory demands of the task can be further increased by having the patient engage in a secondary task while completing the n-back task to simulate the occurrence of interrupting an activity to respond to an additional task and being able to return to the original activity.

Table 12.1. Continued

Therapy	Area of Cognitive Impairment	Specific Examples	Procedure/Treatment
			This treatment is conducted individually and part of the treatment time is spent discussing the patient's performance and helping the patient identify task variables which negatively or positively influenced their performance. The work with the therapist also includes attention to managing frustration and other emotional responses elicited by the task, analyzing attentional difficulties relevant to the patient's everyday functioning, and facilitating the application of strategies learned within the session to everyday functioning

(Source: "Types of Therapies," Military Health System (MHS).)

Section 12.3

Scales and Measurements of Brain Functioning

This section contains text excerpted from the following sources: Text under the heading "How Do Healthcare Providers Diagnose Traumatic Brain Injury (TBI)?" is excerpted from "How Do Health Care Providers Diagnose Traumatic Brain Injury (TBI)?" *Eunice Kennedy Shriver* National Institute of Child Health and Human Development (NICHD), December 1, 2016; Text under the heading "Selected Clinical Measures for Assessing Paediatric Brain Function" is excerpted from "Traumatic Brain Injury in the United States: Assessing Outcomes in Children," Centers for Disease Control and Prevention (CDC), January 22, 2016.

How Do Healthcare Providers Diagnose Traumatic Brain Injury (TBI)?

To diagnose TBI, healthcare providers may use one or more tests that assess a person's physical injuries, brain and nerve functioning, and level of consciousness. Some of these tests are described below.

- Glasgow Coma Scale (GCS)
- Measurements for Level of TBI
- Speech and Language Tests
- Cognition and Neuropsychological Tests
- Imaging Tests
- Tests for Assessing TBI in Military Settings

Glasgow Coma Scale (GCS)

The GCS measures a person's functioning in three areas:

- **Ability to speak,** such as whether the person speaks normally, speaks in a way that doesn't make sense, or doesn't speak at all

- **Ability to open eyes,** including whether the person opens his or her eyes only when asked

- **Ability to move,** ranging from moving one's arms easily to not moving even in response to painful stimulation

A healthcare provider rates a person's responses in these categories and calculates a total score. A score of 13 and higher indicates a mild TBI, 9 through 12 indicates a moderate TBI, and 8 or below indicates severe TBI. However, there may be no correlation between initial GCS score and the person's short- or long-term recovery or abilities.

Measurements for Level of TBI

Healthcare providers sometimes rank the person's level of consciousness, memory loss, and GCS score.

A TBI is considered mild if:

- The person was not unconscious or was unconscious for less than 30 minutes.
- Memory loss lasted less than 24 hours.
- The GCS was 13–15.

A research supported by *Eunice Kennedy Shriver* National Institute of Child Health and Human Development (NICHD) has found, however, that diagnosis of mild TBI (concussion), in practice, uses inconsistent criteria and relies heavily on patients' self-reported symptoms.

A TBI is considered moderate if:

- The person was unconscious for more than 30 minutes and up to 24 hours.
- Memory loss lasted anywhere from 24 hours to 7 days.
- The GCS was 9–12.

A TBI is considered severe if:

- The person was unconscious for more than 24 hours.
- Memory loss lasted more than 7 days.
- The GCS was 8 or lower.

Speech and Language Tests

- A **speech-language pathologist** completes a formal evaluation of speech and language skills, including an oral motor evaluation of the strength and coordination of the muscles that control speech, understanding and use of grammar and vocabulary, as well as reading and writing.

- Social communication skills are evaluated with formal tests and role-playing scenarios.

- If a patient has problems with swallowing, the speech-language pathologist will make recommendations regarding management and treatment to ensure that the individual is able to swallow safely and receive adequate nutrition.

Cognition and Neuropsychological Tests

- Cognition describes the processes of thinking, reasoning, problem solving, information processing, and memory.

  - Most patients with severe TBI suffer from cognitive disabilities, including the loss of many higher level mental skills.

- Neuropsychological assessments are often used to obtain information about cognitive capabilities.

  - These tests are specialized task-oriented evaluations of human brain-behavior relationships, evaluating higher cognitive functioning as well as basic sensory-motor processes.

  - Testing by a neuropsychologist can assess the individual's cognitive, language, behavioral, motor, and executive functions and provide information regarding the need for rehabilitative services.

  - For this assessment, a neuropsychologist reviews the case history and hospital records of the patient, and interviews the patient and his/her family.

  - The neuropsychologist acquires information about the "person" the individual was before the injury, based on aspects like school performance, habits, and lifestyle, in order to detail which abilities remain unchanged as well as areas of the brain that are adversely affected by the injury and how the injury is expected to impact the individual's life.

Imaging Tests

Healthcare providers may also use tests that take images of a person's brain. These include, but are not limited to:

- **Computerized tomography (CT).** A CT (or "cat") scan takes X-rays from many angles to create a complete picture. It can quickly show bleeding in the brain, bruised brain tissue, and other damage.

- **Magnetic resonance imaging (MRI).** MRI uses magnets and radio waves to produce more detailed images than CT scans. An MRI likely would not be used as part of an initial TBI assessment because it takes too long to complete. It may be used in follow-up examinations, though.

- **Intracranial pressure (ICP)** monitoring. Sometimes, swelling of the brain from a TBI can increase pressure inside the skull. The pressure can cause additional damage to the brain. A healthcare provider may insert a probe through the skull to monitor this swelling. In some cases, a shunt or drain is placed into the skull to relieve ICP.

Tests for Assessing TBI in Military Settings

A severe trauma may be obvious in a military situation, but a milder TBI may not be as easy to identify. The U.S. Department of Defense (DOD) and U.S. Department of Veterans Affairs (VA) have therefore established procedures to assess quickly whether the person suffered:

- A loss of consciousness

- Memory problems

- Neurologic symptoms, such as confusion or poor coordination

This assessment, combined with other measures, helps determine the type of care necessary, including evacuation for a higher level of treatment.

Selected Clinical Measures for Assessing Paediatric Brain Function

A wide range of clinical measures is available for assessing outcomes of TBI

Glasgow Coma Scale (GCS)

- Is a useful indicator of severity, but not for children younger than age 5.

- Scores for the same patient vary depending on when they were collected, e.g., GCS scores collected by Emergency Medical Technicians (EMTs) before admission are not as reliable as those collected in the ED or hospital. Centers for Disease Control and Prevention (CDC) TBI surveillance guidelines recommend use of the first GCS after admission to ED or hospital.

Children's Coma Score

- Is a modification of the Glasgow Coma Score designed to be used in children aged 3 years and younger.

- Eye opening and motor response subscales are identical to the GCS, but the verbal response subscale rates behavior/affect in preverbal populations.

- Is unclear how widely this score is being used or whether the score represents a significant improvement in the GCS for use with children. More research on this topic is needed.

Abbreviated Injury Score (AIS) / Injury Severity Score (ISS)

- Are used routinely in the clinical setting.

- Most recent version (AIS 98) is better than previous versions for assessing children.

- Because of the variability within AIS levels, researchers should consider supplementing AIS/ISS with Therapeutic Intensity Level, which is used in some clinical settings to determine severity based on the intensity of treatment required by the patient.

- The AIS score for the head is highly correlated with GCS and is a useful measure of TBI severity.

Loss of Consciousness (LOC)

- Measures the length of time between injury and when the patient regains consciousness.

- Is strongly correlated with outcomes in children and adults and is a key piece of information that should be collected.

Length of Posttraumatic Amnesia (PTA)

- Measures the time from when a patient emerges from coma until he or she is no longer disoriented.

- Appears to be strongly correlated with outcome; however, it is difficult to document consistently and accurately within a hospital protocol.

- Inter-rater reliability is low; that is, different people report different lengths of PTA.

- Despite limitations, PTA should be collected and reported as accurately as possible.

Rancho Los Amigos Scale

- Is a 7-level scale for assessing early recovery in the brain injury rehabilitation setting.

- Rates behavior, cognitive functioning, and response to the environment.

- Levels range from No Response (Level I) through Purposeful-Appropriate Responses (Level VII).

- May be useful for research on outcomes but to date has not been used widely or evaluated for that purpose.

Pediatric Trauma Score (PTS)

- Is a composite injury score in which the injured child receives a score of -1 (severely injured), +1 (moderately injured) or +2 (slightly injured or not injured) in each of six areas—body weight/size, airway, blood pressure, central nervous system activity, open wounds and skeletal injuries.

- Score is not useful for TBI research because it does not separate head injury from injury to other body regions/functions.

Neuropsychological / Psychiatric Tests

- These detailed tests of cognitive and psychological functioning are frequently conducted by trained professionals.

- Results from these tests are important, particularly to document more subtle deficits, but they must be done in a clinical setting.

School Performance Assessments

Assessments of school performance include achievement tests, which measure students' academic performance, and school function assessments, which assess students' ability to behave appropriately in the classroom.

Achievement Tests

- These tests of academic achievement are not sensitive to TBI-related problems.

- Thinking and reasoning are not assessed.

- Bright students may do well based on previous learning, thus masking TBI-related problems.

- Scores may improve even as behavior worsens.

- Achievement test results, if available for review, might provide some useful information about previous performance; however, meeting participants did not strongly recommend including them in studies assessing longer term outcomes of TBI.

School Function Assessments

- These checklists are specifically designed to assess functioning in the classroom setting.

- They are helpful in detecting problems specific to the classroom, including awareness of hygiene and behavior regulation.

- Meeting participants recommended including at least some key items from school function assessments in studies of outcomes of TBI in children and youth.

Section 12.4

Rehabilitative Technology for Brain Disorders

This section contains text excerpted from the following sources: Text in this section begins with excerpts from "Rehabilitative and Assistive Technology," *Eunice Kennedy Shriver* National Institute of Child Health and Human Development (NICHD), December 1, 2016; Text beginning with the heading "How Does Rehabilitative and Assistive Technology Benefit People with Neurological Disabilities?" is excerpted from "How Does Rehabilitative and Assistive Technology Benefit People with Disabilities?" *Eunice Kennedy Shriver* National Institute of Child Health and Human Development (NICHD), December 1, 2016; Text under the heading "How Can Future Rehabilitation Engineering Research Improve the Quality of Life for Individuals?" is excerpted from "Rehabilitation Engineering," National Institute of Biomedical Imaging and Bioengineering (NIBIB), November 2016.

Rehabilitative and assistive technology refers to tools, equipment, or products that can help a person with a disability to function successfully at school, home, work, and in the community. Disabilities are disorders, diseases, health conditions, or injuries that affect an individual's physical, intellectual, or mental well-being. Rehabilitative and assistive technologies can help people with disabilities to function more easily in their everyday lives and can also make it easier for a caregiver to care for a disabled person. The term "rehabilitative technology" is sometimes used to refer to aids used to help people recover their functioning after injury or illness. "Assistive technologies" may be as simple as a magnifying glass to improve visual perception or as complex as a computerized communication system.

Some of these technologies are made possible through rehabilitative engineering research, which is the application of engineering and scientific principles to study how people with disabilities function in society. It includes studying barriers to optimal function and designing solutions so that people with disabilities can interact successfully in their environments.

Rehabilitative and assistive technology refers to tools, equipment, or products that can help a person with a disability to function successfully at school, home, work, and in the community. Disabilities are disorders, diseases, health conditions, or injuries that affect an individual's physical, intellectual, or mental well-being. Rehabilitative and assistive technologies can help people with disabilities to function more easily in their everyday lives and can also make it easier for a caregiver to care for a disabled person. The term "rehabilitative technology" is sometimes used to refer to aids used to help people recover their functioning after injury or illness. "Assistive technologies" may be as simple as a magnifying glass to improve visual perception or as complex as a computerized communication system.

Some of these technologies are made possible through rehabilitative engineering research, which is the application of engineering and scientific principles to study how people with disabilities function in society. It includes studying barriers to optimal function and designing solutions so that people with disabilities can interact successfully in their environments.

How Does Rehabilitative and Assistive Technology Benefit People with Neurological Disabilities?

Deciding which type of rehabilitative or assistive technology would be most helpful for a person with a disability is usually made by the disabled person and his or her family and caregivers, along with a team of professionals and consultants. The team is trained to match particular assistive technologies to specific needs to help the person function more independently. The team may include family doctors, regular and special education teachers, speech-language pathologists, rehabilitation engineers, occupational therapists, and other specialists, including representatives from companies that manufacture assistive technology.

Assistive technology enables students with disabilities to compensate for the impairments they experience. This specialized technology promotes independence and decreases the need for other educational support.

Appropriate assistive technology helps people with disabilities overcome or compensate, at least in part, for their limitations. Rehabilitative technology can help restore function in people who have developed a disability due to disease, injury, or aging. Rehabilitative and assistive technology can enable individuals to:

- Care for themselves and their families

- Work

- Learn in schools and other educational institutions

- Access information through computers and reading

- Enjoy music, sports, travel, and the arts

- Participate fully in community life

Assistive technology also benefits employers, teachers, family members, and everyone who interacts with users of the technology. Increasing opportunities for participation benefits everyone.

What Types of Assistive Devices Are Available?

Health professionals use a variety of names to describe assistive devices:

- **Assistive listening devices (ALDs)** help amplify the sounds you want to hear, especially where there's a lot of background noise. ALDs can be used with a hearing aid or cochlear implant to help a wearer hear certain sounds better.

- **Augmentative and alternative communication (AAC)** devices help people with communication disorders to express themselves. These devices can range from a simple picture board to a computer program that synthesizes speech from text.

- **Alerting devices** connect to a doorbell, telephone, or alarm that emits a loud sound or blinking light to let someone with hearing loss know that an event is taking place.

What Types of Assistive Listening Devices Are Available?

Several types of ALDs are available to improve sound transmission for people with hearing loss. Some are designed for large facilities such as classrooms, theaters, places of worship, and airports. Other types are intended for personal use in small settings and for one-on-one conversations. All can be used with or without hearing aids or a cochlear implant. ALD systems for large facilities include hearing loop systems, frequency-modulated (FM) systems, and infrared systems.

Hearing loop (or induction loop) systems use electromagnetic energy to transmit sound. A hearing loop system involves four parts:

- A sound source, such as a public address system, microphone, or home TV or telephone

- An amplifier

- A thin loop of wire that encircles a room or branches out beneath carpeting

- A receiver worn in the ears or as a headset

Amplified sound travels through the loop and creates an electromagnetic field that is picked up directly by a hearing loop receiver or a telecoil, a miniature wireless receiver that is built into many hearing aids and cochlear implants. To pick up the signal, a listener must be wearing the receiver and be within or near the loop. Because the sound is picked up directly by the receiver, the sound is much clearer, without as much of the competing background noise associated with many listening environments. Some loop systems are portable, making it possible for people with hearing loss to improve their listening environments, as needed, as they proceed with their daily activities. A hearing loop can be connected to a public address system, a television, or any other audio source. For those who don't have hearing aids with embedded telecoils, portable loop receivers are also available.

FM systems use radio signals to transmit amplified sounds. They are often used in classrooms, where the instructor wears a small microphone connected to a transmitter and the student wears the receiver, which is tuned to a specific frequency, or channel. People who have a telecoil inside their hearing aid or cochlear implant may also wear a wire around the neck (called a neckloop) or behind their aid or implant (called a silhouette inductor) to convert the signal into magnetic signals that can be picked up directly by the telecoil. FM systems can transmit signals up to 300 feet and are able to be used in many public places. However, because radio signals are able to penetrate walls, listeners in one room may need to listen to a different channel than those in another room to avoid receiving mixed signals. Personal FM systems operate in the same way as larger scale systems and can be used to help people with hearing loss to follow one-on-one conversations.

Infrared systems use infrared light to transmit sound. A transmitter converts sound into a light signal and beams it to a receiver that is worn by a listener. The receiver decodes the infrared signal back to sound. As with FM systems, people whose hearing aids or cochlear implants have a telecoil may also wear a neckloop or silhouette inductor to convert the infrared signal into a magnetic signal, which can be picked up through their telecoil. Unlike induction loop or FM systems, the infrared signal cannot pass through walls, making it particularly useful in courtrooms, where confidential information is often discussed, and in buildings where competing signals can be a problem, such as classrooms or movie theaters. However, infrared systems cannot be used in environments with too many competing light sources, such as outdoors or in strongly lit rooms.

Personal amplifiers are useful in places in which the above systems are unavailable or when watching TV, being outdoors, or traveling in a car. About the size of a cell phone, these devices increase sound levels and reduce background noise for a listener. Some have directional microphones that can be angled toward a speaker or other source of sound. As with other ALDs, the amplified sound can be picked up by a receiver that the listener is wearing, either as a headset or as earbuds.

What Types of Augmentative and Alternative Communication Devices Are Available for Communicating Face-to-Face?

The simplest AAC device is a picture board or touch screen that uses pictures or symbols of typical items and activities that make up a person's daily life. For example, a person might touch the image of a glass to ask for a drink. Many picture boards can be customized and expanded based on a person's age, education, occupation, and interests.

Keyboards, touch screens, and sometimes a person's limited speech may be used to communicate desired words. Some devices employ a text display. The display panel typically faces outward so that two people can exchange information while facing each other. Spelling and word prediction software can make it faster and easier to enter information.

Speech-generating devices go one step further by translating words or pictures into speech. Some models allow users to choose from several different voices, such as male or female, child or adult, and even some regional accents. Some devices employ a vocabulary of prerecorded words while others have an unlimited vocabulary, synthesizing speech as words are typed in. Software programs that convert personal computers into speaking devices are also available.

What Augmentative and Alternative Communication Devices Are Available for Communicating by Telephone?

For many years, people with hearing loss have used text telephone or telecommunications devices, called TTY or TDD machines, to communicate by phone. This same technology also benefits people with speech difficulties. A TTY machine consists of a typewriter keyboard that displays typed conversations onto a readout panel or printed on paper. Callers will either type messages to each other over the system or, if a call recipient does not have a TTY machine, use the national toll-free telecommunications relay service at 711 to communicate. Through the relay service, a communications assistant serves as a bridge between two callers, reading typed messages aloud to the person with hearing while transcribing what's spoken into type for the person with hearing loss.

With today's new electronic communication devices, however, TTY machines have almost become a thing of the past. People can place phone calls through the telecommunications relay service using almost any device with a keypad, including a laptop, personal digital assistant, and cell phone. Text messaging has also become a popular method of communication, skipping the relay service altogether.

Another system uses voice recognition software and an extensive library of video clips depicting American Sign Language to translate a signer's words into text or computer-generated speech in real time. It is also able to translate spoken words back into sign language or text.

Finally, for people with mild to moderate hearing loss, captioned telephones allow you to carry on a spoken conversation, while providing a transcript of the other person's words on a readout panel or computer screen as back-up.

What Types of Alerting Devices Are Available?

Alerting or alarm devices use sound, light, vibrations, or a combination of these techniques to let someone know when a particular event is occurring. Clocks and wake-up alarm systems allow a person to choose to wake up to flashing lights, horns, or a gentle shaking.

Visual alert signalers monitor a variety of household devices and other sounds, such as doorbells and telephones. When the phone rings, the visual alert signaler will be activated and will vibrate or flash a light to let people know. In addition, remote receivers placed around the house can alert a person from any room. Portable vibrating pagers can let parents and caretakers know when a baby is crying. Some baby monitoring devices analyze a baby's cry and light up a picture to indicate if the baby sounds hungry, bored, or sleepy.

How Can Future Rehabilitation Engineering Research Improve the Quality of Life for Individuals?

Ongoing research in rehabilitation engineering involves the design and development of innovative technologies and techniques that can help people regain physical or cognitive functions. For example:

- **Rehabilitation robotics,** to use robots as therapy aids instead of solely as assistive devices. Smart rehabilitation robotics aid mobility training in individuals suffering from impaired movement, such as following a stroke.

- **Virtual rehabilitation**, which uses virtual reality simulation exercises for physical and cognitive rehabilitation. These tools are entertaining, motivate patients to exercise, and provide objective measures such as range of motion. The exercises can be performed at home by a patient and monitored by a therapist over the Internet (known as tele-rehabilitation), which offers convenience as well as reduced costs.

- **Physical prosthetics,** such as smarter artificial legs with powered ankles, exoskeletons, dextrous upper limbs and hands. This is an area where researchers continue to make advances in design and function to better mimic natural limb movement and user intent.

- **Advanced kinematics,** to analyze human motion, muscle electrophysiology and brain activity to more accurately monitor human functions and prevent secondary injuries.

- **Sensory prosthetics,** such as retinal and cochlear implants to restore some lost function to provide navigation and communication, increasing independence and integration into the community.

- **Brain computer interfaces,** to enable severely impaired individuals to communicate and access information. These technologies use the brain's electrical impulses to allow individuals to move a computer cursor or a robotic arm that can reach and grab items, or send text messages.

- **Modulation of organ function,** as interventions for urinary and fecal incontinence and sexual disorders. Recent developments in neuromodulation of the peripheral nervous system offer the promise to treat organ function in the case of a spinal cord injury.

- **Secondary disorder treatment,** such as pain management.

Part Three

Genetic and Congenital Brain Disorders

Chapter 13

Adrenoleukodystrophy

What Is X-Linked Adrenoleukodystrophy (X-ALD)?

X-ALD is a genetic disease that affects the nervous system and the adrenal glands (small glands located on top of each kidney). People with this disease often have progressive loss of the fatty covering (myelin) that surrounds the nerves in the brain and spinal cord. They may also have a shortage of certain hormones that is caused by damage to the outer layer of the adrenal glands (adrenal cortex). This is called adrenocortical insufficiency, or Addison disease. There are three forms of X-ALD: a childhood cerebral form, an adrenomyeloneuropathy (AMN) type, and an adrenal insufficiency only type. The disease primarily affects males.

What Are the Symptoms of X-ALD?

The signs and symptoms of the disease depend on the specific type. The symptoms of the childhood cerebral form of X-ALD typically begin between ages 4–8 years old. The first noticeable symptom is usually behavior problems in school such as struggling to pay attention. Some boys may have seizures as their first symptom. As the disease progresses, other symptoms may include vomiting, vision loss, learning

This chapter includes text excerpted from "X-Linked Adrenoleukodystrophy," Genetic and Rare Diseases Information Center (GARD), National Center for Advancing Translational Sciences (NCATS), November 8, 2017.

disabilities, trouble eating (dysphagia), deafness, fatigue, and trouble coordinating movements (ataxia).

The symptoms of the AMN type usually begin in early to midadulthood. Symptoms can include leg stiffness, weakness, and pain in the hands, and feet (peripheral neuropathy), muscle spasms, and weakness, and urinary problems or sexual dysfunction.

The adrenal insufficiency only (Addison disease only) type of X-ALD is characterized by men who develop adrenal insufficiency. Symptoms of adrenal insufficiency can develop at any time between childhood and adulthood and include decreased appetite, increased pigment (melanin) in the skin making it appear darker, muscle weakness, and vomiting. Males with the other forms of X-ALD can have adrenal insufficiency in addition to the other symptoms. Some individuals affected with X-ALD can also develop symptoms of mental illness.

What Causes X-ALD?

X-ALD is caused by a mutation (change) in the *ABCD1* gene. This gene provides instructions to make a protein called the adrenoleukodystrophy protein (ALDP). ALDP normally moves a type of fat molecule called very long-chain fatty acids (VLCFA) into a special part of the cell to be broken down. When the *ABCD1* gene is changed, there is too little ALDP in the cells or the ALDP that is made does not work normally. This causes VLCFA to build-up in the body. High levels of VLCFA are thought to be damaging to the outside of the adrenal glands (adrenal cortex) and the fatty covering (myelin) that surrounds the nerve cells in the brain and spinal cord. Researchers believe the damage caused by VLCFA may involve inflammation, especially in the brain.

Is X-ALD Inherited?

X-ALD is inherited in an X-linked manner. This means that the *ABCD1* gene is located on the X chromosome. The X chromosome is one of the sex chromosomes. Each woman has two X chromosomes, and each man has one X chromosome and one Y chromosome. Because men have only one X chromosome, they only have one copy of the *ABCD1* gene. If this gene has a disease-causing change, they will have X-ALD.

Women who have disease-causing changes in one copy of the *ABCD1* gene are known as carriers of the disease. About 80 percent of carriers do not have signs or symptoms of X-ALD because they have another working copy of *ABCD1*. However, about 20 percent of female carriers have symptoms that are similar to the adrenomyeloneuropathy (AMN) type of X-ALD.

If a male is diagnosed with X-ALD, it is likely that his mother is a carrier of the disease. However, about 5 percent of cases of X-ALD are caused by a new genetic change *(de novo)* in the individual. In these situations, the mother is not a carrier of the disease, and other family members are not at risk to have children with X-ALD. Therefore, when a male is diagnosed with X-ALD, it is important to determine if his mother is a carrier by testing her VLCFA levels or by genetic testing.

If a woman is found to be a carrier of X-ALD, for each of her children there is a 50 percent chance that he or she will inherit the change in *ABCD1*. This means that for each son, there is a 50 percent chance that he will be affected with X-ALD. For each daughter, there is a 50 percent chance that she will be a carrier of the disease like her mother.

X-ALD shows a characteristic known as variable expressivity. This means that the exact symptoms of each person with X-ALD can differ, even within the same family. For example, some boys may have the childhood cerebral form of X-ALD, while other members of the same family may have the adrenal insufficiency only type. It is not known what causes variable expressivity of the disease to occur. The symptoms cannot be predicted by levels of a very long-chain fatty acid (VLCFA) or by looking at the exact genetic change (mutation) in each individual.

How Is X-ALD Diagnosed?

X-ALD is suspected when a doctor observes signs and symptoms of the disease. X-ALD should be considered as a possible cause of symptoms in four situations:

- Boys with attention deficit disorder (ADD) who also have signs of neurological problems.
- Young men with progressive trouble walking or coordinating movements.
- All males with adrenal insufficiency (Addison disease), even in the absence of other symptoms.
- Adult women with progressive muscle weakness or wasting.

If a diagnosis of X-ALD is suspected, a blood test of very long-chain fatty acids will detect elevated levels in 99 percent of males. Genetic testing can be used to confirm the diagnosis. After diagnosis, a brain magnetic resonance imaging (MRI) can be completed to determine the extent of the disease. A brain MRI will be abnormal even if symptoms of the disease are not very severe.

What Is the Treatment for X-ALD?

The treatment for X-ALD depends on the signs and symptoms present in each person. For individuals who have adrenal insufficiency, corticosteroids are used to normalize hormone levels. Physical therapy may be helpful for men with the AMN form of the disease. Individuals who have neurological symptoms may be eligible for a bone marrow transplant. However, this treatment has risks. It is only recommended for boys who have evidence of neurological disease based on a brain MRI but do not yet have disease that has progressed to showing severe symptoms.

For boys who do not yet have symptoms of X-ALD, treatment with Lorenzo's oil may help to slow down the progression of the disease. However, this treatment is experimental, and the treatment's exact benefit has not been definitively shown. Clinical trials investigating treatment with gene therapy are underway and have shown some preliminary success.

What Is the Prognosis for X-ALD?

The long-term outlook for people affected by X-ALD depends on the exact type of the disease that each person has. The childhood cerebral form of the disease is progressive. Boys with this form of the disease often pass away within a few years of beginning to show symptoms. The other forms of X-ALD are less severe. The disease for these individuals may be slowly progressive, or it may not affect a person's lifespan at all.

It is important to remember that the exact signs and symptoms of a person with X-ALD cannot be predicted by the signs and symptoms of other members of the family. Therefore, the long-term outlook for individuals who have X-ALD within the same family can be very different.

Chapter 14

Batten Disease (Neuronal Ceroid Lipofuscinoses)

What Is Batten Disease?

Batten disease is a fatal, inherited disorder of the nervous system that typically begins in childhood. Early symptoms of this disorder usually appear between the ages of 5–10 years, when parents or physicians may notice a previously normal child has begun to develop vision problems or seizures. In some cases the early signs are subtle, taking the form of personality and behavior changes, slow learning, clumsiness, or stumbling. Over time, affected children suffer cognitive impairment (CI), worsening seizures, and progressive loss of sight and motor skills. Eventually, children with Batten disease become blind, bedridden, and demented. Batten disease is often fatal by the late teens or twenties.

Batten disease is named after the British pediatrician who first described it in 1903. Also known as Spielmeyer-Vogt-Sjogren-Batten disease, it is the most common form of a group of disorders called the neuronal ceroid lipofuscinoses, or NCLs. Although Batten disease originally referred specifically to the juvenile form of NCL (JNCL), the term Batten disease is increasingly used by pediatricians to describe all forms of NCL.

This chapter includes text excerpted from "Batten Disease Fact Sheet," National Institute of Neurological Disorders and Stroke (NINDS), May 10, 2017.

What Are the Other Forms of NCL?

There are four other main types of NCL, including three forms that begin earlier in childhood and a very rare form that strikes adults. The symptoms of these childhood types are similar to those caused by Batten disease, but they become apparent at different ages and progress at different rates.

- **Congenital NCL** is a very rare and severe form of NCL. Babies have abnormally small heads (microcephaly) and seizures, and die soon after birth.

- **Infantile NCL** (INCL or Santavuori-Haltia disease) begins between about ages 6 months and 2 years and progresses rapidly. Affected children fail to thrive and have microcephaly. Also typical are short, sharp muscle contractions called myoclonic jerks. These children usually die before age 5, although some have survived in a vegetative state a few years longer.

- **Late infantile NCL** (LINCL, or Jansky-Bielschowsky disease) begins between ages 2–4. The typical early signs are loss of muscle coordination (ataxia) and seizures that do not respond to drugs. This form progresses rapidly and ends in death between ages 8–12.

- **Adult NCL** (also known as Kufs disease, Parry disease, and ANCL) generally begins before age 40, causes milder symptoms that progress slowly, and does not cause blindness. Although age of death varies among affected individuals, this form does shorten life expectancy.

There are also "variant" forms of late infantile NCL (vLINCL) that do not precisely conform to classical late infantile NCL.

How Many People Have These Disorders?

Batten disease and other forms of NCL are relatively rare, occurring in an estimated 2–4 of every 100,000 live births in the United States. These disorders appear to be more common in Finland, Sweden, other parts of northern Europe, and Newfoundland, Canada. Although NCLs are classified as rare diseases, they often strike more than one person in families that carry the defective genes.

How Are NCLs Inherited?

Childhood NCLs are autosomal recessive disorders (ARD); that is, they occur only when a child inherits two copies of the defective gene, one from each parent. When both parents carry one defective gene, each of their children faces a one in four chance of developing NCL. At the same time, each child also faces a one in two chance of inheriting just one copy of the defective gene. Individuals who have only one defective gene are known as carriers, meaning they do not develop the disease, but they can pass the gene on to their own children. Because the mutated genes that are involved in certain forms of Batten disease are known, carrier detection is possible in some instances.

Adult NCL may be inherited as an autosomal recessive or, less often, as an autosomal dominant disorder. In autosomal dominant inheritance, all people who inherit a single copy of the disease gene develop the disease. As a result, there are no unaffected carriers of the gene.

What Causes These Diseases?

Symptoms of Batten disease and other NCLs are linked to a buildup of substances called lipofuscins (lipopigments) in the body's tissues. These lipopigments are made up of fats and proteins. Their name comes from the technical word lipo, which is short for "lipid" or fat, and from the term pigment, used because they take on a greenish yellow color when viewed under an ultraviolet light microscope. The lipopigments build-up in cells of the brain and the eye as well as in skin, muscle, and many other tissues. The substances are found inside a part of cells called lysosomes. Lysosomes are responsible for getting rid of things that become damaged or are no longer needed and must be cleared from inside the cell. The accumulated lipopigments in Batten disease and the other NCLs form distinctive shapes that can be seen under an electron microscope. Some look like half moons, others like fingerprints. These deposits are what doctors look for when they examine a skin sample to diagnose Batten disease. The specific appearance of the lipopigment deposits can be useful in guiding further diagnostic tests that may identify the specific gene defect.

To date, eight genes have been linked to the varying forms of NCL. Mutations of other genes in NCL are likely since some individuals do not have mutations in any of the known genes. More than one gene may be associated with a particular form of NCL. The known NCL genes are:

Ceroid-lipofuscinosis *CLN1* encodes an enzyme called palmitoyl protein thioesterase 1 (*PPT1*) that is insufficiently active in Infantile NCL.

CLN 2 produces an enzyme called tripeptidyl peptidase 1 (*TPP1*)—an acid protease that degrades proteins. The enzyme is insufficiently active in Late Infantile NCL (also referred to as CLN2).

CLN3 mutation is the major cause of Juvenile NCL. The gene codes for a protein called CLN3 or battenin, which is found in the membranes of the cell (most predominantly in lysosomes and in related structures called endosomes). The protein's function is currently unknown.

CLN5, which causes variant Late Infantile NCL (vLINCL, also referred to as CLN5), produces a lysosomal protein called CLN5, whose function has not been identified.

CLN6, which also causes Late Infantile NCL, encodes a protein called CLN6 or linclin. The protein is found in the membranes of the cell (most predominantly in a structure called the endoplasmic reticulum). Its function has not been identified.

MFSD8, seen in variant Late Infantile NCL (also referred to as CLN7), encodes the MFSD8 protein that is a member of a protein family called the major facilitator superfamily. This superfamily is involved with transporting substances across the cell membranes. The precise function of MFSD8 has not been identified.

CLN8 causes progressive epilepsy with mental retardation. The gene encodes a protein also called CLN8, which is found in the membranes of the cell—most predominantly in the endoplasmic reticulum. The protein's function has not been identified.

CTSD, involved with Congenital NCL (also referred to as CLN10), encodes cathepsin D, a lysosomal enzyme that breaks apart other proteins. A deficiency of cathepsin D causes the disorder.

How Are These Disorders Diagnosed?

Because vision loss is often an early sign, Batten disease may be first suspected during an eye exam. An eye doctor can detect a loss of cells within the eye that occurs in the childhood forms of NCL. However, because such cell loss occurs in other eye diseases, the disorder cannot be diagnosed by this sign alone. Often an eye specialist or other physician who suspects NCL may refer the child to a neurologist for additional testing.

In order to diagnose NCL, the neurologist needs the individual's medical and family history and information from various laboratory tests. Diagnostic tests used for NCLs include:

- **Blood or urine tests.** These tests can detect abnormalities that may indicate Batten disease. For example, elevated levels of a chemical called dolichol are found in the urine of many individuals with NCL. The presence of vacuolated lymphocytes—white blood cells that contain holes or cavities (observed by microscopic analysis of blood smears)—when combined with other findings that indicate NCL, is suggestive for the juvenile form caused by *CLN3* mutations.

- **Skin or tissue sampling.** The doctor can examine a small piece of tissue under an electron microscope. The powerful magnification of the microscope helps the doctor spot typical NCL deposits. These deposits are common in skin cells, especially those from sweat glands.

- **Electroencephalogram or EEG.** An EEG uses special patches placed on the scalp to record electrical currents inside the brain. This helps doctors see telltale patterns in the brain's electrical activity that suggest an individual has seizures.

- **Electrical studies of the eyes.** These tests, which include visual evoked responses and electroretinograms, can detect various eye problems common in childhood NCLs.

- **Diagnostic imaging using computed tomography (CT) or magnetic resonance imaging (MRI).** Diagnostic imaging can help doctors look for changes in the brain's appearance. CT uses X-rays and a computer to create a sophisticated picture of the brain's tissues and structures, and may reveal brain areas that are decaying, or "atrophic," in persons with NCL. MRI uses a combination of magnetic fields and radio waves, instead of radiation, to create a picture of the brain.

- **Measurement of enzyme activity.** Measurement of the activity of palmitoyl protein thioesterase involved in CLN1, the acid protease involved in CLN2, and, though more rare, cathepsin D activity involved in CLN10, in white blood cells or cultured skin fibroblasts (cells that strengthen skin and give it elasticity) can be used to confirm or rule out these diagnoses.

- **Deoxyribonucleic acid (DNA) analysis.** If families where the mutation in the gene for CLN3 is known, DNA analysis can be used to confirm the diagnosis or for the prenatal diagnosis of this form of Batten disease. When the mutation is known, DNA analysis can also be used to detect unaffected carriers of this condition for genetic counseling. If a family mutation has not previously been identified or if the common mutations are not present, recent molecular advances have made it possible to sequence all of the known *NCL* genes, increasing the chances of finding the responsible mutation(s).

Is There Any Treatment?

The U.S. Food and Drug Administration (FDA) approved cerliponase alfa as a treatment for slow loss of walking ability (ambulation) in children 3 years of age and older with late infantile neuronal ceroid lipofuscinosis type 2 (CLN2). No specific treatment is known that can reverse the symptoms of Batten disease or other NCLs. However, seizures can sometimes be reduced or controlled with anticonvulsant drugs, and other medical problems can be treated appropriately as they arise. At the same time, physical and occupational therapy may help patients retain function as long as possible.

Some reports have described a slowing of the disease in children with Batten disease who were treated with vitamins C and E, and with diets low in vitamin A. However, these treatments did not prevent the fatal outcome of the disease.

Support and encouragement can help patients and families cope with the profound disability and dementia caused by NCLs. Often, support groups enable affected children, adults, and families to share common concerns and experiences.

Meanwhile, scientists pursue medical research that could someday yield an effective treatment.

Chapter 15

Cerebral Autosomal Dominant Arteriopathy with Sub-Cortical Infarcts and Leukoencephalopathy (CADASIL)

Cerebral autosomal dominant arteriopathy with subcortical infarcts and leukoencephalopathy (CADASIL) is an inherited disease of the blood vessels that occurs when the thickening of blood vessel walls blocks the flow of blood to the brain. The disease primarily affects the small blood vessels in the white matter of the brain. CADASIL is characterized by migraine headaches and multiple strokes, which progresses to dementia. Other symptoms include white matter lesions throughout the brain, cognitive deterioration (CI), seizures, vision problems, and psychiatric problems such as severe depression and changes in behavior and personality. Individuals may also be at higher risk of heart attack. Symptoms and disease onset vary widely, with signs typically appearing in the mid-30s. Some individuals may not

This chapter includes text excerpted from "CADASIL," Genetic and Rare Diseases Information Center (GARD), National Center for Advancing Translational Sciences (NCATS), October 19, 2015.

show signs of the disease until later in life. CADASIL is caused by a change (or mutation) in a gene called *NOTCH3* and is inherited in an autosomal dominant manner.

Symptoms

Strokes are the main feature of CADASIL and often occur repeatedly. Strokes may lead to severe disability such as an inability to walk and urinary incontinence. The average age at onset for stroke-like episodes is 46 years.

A decline in thinking ability (cognitive deficit) is the second most common feature and occurs in over half of affected people. This may begin as early as 35 years of age. CADASIL typically causes a slow decline in thought processes, and approximately 75 percent of affected people eventually develop dementia (including significant difficulty with reasoning and memory). Thirty percent of people with CADASIL also experience psychiatric issues, varying from personality changes to severe depression.

Migraines with aura occur in about 35 percent of people with CADASIL, with the first attack occurring at an average age of 26 years. Epilepsy is present in 10 percent of affected people and usually presents at middle age.

Cause

CADASIL is caused by a mutation in the *NOTCH3* gene. The *NOTCH3* gene gives the body instructions to make the *Notch3* receptor protein, needed for normal function and survival of vascular smooth muscle cells. Mutations in *NOTCH3* cause the body to make an abnormal protein, thus impairing the function and survival of vascular smooth muscle cells and causing these cells to self-destruct. The loss of vascular smooth muscle cells in the brain causes blood vessel damage that leads to the characteristic features of CADASIL.

Inheritance

CADASIL is inherited in an autosomal dominant manner. This means that having a mutation in only one copy of the responsible gene in each cell is enough to cause CADASIL. In most cases, an affected person inherits the mutated gene from an affected parent. In rare cases, CADASIL may result from having a new mutation in the gene, in which case it is not inherited from a parent.

When a person with an autosomal dominant condition has children, each child has a 50 percent (1 in 2) chance to inherit the mutated copy of the gene.

Diagnosis

Making a diagnosis for a genetic or rare disease can often be challenging. Healthcare professionals typically look at a person's medical history, symptoms, physical exam, and laboratory test results in order to make a diagnosis.

Treatment

There is currently no treatment for CADASIL that is proven to be effective. While antiplatelet treatment is often used, it is also not proven to be useful. Migraine should be treated both symptomatically and prophylactically (with preventative methods), depending on the frequency of symptoms. When hypertension, diabetes or hypercholesterolemia (high cholesterol) are also present, they should be treated. Supportive care, including practical help, emotional support, and counseling, is useful for affected people and their families. Smoking increases the risk of stroke, so affected people who smoke should quit.

Prognosis

Symptoms of CADASIL usually progress slowly. By age 65, most people have severe cognitive problems and dementia. Some people lose the ability to walk, and most become completely dependent on the care of others due to multiple strokes.

Chapter 16

Mental Health Disorders Rooted in Genetic Brain Disorders

Mental disorders are health conditions that affect how a person thinks, feels, and acts. These disorders can impact a person's life in significant ways, including how he or she copes with life, earns a living, and relates to others.

"Why did this happen?" That is a common question that patients and their families have following a psychotic episode, suicide attempt, or the diagnosis of any serious mental disorder.

Research conducted and funded by the National Institute of Mental Health (NIMH) has found that many mental disorders are caused by a combination of biological, environmental, psychological, and genetic factors. In fact, a growing body of research has found that certain genes and gene variations are associated with mental disorders. So what is the best way to "look at your genes" and determine your own personal risk?

Your Family Health History

Your family history is one of your best clues about your risk of developing mental disorders and many other common illnesses. Certain

This chapter includes text excerpted from "Looking at My Genes: What Can They Tell Me about My Mental Health?" National Institute of Mental Health (NIMH), 2017.

mental illnesses tend to run in families, and having a close relative with a mental disorder could mean you are at a higher risk.

If a family member has a mental disorder, it does not necessarily mean you will develop one. Many other factors also play a role. But knowing your family mental health history can help you determine whether you are at a higher risk for certain disorders, help your doctor recommend actions for reducing your risk, and enable both you and your doctor to look for early warning signs.

To gain a better understanding of your family health history, it may help to:

Talk to Your Blood Relatives

The first step in creating a family health history is to talk to your blood relatives. The most helpful information comes from "first-degree" relatives—parents, brothers and sisters, and children. Information from "second-degree" relatives, such as nieces, nephews, half-brothers, half-sisters, grandparents, aunts, and uncles, can also be helpful.

Don't worry if you cannot get complete information on every relative. Some people may not want to talk. Others may be unable to remember information accurately. That's okay. Whatever information you can collect will be helpful.

As a family grows or family members are diagnosed with health conditions, new or updated information can be added. It may take a little time and effort, but this lasting legacy can improve the health of your family for generations to come.

Talk to a Mental Health Professional

If you have mental illness in your family, you may want to consult with a mental health professional who can help you understand risk factors and preventive factors. The NIMH Help for Mental Illness webpage (www.nimh.nih.gov/health/find-help/index.shtml) provides a number of resources for finding immediate help, locating a healthcare provider or treatment, and participating in clinical trials.

Your Genes

Genes are segments of deoxyribonucleic acid (DNA) found in every cell and are passed down from parents to children at conception. Some diseases—such as sickle cell anemia (SCA) or cystic fibrosis (CF)—are caused by genetic mutation(s), or a permanent change in one or more specific genes.

In other diseases, including many brain disorders, gene variants play a role in increasing or decreasing a person's risk of developing a disease or condition. Research is advancing our understanding of the role of genetics in mental health. Although there are common genetic variants associated with rare disorders like Fragile X or Rett syndrome (RS), no gene variants can predict with certainty that a person will develop a mental disorder. In most cases, even the genetic variant with the most supporting research raise a person's risk by only very small amounts. Knowing that you have one of these gene variants won't tell you nearly as much about your risk as your family history can.

Chapter 17

Other Inherited Neurological Disorders

Chapter Contents

Section 17.1

Aicardi Syndrome

This section contains text excerpted from the following sources:
Text in this section begins with excerpts from "Aicardi Syndrome,"
Genetics Home Reference (GHR), National Institutes of Health (NIH),
February 20, 2018; Text beginning with the heading "What Is the
Treatment for Aicardi Syndrome?" is excerpted from
"Aicardi Syndrome Information Page," National Institute of
Neurological Disorders and Stroke (NINDS), May 23, 2017.

Aicardi syndrome is a disorder that occurs almost exclusively in females. It is characterized by three main features that occur together in most affected individuals. People with Aicardi syndrome have absent or underdeveloped tissue connecting the left and right halves of the brain (agenesis or dysgenesis of the corpus callosum). They have seizures beginning in infancy (infantile spasms), which tend to progress to recurrent seizures (epilepsy) that can be difficult to treat. Affected individuals also have chorioretinal lacunae, which are defects in the light-sensitive tissue at the back of the eye (retina).

People with Aicardi syndrome often have additional brain abnormalities, including asymmetry between the two sides of the brain, brain folds and grooves that are small in size or reduced in number, cysts, and enlargement of the fluid-filled cavities (ventricles) near the center of the brain. Some have an unusually small head (microcephaly). Most affected individuals have moderate to severe developmental delay and intellectual disability, although some people with this disorder have milder disability.

In addition to chorioretinal lacunae, people with Aicardi syndrome may have other eye abnormalities such as small or poorly developed eyes (microphthalmia) or a gap or hole (coloboma) in the optic nerve, a structure that carries information from the eye to the brain. These eye abnormalities may cause blindness in affected individuals. Some people with Aicardi syndrome have unusual facial features including a short area between the upper lip and the nose (philtrum), a flat nose with an upturned tip, large ears, and sparse eyebrows. Other features of this condition include small hands, hand malformations, and spinal and rib abnormalities leading to progressive abnormal curvature of the spine (scoliosis). They often have gastrointestinal problems such as constipation or diarrhea, gastroesophageal reflux disease (GERD), and difficulty feeding.

The severity of Aicardi syndrome varies. Some people with this disorder have very severe epilepsy and may not survive past childhood. Less severely affected individuals may live into adulthood with milder signs and symptoms.

What Is the Treatment for Aicardi Syndrome?

There is no cure for Aicardi syndrome nor is there a standard course of treatment. Treatment generally involves medical management of seizures and programs to help parents and children cope with developmental delays. Long-term management by a pediatric neurologist with expertise in the management of infantile spasms is recommended.

What Is the Prognosis for Aicardi Syndrome?

The prognosis for girls with Aicardi syndrome varies according to the severity of their symptoms. There is an increased risk for death in childhood and adolescence, but survivors into adulthood have been described.

Section 17.2

Alpers-Huttenlocher Syndrome

This section contains text excerpted from the following sources: Text in this section begins with excerpts from "Alpers-Huttenlocher Syndrome," Genetics Home Reference (GHR), National Institutes of Health (NIH), January 16, 2018; Text beginning with the heading "What Is the Treatment for AHS?" is excerpted from "Alpers' Disease Information Page," National Institute of Neurological Disorders and Stroke (NINDS), September 18, 2011. Reviewed February 2018.

Alpers-Huttenlocher syndrome (AHS) is one of the most severe of a group of conditions called the polymerase gamma (POLG)-related disorders. The conditions in this group feature a range of similar signs and symptoms involving muscle-, nerve-, and brain-related functions. Alpers-Huttenlocher syndrome typically becomes apparent in children between ages 2–4. People with this condition usually have three characteristic features: recurrent seizures that do not improve with treatment (intractable epilepsy), loss of mental and movement abilities (psychomotor regression), and liver disease.

People with AHS usually have additional signs and symptoms. Most have problems with coordination and balance (ataxia) and disturbances in nerve function (neuropathy). Neuropathy can lead to abnormal or absent reflexes (areflexia). In addition, affected individuals may develop weak muscle tone (hypotonia) that worsens until they lose the ability to control their muscles and movement. Some people with AHS lose the ability to walk, sit, or feed themselves. Other movement-related symptoms in affected individuals can include involuntary muscle twitches (myoclonus), uncontrollable movements of the limbs (choreoathetosis), or a pattern of movement abnormalities known as parkinsonism.

Affected individuals may have other brain-related signs and symptoms. Migraine headaches, often with visual sensations or auras, are common. Additionally, people with this condition may have decreased brain function that is demonstrated as sleepiness, inability to concentrate, irritability, or loss of language skills or memory. Some people with the condition may lose their eyesight or hearing. People with AHS can survive from a few months to more than 10 years after the condition first appears.

What Is the Treatment for AHS?

There is no cure for Alpers disease and no way to slow its progression. Treatment is symptomatic and supportive. Anticonvulsants may be used to treat the seizures, but at times the seizures do not respond well to therapy, even at high doses. Therefore, the benefit of seizure control should be weights against what could be excessive sedation from the anticonvulsant. Valproate should not be used since it can increase the risk of liver failure. Physical therapy may help to relieve spasticity and maintain or increase muscle tone.

What Is the Prognosis for AHS?

The prognosis for individuals with Alpers disease is poor. Those with the disease usually die within their first decade of life. Continuous, unrelenting seizures often lead to death. Liver failure and cardiorespiratory failure due to brain, spinal cord, and nerve involvement may also occur.

Section 17.3

Gerstmann-Straussler-Scheinker (GSS) Disease

This section includes text excerpted from "Gerstmann-Straussler-Scheinker Disease," Genetic and Rare Diseases Information Center (GARD), National Center for Advancing Translational Sciences (NCATS), December 7, 2016.

The disease Gerstmann-Straussler-Scheinker (GSS) is a type of prion disease. The diseases caused by prions are a group of conditions that affect the nervous system. The main feature of the disease is a progressive degeneration of the cerebellum (the part of the brain that controls coordination, balance, and muscle tone), as well as different degrees of dementia. Signs and symptoms usually develop between the ages of 35–50 and may include weakness in the legs, decreased reflexes, abnormal sensations, incoordination (ataxia) progressive, cognitive dysfunction, speech disorders, and muscle rigidity (spasticity). On average, people affected by the disease survive approximately 60 months (range of 2–10 years) after diagnosis. It is caused by changes (mutations) at gene *PRNP* and the inheritance is autosomal dominant. The treatment is based on the signs and symptoms present in each person.

What Are the Symptoms of GSS Disease?

Signs and symptoms of GSS disease usually develop between the ages of 35–50 years. There may be:

• Ataxia progressive, such as clumsiness, instability and difficulty walking

- Cognitive dysfunction with slow thinking and various degrees of dementia (more mild or more severe)

- Difficult to talk (dysarthria)

- Abnormal movements of the eyes (nystagmus)

- Muscular stiffness (spasticity)

- Visual disturbances that can lead to blindness

- Difficulty to swallow

- Deafness

- Parkinsonian symptoms (present in some families)

What Causes GSS Disease?

GSS disease is usually caused by certain changes (mutations) at gene *PRNP*. This gene encodes a protein called prion. Although the exact function of this protein is unknown, it seems to have an important role in the human brain and other tissues throughout the body. Mutations in the *PRNP* gene result in the production of an abnormally shaped prion protein. The abnormal protein accumulates in the brain, forming lumps that damage or destroy neurons. This loss of cells of the brain leads to the signs and symptoms of GSS disease.

Is GSS Disease Inherited?

GGS is inherited in a autosomal dominant. Each cell of the body has two copies of each gene. In autosomal dominant diseases, for a person to be affected, only a change is needed (mutation) in one of the copies of the gene responsible for the disease. In some cases, an affected person inherits the mutation from an affected parent or an affected mother. Other cases may be the result of new mutations *(de novo)* in the gene. These cases occur in people with no history of the disease in their family. A person with GSS has a probability 50 percent in each pregnancy to pass the mutated gene to your child.

What Is the Diagnosis for GSS Disease?

The diagnosis of GSS disease is based on a combination of the following:

- Characteristic signs and symptoms

- Findings in the nervous system, such as multiple amyloid plaques (lumps that form in the brain and cause death of cells nervous and the progressive symptoms of the disease)

- A family history consistent with inheritance autosomal dominant

- Genetic test showing a mutation cause of the disease in the gene *PRNP* (establishes and confirms the diagnosis).

Genetic testing for family members at risk who do not yet have symptoms of the disease are possible if the mutation causing the disease in the family is known. This test is not useful for predicting the age of onset, severity, type of symptoms, or rate of progression. Genetic tests to find out if there is the mutation causing the disease, in people who do not have clear symptoms of the disease are called "predictive tests."

Exams

- The Genetic Testing Registry (GTR) has a list of laboratories that offer the genetic test for this disease. Most of the time the laboratories do not accept direct contact with patients and their families only with a health professional. A genetic professional can guide you to know if you need to do the genetic examination.

What Is the Treatment for GSS Disease?

The treatment of GSS disease is only to improve the signs and symptoms present in each person. Currently there is no cure for the disease and there are no known treatments to slow down its progression.

There have been several reports of cases in which several types of medications have been used (amantadine, vidarabine, metisoprinol, doxycycline, acyclovir, interferon, polianions, and amphotericin B) but none have been confirmed as truly effective, however, there are several laboratory studies that are seeking treatment.

The National Prion Disease Surveillance Center (NPDPSC) is responsible for collecting and recording all cases of prion disease in the United States. They must be notified regarding all cases of suspected prion disease in the United States.

What Is the Forecast on GSS Disease?

Currently the forecast for people with GSS disease is not good. On average, people affected by the disease survive approximately

217

60 months (range of 2–10 years) after diagnosis. In the last stages, affected people are usually in bed due to the ataxia severe, cannot eat well due to lack of coordination in swallowing, and cannot speak well. The studies that are being done are trying to find an effective treatment that can improve the prognosis.

Section 17.4

Infantile Neuroaxonal Dystrophy (INAD)

This section contains text excerpted from the following sources: Text in this section begins with excerpts from "Infantile Neuroaxonal Dystrophy," Genetics Home Reference (GHR), National Institutes of Health (NIH), February 20, 2018; Text beginning with the heading "What Is the Treatment for INAD?" is excerpted from "Infantile Neuroaxonal Dystrophy Information Page," National Institute of Neurological Disorders and Stroke (NINDS), May 24, 2017.

Infantile neuroaxonal dystrophy (INAD) is a disorder that primarily affects the nervous system. Individuals with INAD typically do not have any symptoms at birth, but between the ages of about 6 and 18 months they begin to experience delays in acquiring new motor and intellectual skills, such as crawling or beginning to speak. Eventually they lose previously acquired skills (developmental regression). In some cases, signs and symptoms of INAD first appear later in childhood or during the teenage years and progress more slowly.

Children with INAD experience progressive difficulties with movement. They generally have muscles that are at first weak and "floppy" (hypotonic), and then gradually become very stiff (spastic). Eventually, affected children lose the ability to move independently. Lack of muscle strength causes difficulty with feeding. Muscle weakness can also result in breathing problems that can lead to frequent infections, such as pneumonia. Seizures occur in some affected children.

Rapid, involuntary eye movements (nystagmus), eyes that do not look in the same direction (strabismus), and vision loss due to deterioration (atrophy) of the nerve that carries information from the eye to the brain (the optic nerve) often occur in INAD. Hearing loss may also develop. Children with this disorder experience progressive deterioration of cognitive functions (dementia), and they eventually lose awareness of their surroundings.

INAD is characterized by the development of swellings called spheroid bodies in the axons, the fibers that extend from nerve cells (neurons) and transmit impulses to muscles and other neurons. In some individuals with INAD, abnormal amounts of iron accumulate in a specific region of the brain called the basal ganglia. The relationship of these features to the symptoms of INAD is unknown.

What Is the Treatment for INAD?

There is no cure for INAD and no treatment that can stop the progress of the disease. Treatment is symptomatic and supportive. Doctors can prescribe medications for pain relief and sedation. Physiotherapists and other physical therapists can teach parents and caregivers how to position and seat their child, and to exercise arms and legs to maintain comfort.

What Is the Prognosis for INAD?

INAD is a progressive disease. Once symptoms begin, they will worsen over time. Generally, a baby's development starts to slow down between the ages of 6 months to 3 years. The first symptoms may be slowing of motor and mental development, followed by loss or regression of previously acquired skills. Rapid, wobbly eye movements and squints may be the first symptoms, followed by floppiness in the body and legs (more than in the arms). For the first few years, a baby with INAD will be alert and responsive, despite being increasingly physically impaired. Eventually, because of deterioration in vision, speech, and mental skills, the child will lose touch with its surroundings. Death usually occurs between the ages of 5–10 years.

Section 17.5

Leigh Disease

This section includes text excerpted from "Leigh's Disease
Information Page," National Institute of Neurological
Disorders and Stroke (NINDS), July 7, 2017.

Leigh disease is a rare inherited neurometabolic disorder that
affects the central nervous system (CNS). This progressive disorder
begins in infants between the ages of three months and two years.
Rarely, it occurs in teenagers and adults. Leigh disease can be caused
by mutations in mitochondrial deoxyribonucleic acid (mDNA) or by
deficiencies of an enzyme called pyruvate dehydrogenase (PDH).

Symptoms of Leigh disease usually progress rapidly. The earliest
signs may be poor sucking ability, and the loss of head control and
motor skills. These symptoms may be accompanied by loss of appetite,
vomiting, irritability, continuous crying, and seizures. As the disorder
progresses, symptoms may also include generalized weakness, lack of
muscle tone, and episodes of lactic acidosis, which can lead to impairment of respiratory and kidney function.

In Leigh disease, genetic mutations in mitochondrial DNA interfere
with the energy sources that run cells in an area of the brain that plays
a role in motor movements. The primary function of mitochondria is to
convert the energy in glucose and fatty acids into a substance called
adenosine triphosphate (ATP). The energy in ATP drives virtually all
of a cell's metabolic functions. Genetic mutations in mitochondrial
DNA, therefore, result in a chronic lack of energy in these cells, which
in turn affects the central nervous system and causes progressive
degeneration of motor functions.

There is also a form of Leigh disease (called X-linked Leigh disease)
which is the result of mutations in a gene that produces another group
of substances that are important for cell metabolism. This gene is only
found on the X chromosome.

What Is the Treatment for Leigh Disease?

The most common treatment for Leigh disease is thiamine or
vitamin B1. Oral sodium bicarbonate or sodium citrate may also be

prescribed to manage lactic acidosis. Researchers are currently testing dichloroacetate to establish its effectiveness in treating lactic acidosis. In individuals who have the X-linked form of Leigh disease, a high-fat, low-carbohydrate diet may be recommended.

What Is the Prognosis for Leigh Disease?

The prognosis for individuals with Leigh disease is poor. Individuals who lack mitochondrial complex intravenous (IV) activity and those with pyruvate dehydrogenase deficiency tend to have the worst prognosis and die within a few years. Those with partial deficiencies have a better prognosis, and may live to be 6 or 7 years of age. Some have survived to their midteenage years.

Chapter 18

Birth Defects That Affect the Brain

Chapter Contents

Section 18.1

Agenesis of the Corpus Callosum

This section includes text excerpted from "Agenesis of the Corpus Callosum Information Page," National Institute of Neurological Disorders and Stroke (NINDS), May 23, 2017.

Agenesis of the corpus callosum (ACC) is one of several disorders of the corpus callosum, the structure that connects the two hemispheres (left and right) of the brain. In ACC the corpus callosum is partially or completely absent. It is caused by a disruption of brain cell migration during fetal development. ACC can occur as an isolated condition or in combination with other cerebral abnormalities, including Arnold-Chiari malformation, Dandy–Walker syndrome (DWS), schizencephaly (clefts or deep divisions in brain tissue), and holoprosencephaly (failure of the forebrain to divide into lobes.) Girls may have a gender-specific condition called Aicardi syndrome, which causes severe cognitive impairment and developmental delays, seizures, abnormalities in the vertebra of the spine, and lesions on the retina of the eye. ACC can also be associated with malformations in other parts of the body, such as midline facial defects. The effects of the disorder range from subtle or mild to severe, depending on associated brain abnormalities. Children with the most severe brain malformations may have intellectual impairment, seizures, hydrocephalus, and spasticity. Other disorders of the corpus callosum include dysgenesis, in which the corpus callosum is developed in a malformed or incomplete way, and hypoplasia, in which the corpus callosum is thinner than usual. Individuals with these disorders have a higher risk of hearing deficits and cardiac abnormalities than individuals with the normal structure. It is estimated that at least one in 4,000 individuals has a disorder of the corpus callosum.

Treatment

There is no standard course of treatment for ACC. Treatment usually involves management of symptoms and seizures if they occur. Associated difficulties are much more manageable with early recognition and therapy, especially therapies focusing on left/right coordination. Early diagnosis and interventions are currently the best treatments to improve social and developmental outcomes.

Prognosis

Prognosis depends on the extent and severity of malformations. Intellectual impairment does not worsen. Individuals with a disorder of the corpus callosum typically have delays in attaining developmental milestones such as walking, talking, or reading; challenges with social interactions; clumsiness and poor motor coordination, particularly on skills that require coordination of left and right hands and feet (such as swimming, bicycle riding, and driving; and mental and social processing problems that become more apparent with age, with problems particularly evident from junior high school into adulthood.

Section 18.2

Arteriovenous Malformations and Other Vascular Lesions

This section includes text excerpted from "Arteriovenous Malformations and Other Vascular Lesions of the Central Nervous System Fact Sheet," National Institute of Neurological Disorders and Stroke (NINDS), September 2015.

What Are Arteriovenous Malformations?

Arteriovenous malformations (AVMs) are abnormal, snarled tangles of blood vessels that cause multiple irregular connections between the arteries and veins. These malformations most often occur in the spinal cord and in any part of the brain or on its surface, but can develop elsewhere in the body.

Normally, arteries carry oxygen-rich blood away from the heart to the body's cells, organs, and tissues; veins return blood with less oxygen to the lungs and heart. But in an AVM, the absence of capillaries—a network of small blood vessels that connect arteries to veins and deliver oxygen to cells—creates a shortcut for blood to pass directly from arteries to veins and bypass tissue, which can lead to tissue damage and the death of nerve cells and other cells. Over time, some AVMs get progressively larger as the amount of blood flow increases.

In some cases, a weakened blood vessel may burst, spilling blood into the brain (hemorrhage) that can cause stroke and brain damage. Other neurological problems include headache, weakness, seizures, pain, and problems with speech, vision, or movement. In most cases, people with neurological AVMs experience few, if any, significant symptoms.

It is unclear why AVMs form. Most often AVMs are congenital, but they can appear sporadically. In some cases the AVM may be inherited, but it is more likely that other inherited conditions increase the risk of having an AVM. The malformations tend to be discovered only incidentally, usually during treatment for an unrelated disorder or at autopsy. It is estimated that brain AVMs occur in less than one percent of the general population; each year about one percent of those with AVMs will die as a direct result of the AVM.

Treatment options depend on the type of AVM, its location, noticeable symptoms, and the general health condition of the individual.

What Are the Symptoms?

Symptoms can vary greatly in severity; in some people the severity of symptoms becomes debilitating or even life-threatening.

Seizures and headaches that may be severe are the most generalized symptoms of AVMs, but no particular type of seizure or headache pattern has been identified. Seizures can be focal (meaning they involve a small part of the brain) or generalized (widespread), involving convulsions, a loss of control over movement, or a change in a person's level of consciousness. Headaches can vary greatly in frequency, duration, and intensity, sometimes becoming as severe as migraines. Pain may be on either one side of the head or on both sides. Sometimes a headache consistently affecting one side of the head may be closely linked to the site of an AVM. Most often, the location of the pain is not specific to the malformation and may encompass most of the head.

AVMs also can cause a wide range of more specific neurological symptoms that vary from person to person, depending primarily upon the location of the AVM. Such symptoms may include:

- muscle weakness or paralysis in one part of the body

- a loss of coordination (ataxia) that can lead to such problems as gait disturbances

- difficulties carrying out tasks that require planning (apraxia)

- back pain or weakness in the lower extremities caused by a spinal AVM

- dizziness

- visual problems such as a loss of part of the visual field, inability to control eye movement, or swelling of a part of the optic nerve

- difficulty speaking or understanding language (aphasia)

- abnormal sensations such as numbness, tingling, or spontaneous pain

- memory deficits

- confusion, hallucinations, or dementia

AVMs may also cause subtle learning or behavioral disorders in some people during their childhood or adolescence, long before more obvious symptoms become evident.

Symptoms caused by AVMs can appear at any age. Because the abnormalities tend to result from a slow buildup of neurological damage over time, they are most often noticed when people are in their twenties or older. If AVMs do not become symptomatic by the time people reach their late forties or early fifties, they tend to remain stable and are less likely to produce symptoms. Some pregnant women may experience a sudden onset or worsening of symptoms due to accompanying cardiovascular changes, especially increases in blood volume and blood pressure.

Although most neurological AVMs have very few, if any, significant symptoms, one particularly severe type of AVM causes symptoms to appear at, or very soon after, birth. Called a vein of Galen defect after the major blood vessel involved, this lesion is located deep inside the brain. It is frequently associated with hydrocephalus (an accumulation of fluid within certain spaces in the brain, often with visible enlargement of the head), swollen veins visible on the scalp, seizures, failure to thrive, and congestive heart failure. Children born with this condition who survive past infancy often remain developmentally impaired.

227

How Do AVMs Damage the Brain and Spinal Cord?

AVMs damage the brain or spinal cord through three basic mechanisms: by reducing the amount of oxygen reaching neurological tissues; by causing bleeding (hemorrhage) into surrounding tissues; and by compressing or displacing parts of the brain or spinal cord.

- AVMs affect oxygen delivery to the brain or spinal cord by altering normal patterns of blood flow using the arteries, veins, and capillaries. In AVMs arteries pump blood directly into veins through a passageway called afistula. Since the network of capillaries is bypassed, the rate of blood flow is uncontrolled and too rapid to allow oxygen to be dispersed to surrounding tissues. As a result, the cells that make up these tissues become oxygen-depleted and begin to deteriorate, sometimes dying off completely.

- This abnormally rapid rate of blood flow frequently causes blood pressure inside the vessels located in the central portion of an AVM directly adjacent to the fistula—an area doctors refer to as the nidus—to rise to dangerously high levels. The arteries feeding blood into the AVM often become swollen and distorted; the veins that drain blood away from it often become abnormally constricted (a condition called stenosis). Also, the walls of the involved arteries and veins are often abnormally thin and weak. Aneurysms—balloon-like bulges in blood vessel walls that are susceptible to rupture—may develop in association with approximately half of all neurological AVMs due to this structural weakness.

- Bleeding into the brain, called intracranial hemorrhage, can result from the combination of high internal pressure and vessel wall weakness. Such hemorrhages are often microscopic in size (called microbleeds), causing limited damage and few significant symptoms. (Generally, microbleeds do not have short-term consequences on brain function, but microbleeds over time can lead to an increased risk of dementia and cognitive disruption.) Even many nonsymptomatic AVMs show evidence of past bleeding. But massive hemorrhages can occur if the physical stresses caused by extremely high blood pressure, rapid blood flow rates, and vessel wall weakness are great enough. If a large enough volume of blood escapes from a ruptured AVM into the surrounding brain, the result can be a catastrophic stroke. AVMs account for approximately two percent of all hemorrhagic strokes that occur each year.

- Even in the absence of bleeding or significant oxygen depletion, large AVMs can damage the brain or spinal cord simply by their presence. They can range in size from a fraction of an inch to more than 2.5 inches in diameter, depending on the number and size of the blood vessels making up the lesion. The larger the lesion, the greater the amount of pressure it exerts on surrounding brain or spinal cord structures. The largest lesions may compress several inches of the spinal cord or distort the shape of an entire hemisphere of the brain. Such massive AVMs can constrict the flow of cerebrospinal fluid—a clear liquid that normally nourishes and protects the brain and spinal cord—by distorting or closing the passageways and open chambers (ventricles) inside the brain that allow this fluid to circulate freely. As cerebrospinal fluid accumulates, hydrocephalus results. This fluid buildup further increases the amount of pressure on fragile neurological structures, adding to the damage caused by the AVM itself.

Where Do Neurological AVMs Tend to Form?

AVMs can form virtually anywhere in the brain or spinal cord—wherever arteries and veins exist. Some are formed from blood vessels located in the dura mater or in the pia mater, the outermost and innermost, respectively, of the three membranes surrounding the brain and spinal cord. (The third membrane, called the arachnoid, lacks blood vessels.) AVMs of the dura mater affect the function of the spinal cord by transmitting excess pressure to the venous system of the spinal cord. AVMs of the spinal cord affect the function of the spinal cord by hemorrhage, by reducing blood flow to the spinal cord, or by causing excess venous pressure. Spinal AVMs frequently cause attacks of sudden, severe back pain, often concentrated at the roots of nerve fibers where they exit the vertebrae, with pain that is similar to that caused by a slipped disk. These lesions also can cause sensory disturbances, muscle weakness, or paralysis in the parts of the body served by the spinal cord or the damaged nerve fibers. A spinal cord AVM can lead to degeneration of the nerve fibers within the spinal cord below the level of the lesion, causing widespread paralysis in parts of the body controlled by those nerve fibers.

AVMs on the surface of the cerebral hemispheres—the uppermost portions of the brain—exert pressure on the cerebral cortex, the brain's "gray matter." Depending on their location, these AVMs may damage portions of the cerebral cortex involved with thinking, speaking, understanding language, hearing, taste, touch, or initiating and controlling voluntary movements. AVMs located on the frontal lobe close to the optic nerve or on the occipital lobe (the rear portion of the cerebrum where images are processed) may cause a variety of visual disturbances.

AVMs also can form from blood vessels located deep inside the interior of the cerebrum (the main portion of the brain). These AVMs may compromise the functions of three vital structures: the thalamus, which transmits nerve signals between the spinal cord and upper regions of the brain; the basal ganglia surrounding the thalamus, which coordinate complex movements and plays a role in learning and memory; and the hippocampus, which plays a major role in memory.

AVMs can affect other parts of the brain besides the cerebrum. The hindbrain is formed from two major structures: the cerebellum, which is nestled under the rear portion of the cerebrum, and the brainstem, which serves as the bridge linking the upper portions of the brain with the spinal cord. These structures control finely coordinated movements, maintain balance, and regulate some functions of internal organs, including those of the heart and lungs. AVM damage to these parts of the hindbrain can result in dizziness, giddiness, vomiting, a loss of the ability to coordinate complex movements such as walking, or uncontrollable muscle tremors.

What Are the Health Consequences of AVMs?

The greatest potential danger posed by AVMs is hemorrhage. Most episodes of bleeding remain undetected at the time they occur because they are not severe enough to cause significant neurological damage. But massive, even fatal, bleeding episodes do occur. Whenever an AVM is detected, the individual should be carefully and consistently monitored for any signs of instability that may indicate an increased risk of hemorrhage.

A few physical characteristics appear to indicate a greater-than-usual likelihood of clinically significant hemorrhage:

- Smaller AVMs have a greater likelihood of bleeding than do larger ones.

- Impaired drainage by unusually narrow or deeply situated veins increases the chances of hemorrhage.

- Pregnancy appears to increase the likelihood of clinically significant hemorrhage, mainly because of increases in blood pressure and blood volume.

- AVMs that have hemorrhaged once are about nine times more likely to bleed again during the first year after the initial hemorrhage than are lesions that have never bled.

The damaging effects of a hemorrhage are related to lesion location. Bleeding from AVMs located deep inside the interior tissues, or parenchyma, of the brain typically causes more severe neurological damage than does hemorrhage by lesions that have formed in the dural or pial membranes or on the surface of the brain or spinal cord. (Deeply located bleeding is usually referred to as an intracerebral or parenchymal hemorrhage; bleeding within the membranes or on the surface of the brain is known as subdural or subarachnoid hemorrhage.) Therefore, location is an important factor to consider when weighing the relative risks surgery to treat AVMs.

What Other Types of Vascular Lesions Affect the Central Nervous System (CNS)?

Besides AVMs, three other main types of vascular lesion can arise in the brain or spinal cord: cavernous malformations, capillary telangiectases, and venous malformations. These lesions may form virtually anywhere within the CNS, but unlike AVMs, they are not caused by high-velocity blood flow from arteries into veins. Instead of a combination of arteries and veins, these low-flowing lesions involve only one type of blood vessel. These lesions are less unstable than AVMs and do not pose the same relatively high risk of significant hemorrhage. In general, low-flow lesions tend to cause fewer troubling neurological symptoms and require less aggressive treatment than do AVMs.

Cavernous malformations are formed from groups of tightly packed, abnormally thin-walled, small blood vessels that displace normal neurological tissue in the brain or spinal cord. The vessels are filled with slow-moving or stagnant blood that is usually clotted or in a state of decomposition. Like AVMs, cavernous malformations can range in size from a few fractions of an inch to several inches in diameter, depending on the number of blood vessels involved. Some people develop multiple lesions. Although cavernous malformations usually do not hemorrhage as severely as AVMs do, they sometimes leak blood into surrounding tissues because the walls of the involved blood vessels are extremely fragile. Although they are often not as symptomatic as AVMs, cavernous malformations can cause seizures in some people. After AVMs, cavernous malformations are the type of vascular lesion most likely to require treatment.

Capillary telangiectases are groups of abnormally swollen capillaries and usually measure less than an inch in diameter. Telangiectases are usually benign and rarely cause extensive damage to surrounding brain or spinal cord tissues. Any isolated hemorrhages that occur are microscopic in size. However, in some inherited disorders in which people develop large numbers of these lesions, telangiectases can contribute to the development headaches or seizures.

Venous malformations consist of abnormally enlarged veins. The structural defect usually does not interfere with the function of the blood vessels, and venous malformations rarely hemorrhage. As with telangiectases, most venous malformations do not produce symptoms, remain undetected, and follow a benign course.

What Causes Vascular Lesions?

The cause of vascular anomalies of the CNS is not yet well understood. Scientists believe the anomalies most often result from mistakes that occur during embryonic or fetal development. These mistakes may be linked to genetic mutations in some cases. A few types of vascular malformations are known to be hereditary and thus are known to have a genetic basis. Some evidence also suggests that at least some of these lesions are acquired later in life as a result of injury to the CNS.

During fetal development, new blood vessels continuously form and then disappear as the human body changes and grows. These changes in the body's vascular map continue after birth and are controlled by angiogenic factors, chemicals produced by the body that stimulate new blood vessel formation and growth. Researchers have identified changes in the chemical structures of various angiogenic factors in some people who have AVMs or other vascular abnormalities of the CNS. However, it is not yet clear how these chemical changes actually cause changes in blood vessel structure.

By studying patterns of occurrence in families, researchers have established that one type of cavernous malformation involving multiple lesion formation is caused by a genetic mutation in chromosome 7. This genetic mutation appears in many ethnic groups, but it is especially frequent in a large population of Hispanic Americans living in the Southwest; these individuals share a common ancestor in whom the genetic change occurred. Some other types of vascular defects of the CNS are part of larger medical syndromes known to be hereditary. They include hereditary hemorrhagic telangiectasia (HHT), Sturge-Weber syndrome (SWS), and Klippel-Trenaunay syndrome (KTS).

How Are AVMs and Other Vascular Lesions Detected?

One of the more distinctive signs clinicians use to diagnose an AVM is an auditory phenomenon called a bruit—a rhythmic, whooshing sound caused by excessively rapid blood flow through the arteries and veins of an AVM. The sound is similar to that made by a torrent of water rushing through a narrow pipe. A bruit can sometimes become a symptom when it is especially severe. When audible to individuals, the bruit may compromise hearing, disturb sleep, or cause significant psychological distress.

An array of imaging technologies can be used to uncover the presence of AVMs. Cerebral angiography, also called cerebral arteriography, provides the most accurate pictures of blood vessel structure in brain AVMs. A special water-soluble dye, called a contrast agent, is injected into an artery and highlights the structure of blood vessels so that it can be seen on X-rays. CT scans (computed axial tomography) use X-rays to create an image of the head, brain, or spinal cord and are especially useful in revealing the presence of hemorrhage. MRI (magnetic resonance imaging) uses magnetic fields and radio waves to create detailed images that can show subtle changes in neurological tissues. Magnetic resonance angiography (MRA) can record the pattern and velocity of blood flow through vascular lesions as well as the flow of cerebrospinal fluid throughout the brain and spinal cord. Transcranial Doppler (TCD) ultrasound can diagnose medium-size to large AVMS and also detect the presence and extent of hemorrhage. It evaluates blood flow through the brain by directing high-frequency sound waves through the skull at particular arteries. The resulting sound wave signals that bounce back from blood cells are interpreted by a computer to make an image of the velocity of blood flow.

How Are AVMs and Other Vascular Lesions Treated?

There are several options for treating AVMs. Although medication can often lessen general symptoms such as headache, back pain, and seizures caused by AVMs and other vascular lesions, the definitive treatment for AVMs is either surgery or focused radiation therapy. Venous malformations and capillary telangiectases rarely require surgery. Cavernous malformations are usually well defined enough for surgical removal, but surgery on these lesions is less common than for AVMs because they do not pose the same risk of hemorrhage.

Because so many variables are involved in treating AVMs, doctors must assess the danger posed to individuals largely on a case-by-case basis. A hemorrhage from an untreated AVM can cause serious neurological deficits or death, leading many clinicians to recommend surgical intervention whenever the physical characteristics of an AVM appear to indicate a greater-than-usual likelihood of significant bleeding and subsequent neurological damage. However, surgery on any part of the CNS carries some risk of serious complications or death. There is no easy formula that can allow physicians and individuals to reach a decision on the best course of therapy.

An AVM grading system developed in the mid-1980s can help healthcare professionals estimate the risk of surgery based on the size of the AVM, location in the brain and surrounding tissue involvement, and any leakage.

Three surgical options are used to treat AVMs: conventional surgery, endovascular embolization, and radiosurgery. The choice of treatment depends largely on the size and location of an AVM. Endovascular embolization and radiosurgery are less invasive than conventional surgery and offer safer treatment options for some AVMs located deep inside the brain.

- **Conventional surgery** involves entering the brain or spinal cord and removing the central portion of the AVM, including the fistula, while causing as little damage as possible to surrounding neurological structures. This surgery is most appropriate when an AVM is located in a superficial portion of the brain or spinal cord and is relatively small in size. AVMs located deep inside the brain generally cannot be approached through conventional surgical techniques because there is too great a possibility that functionally important brain tissue will be damaged or destroyed.

- In **endovascular embolization** the surgeon guides a catheter though the arterial network until the tip reaches the site of the AVM. The surgeon then injects a substance (such as fast-drying glue-like substances, fibered titanium coils, and tiny balloons) that will travel through blood vessels and create an artificial blood clot in the center of an AVM. Since embolization usually does not permanently obliterate the AVM, it is usually used as an adjunct to surgery or to radiosurgery to reduce the blood flow through the AVM and make the surgery safer.

- **Radiosurgery** is an even less invasive therapeutic approach often used to treat small AVMs that haven't ruptured. A beam of highly focused radiation is aimed directly on the AVM and damages the walls of the blood vessels making up the lesion. Over the course of the next several months, the irradiated vessels gradually degenerate and eventually close, leading to the resolution of the AVM.

Embolization frequently proves incomplete or temporary, although new embolization materials have led to improved results. Radiosurgery often has incomplete results as well, particularly when an AVM is large, and it poses the additional risk of radiation damage to surrounding normal tissues. Even when successful, complete closure of an AVM takes place over the course of many months following radiosurgery. During that period, the risk of hemorrhage is still present. However, both techniques can treat deeply situated AVMs that had previously been inaccessible. And in many individuals, staged embolization followed by conventional surgical removal or by radiosurgery is now performed, resulting in further reductions in death and complication rates.

Section 18.3

Moebius Syndrome

This section contains text excerpted from the following sources: Text under the heading "What Is Moebius Syndrome?" is excerpted from "Moebius Syndrome," Genetics Home Reference (GHR), National Institutes of Health (NIH), April 2016; Text beginning with the heading "Four Categories of Moebius Syndrome" is excerpted from "Moebius Syndrome Information Page," National Institute of Neurological Disorders and Stroke (NINDS), May 25, 2017.

What Is Moebius Syndrome?

Moebius syndrome is a rare neurological condition that primarily affects the muscles that control facial expression and eye movement. The signs and symptoms of this condition are present from birth.

Weakness or paralysis of the facial muscles is one of the most common features of Moebius syndrome. Affected individuals lack facial expressions; they cannot smile, frown, or raise their eyebrows. The muscle weakness also causes problems with feeding that become apparent in early infancy.

Many people with Moebius syndrome are born with a small chin (micrognathia) and a small mouth (microstomia) with a short or unusually shaped tongue. The roof of the mouth may have an abnormal opening (cleft palate) or be high and arched. These abnormalities contribute to problems with speech, which occur in many children with Moebius syndrome. Dental abnormalities, including missing and misaligned teeth, are also common.

Moebius syndrome also affects muscles that control back and forth eye movement. Affected individuals must move their head from side to side to read or follow the movement of objects. People with this disorder have difficulty making eye contact, and their eyes may not look in the same direction (strabismus). Additionally, the eyelids may not close completely when blinking or sleeping, which can result in dry or irritated eyes.

Other features of Moebius syndrome can include bone abnormalities in the hands and feet, weak muscle tone (hypotonia), and hearing loss. Affected children often experience delayed development of motor skills (such as crawling and walking), although most eventually acquire these skills.

Some research studies have suggested that children with Moebius syndrome are more likely than unaffected children to have characteristics of autism spectrum disorders (ASD), which are a group of conditions characterized by impaired communication and social interaction. However, studies have questioned this association. Because people with Moebius syndrome have difficulty with eye contact and speech due to their physical differences, autism spectrum disorders can be difficult to diagnose in these individuals. Moebius syndrome may also be associated with a somewhat increased risk of intellectual disability; however, most affected individuals have normal intelligence.

Four Categories of Moebius Syndrome

There are four recognized categories of Moebius syndrome:

- Group I, characterized by small or absent brainstem nuclei that control the cranial nerves;

- Group II, characterized by loss and degeneration of neurons in the facial peripheral nerve;

- Group III, characterized by loss and degeneration of neurons and other brain cells, microscopic areas of damage, and hardened tissue in the brainstem nuclei, and,

- Group IV, characterized by muscular symptoms in spite of a lack of lesions in the cranial nerve.

Treatment

There is no specific course of treatment for Moebius syndrome. Treatment is supportive and in accordance with symptoms. Infants may require feeding tubes or special bottles to maintain sufficient nutrition. Surgery may correct crossed eyes and improve limb and jaw deformities. Physical and speech therapy often improves motor skills and coordination, and leads to better control of speaking and eating abilities. Plastic reconstructive surgery may be beneficial in some individuals. Nerve and muscle transfers to the corners of the mouth have been performed to provide limited ability to smile.

Prognosis

There is no cure for Moebius syndrome. In spite of the impairments that characterize the disorder, proper care and treatment give many individuals a normal life expectancy.

Section 18.4

Neuronal Migration Disorders

This section includes text excerpted from "Neuronal Migration Disorders Information Page," National Institute of Neurological Disorders and Stroke (NINDS), May 25, 2017.

Neuronal migration disorders (NMDs) are a group of birth defects caused by the abnormal migration of neurons in the developing brain and nervous system. In the developing brain, neurons must migrate from the areas where they are born to the areas where they will settle into their proper neural circuits. Neuronal migration, which occurs as early as the second month of gestation, is controlled by a complex assortment of chemical guides and signals. When these signals are absent or incorrect, neurons do not end up where they belong. This can result in structurally abnormal or missing areas of the brain in the cerebral hemispheres, cerebellum, brainstem, or hippocampus. The structural abnormalities found in NMDs include schizencephaly, porencephaly, lissencephaly, agyria, macrogyria, polymicrogyria (PMG), pachygyria, microgyria, micropolygyria, neuronal heterotopias (including band heterotopia), agenesis of the corpus callosum (ACC), and agenesis of the cranial nerves. Symptoms vary according to the abnormality, but often feature poor muscle tone and motor function, seizures, developmental delays, impaired cognitive development, failure to grow and thrive, difficulties with feeding, swelling in the extremities, and a smaller than normal head. Most infants with an NMD appear normal, but some disorders have characteristic facial or skull features that can be recognized by a neurologist. Several genetic abnormalities in children with NMDs have been identified. Defects in genes that are involved in neuronal migration have been associated with NMDs, but the role they play in the development of these disorders is not yet well-understood. More than 25 syndromes resulting from abnormal neuronal migration have been described. Among them are syndromes with several different patterns of inheritance; genetic counseling thus differs greatly between syndromes.

Treatment

Treatment is symptomatic, and may include antiseizure medication and special or supplemental education consisting of physical, occupational, and speech therapies.

Prognosis

The prognosis for children with NMDs varies depending on the specific disorder and the degree of brain abnormality and subsequent neurological signs and symptoms.

Section 18.5

Zika and Microcephaly

This section includes text excerpted from "Zika Virus—Microcephaly and Other Birth Defects," Centers for Disease Control and Prevention (CDC), February 6, 2018.

Zika and Microcephaly

Microcephaly is a birth defect in which a baby's head is smaller than expected when compared to babies of the same sex and age. Babies with microcephaly often have smaller brains that might not have developed properly.

Zika virus infection during pregnancy is a cause of microcephaly. During pregnancy, a baby's head grows because the baby's brain grows. Microcephaly can occur because a baby's brain has not developed properly during pregnancy or has stopped growing after birth.

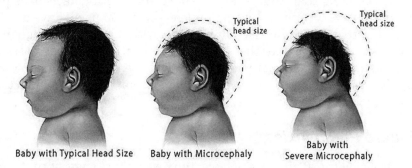

Baby with Typical Head Size   Baby with Microcephaly   Baby with Severe Microcephaly

Figure 18.1. *Typical Head Size, Microcephaly, and Severe Microcephaly Comparison*

(Source: "Facts about Microcephaly," Centers for Disease Control and Prevention (CDC).)

Congenital Zika Syndrome

Congenital Zika syndrome is a unique pattern of birth defects found among fetuses and babies infected with Zika virus during

239

pregnancy. Congenital Zika syndrome is described by the following five features:

- Severe microcephaly where the skull has partially collapsed

- Decreased brain tissue with a specific pattern of brain damage

- Damage (i.e., scarring, pigment changes) to the back of the eye

- Joints with limited range of motion, such as clubfoot

- Too much muscle tone restricting body movement soon after birth

Babies who were infected with Zika before birth may have damage to their eyes and/or the part of their brain that is responsible for vision, which may affect their visual development. Both babies with and without microcephaly can have eye problems. If your baby was born with congenital Zika infection, he or she should receive the recommended screenings and tests to check for eye and other health problems, even if your baby appears healthy.

Not all babies born with congenital Zika infection will have all of these problems. Some infants with congenital Zika virus infection who do not have microcephaly at birth may later experience slowed head growth and develop postnatal microcephaly.

Recognizing that Zika is a cause of certain birth defects does not mean that every pregnant woman infected with Zika will have a baby with a birth defect. It means that infection with Zika during pregnancy increases the chances for these problems. Scientists continue to study how Zika virus affects mothers and their children to better understand the full range of potential health problems that Zika virus infection during pregnancy may cause.

Future Pregnancies

Based on the available evidence, the researchers suggest that Zika virus infection in a woman who is not pregnant would not pose a risk for birth defects in future pregnancies after the virus has cleared from her blood. From what the researchers know about similar infections, once a person has been infected with Zika virus, he or she is likely to be protected from a future Zika infection.

Chapter 19

Cephalic Disorders

What Are Cephalic Disorders?

Cephalic disorders are congenital conditions that stem from damage to, or abnormal development of, the budding nervous system. Cephalic is a term that means "head" or "head end of the body." Congenital means the disorder is present at, and usually before, birth.

Cephalic disorders are not necessarily caused by a single factor but may be influenced by hereditary or genetic conditions or by environmental exposures during pregnancy such as medication taken by the mother, maternal infection, or exposure to radiation. Some cephalic disorders occur when the cranial sutures (the fibrous joints that connect the bones of the skull) join prematurely. Most cephalic disorders are caused by a disturbance that occurs very early in the development of the fetal nervous system.

The human nervous system develops from a small, specialized plate of cells on the surface of the embryo. Early in development, this plate of cells forms the neural tube, a narrow sheath that closes between the 3rd and 4th weeks of pregnancy to form the brain and spinal cord of the embryo. Four main processes are responsible for the development of the nervous system: cell proliferation, the process in which nerve cells divide to form new generations of cells; cell migration, the process in which nerve cells move from their place of origin to the place where they will remain for life; cell differentiation, the process during

This chapter includes text excerpted from "Cephalic Disorders Fact Sheet," National Institute of Neurological Disorders and Stroke (NINDS), September 2003. Reviewed February 2018.

which cells acquire individual characteristics; and cell death, a natural process in which cells die. Understanding the normal development of the human nervous system may lead to a better understanding of cephalic disorders.

Damage to the developing nervous system is a major cause of chronic, disabling disorders, and sometimes, death in infants, children, and even adults. The degree to which damage to the developing nervous system harms the mind and body varies enormously. Many disabilities are mild enough to allow those afflicted to eventually function independently in society. Others are not. Some infants, children, and adults die, others remain totally disabled, and an even larger population is partially disabled, functioning well below normal capacity throughout life.

What Are the Different Kinds of Cephalic Disorders?

Anencephaly is a neural tube defect that occurs when the cephalic (head) end of the neural tube fails to close, usually between the 23rd and 26th days of pregnancy, resulting in the absence of a major portion of the brain, skull, and scalp. Infants with this disorder are born without a forebrain—the largest part of the brain consisting mainly of the cerebrum, which is responsible for thinking and coordination. The remaining brain tissue is often exposed—not covered by bone or skin.

Infants born with anencephaly are usually blind, deaf, unconscious, and unable to feel pain. Although some individuals with anencephaly may be born with a rudimentary brainstem, the lack of a functioning cerebrum permanently rules out the possibility of ever gaining consciousness. Reflex actions such as breathing and responses to sound or touch may occur. The disorder is one of the most common disorders of the fetal central nervous system. Approximately 1,000–2,000 American babies are born with anencephaly each year. The disorder affects females more often than males.

The cause of anencephaly is unknown. Although it is believed that the mother's diet and vitamin intake may play a role, scientists agree that many other factors are also involved.

There is no cure or standard treatment for anencephaly and the prognosis for affected individuals is poor. Most infants do not survive infancy. If the infant is not stillborn, then he or she will usually die within a few hours or days after birth. Anencephaly can often be diagnosed before birth through an ultrasound examination.

Studies have shown that the addition of folic acid to the diet of women of child-bearing age may significantly reduce the incidence of neural tube defects. Therefore it is recommended that all women of child-bearing age consume 0.4 mg of folic acid daily.

Colpocephaly is a disorder in which there is an abnormal enlargement of the occipital horns—the posterior or rear portion of the lateral ventricles (cavities or chambers) of the brain. This enlargement occurs when there is an underdevelopment or lack of thickening of the white matter in the posterior cerebrum. Colpocephaly is characterized by microcephaly (abnormally small head) and delayed development. Other features may include motor abnormalities, muscle spasms, and seizures.

Although the cause is unknown, researchers believe that the disorder results from an intrauterine disturbance that occurs between the 2nd and 6th months of pregnancy. Colpocephaly may be diagnosed late in pregnancy, although it is often misdiagnosed as hydrocephalus (excessive accumulation of cerebrospinal fluid in the brain). It may be more accurately diagnosed after birth when signs of microcephaly, delayed development, and seizures are present.

There is no definitive treatment for colpocephaly. Anticonvulsant medications can be given to prevent seizures, and doctors try to prevent contractures (shrinkage or shortening of muscles). The prognosis for individuals with colpocephaly depends on the severity of the associated conditions and the degree of abnormal brain development. Some children benefit from special education.

Holoprosencephaly (HPE) is a disorder characterized by the failure of the prosencephalon (the forebrain of the embryo) to develop. During normal development the forebrain is formed and the face begins to develop in the 5th and 6th weeks of pregnancy. HPE is caused by a failure of the embryo's forebrain to divide to form bilateral cerebral hemispheres (the left and right halves of the brain), causing defects in the development of the face and in brain structure and function.

There are three classifications of HPE. Alobar holoprosencephaly, the most serious form in which the brain fails to separate, is usually associated with severe facial anomalies. Semilobar holoprosencephaly, in which the brain's hemispheres have a slight tendency to separate, is an intermediate form of the disease. Lobar holoprosencephaly, in which there is considerable evidence of separate brain hemispheres, is the least severe form. In some cases of lobar holoprosencephaly, the patient's brain may be nearly normal.

HPE, once called arhinencephaly, consists of a spectrum of defects or malformations of the brain and face. At the most severe end of this spectrum are cases involving serious malformations of the brain, malformations so severe that they are incompatible with life and often cause spontaneous intrauterine death. At the other end of the spectrum are individuals with facial defects—which may affect the eyes, nose, and upper lip—and normal or near-normal brain development. Seizures and cognitive impairment and development may occur.

The most severe of the facial defects (or anomalies) is cyclopia, an abnormality characterized by the development of a single eye, located in the area normally occupied by the root of the nose, and a missing nose or a nose in the form of a proboscis (a tubular appendage) located above the eye.

Ethmocephaly is the least common facial anomaly. It consists of a proboscis separating narrow-set eyes with an absent nose and microphthalmia (abnormal smallness of one or both eyes). Cebocephaly, another facial anomaly, is characterized by a small, flattened nose with a single nostril situated below incomplete or underdeveloped closely set eyes.

The least severe in the spectrum of facial anomalies is the median cleft lip, also called premaxillary agenesis. Although the causes of most cases of holoprosencephaly remain unknown, researchers know that approximately one-half of all cases have a chromosomal cause. Such chromosomal anomalies as Patau syndrome (trisomy 13) and Edwards' syndrome (trisomy 18) have been found in association with HPE. There is an increased risk for the disorder in infants of diabetic mothers.

There is no treatment for HPE and the prognosis for individuals with the disorder is poor. Most of those who survive show no significant developmental gains. For children who survive, treatment is symptomatic. Although it is possible that improved management of diabetic pregnancies may help prevent holoprosencephaly, there is no means of primary prevention.

Hydranencephaly is a rare condition in which the cerebral hemispheres are absent and replaced by sacs filled with cerebrospinal fluid. Usually the cerebellum and brainstem are formed normally. An infant with hydranencephaly may appear normal at birth. The infant's head size and spontaneous reflexes such as sucking, swallowing, crying, and moving the arms and legs may all seem normal. However, after a few weeks the infant usually becomes irritable and has increased muscle tone (hypertonia). After several months of life, seizures and hydrocephalus may develop. Other symptoms may include visual impairment, lack of growth, deafness, blindness, spastic quadriparesis (paralysis), and intellectual deficits.

Hydranencephaly is an extreme form of porencephaly (a rare disorder characterized by a cyst or cavity in the cerebral hemispheres) and may be caused by vascular insult (such as stroke) or injuries, infections, or traumatic disorders after the 12th week of pregnancy.

Diagnosis may be delayed for several months because the infant's early behavior appears to be relatively normal. Transillumination, an examination in which light is passed through body tissues, usually confirms the diagnosis. Some infants may have additional abnormalities at birth, including seizures, myoclonus (involuntary sudden, rapid jerks), and respiratory problems.

There is no standard treatment for hydranencephaly. Treatment is symptomatic and supportive. Hydrocephalus may be treated with a shunt.

The outlook for children with hydranencephaly is generally poor, and many children with this disorder die before age 1. However, in rare cases, children with hydranencephaly may survive for several years or more.

Iniencephaly is a rare neural tube defect that combines extreme retroflexion (backward bending) of the head with severe defects of the spine. The affected infant tends to be short, with a disproportionately large head. Diagnosis can be made immediately after birth because the head is so severely retroflexed that the face looks upward. The skin of the face is connected directly to the skin of the chest and the scalp is directly connected to the skin of the back. Generally, the neck is absent.

Most individuals with iniencephaly have other associated anomalies such as anencephaly, cephalocele (a disorder in which part of the cranial contents protrudes from the skull), hydrocephalus, cyclopia, absence of the mandible (lower jaw bone), cleft lip and palate, cardiovascular disorders (CVD), diaphragmatic hernia, and gastrointestinal malformation. The disorder is more common among females.

The prognosis for those with iniencephaly is extremely poor. Newborns with iniencephaly seldom live more than a few hours. The distortion of the fetal body may also pose a danger to the mother's life.

Lissencephaly, which literally means "smooth brain," is a rare brain malformation characterized by microcephaly and the lack of normal convolutions (folds) in the brain. It is caused by defective neuronal migration, the process in which nerve cells move from their place of origin to their permanent location.

The surface of a normal brain is formed by a complex series of folds and grooves. The folds are called gyri or convolutions, and the grooves are called sulci. In children with lissencephaly, the normal convolutions are absent or only partly formed, making the surface of the brain smooth.

Symptoms of the disorder may include unusual facial appearance, difficulty swallowing, failure to thrive, and severe psychomotor retardation. Anomalies of the hands, fingers, or toes, muscle spasms, and seizures may also occur.

Lissencephaly may be diagnosed at or soon after birth. Diagnosis may be confirmed by ultrasound, computed tomography (CT), or magnetic resonance imaging (MRI).

Lissencephaly may be caused by intrauterine viral infections or viral infections in the fetus during the first trimester, insufficient blood supply to the baby's brain early in pregnancy, or a genetic disorder. There are two distinct genetic causes of lissencephaly—X-linked and chromosome 17-linked.

The spectrum of lissencephaly is only now becoming more defined as neuroimaging and genetics has provided more insights into migration disorders. Other causes which have not yet been identified are likely as well.

Lissencephaly may be associated with other diseases including isolated lissencephaly sequence, Miller-Dieker syndrome (MDS), and Walker-Warburg syndrome (WWS).

Treatment for those with lissencephaly is symptomatic and depends on the severity and locations of the brain malformations. Supportive care may be needed to help with comfort and nursing needs. Seizures may be controlled with medication and hydrocephalus may require shunting. If feeding becomes difficult, a gastrostomy tube may be considered.

The prognosis for children with lissencephaly varies depending on the degree of brain malformation. Many individuals show no significant development beyond a 3- to 5-month-old level. Some may have near-normal development and intelligence. Many will die before the age of 2. Respiratory problems are the most common causes of death.

Megalencephaly, also called macrencephaly, is a condition in which there is an abnormally large, heavy, and usually malfunctioning brain. By definition, the brain weight is greater than average for the age and gender of the infant or child. Head enlargement may be evident at birth or the head may become abnormally large in the early years of life.

Megalencephaly is thought to be related to a disturbance in the regulation of cell reproduction or proliferation. In normal development, neuron proliferation—the process in which nerve cells divide to form new generations of cells—is regulated so that the correct number of cells is formed in the proper place at the appropriate time.

Symptoms of megalencephaly may include delayed development, convulsive disorders, corticospinal (brain cortex and spinal cord) dysfunction, and seizures. Megalencephaly affects males more often than females.

The prognosis for individuals with megalencephaly largely depends on the underlying cause and the associated neurological disorders. Treatment is symptomatic. Megalencephaly may lead to a condition called macrocephaly. Unilateral megalencephaly or hemimegalencephaly is a rare condition characterized by the enlargement of one-half of the brain. Children with this disorder may have a large, sometimes asymmetrical head. Often they suffer from intractable seizures and mental retardation. The prognosis for those with hemimegalencephaly is poor.

Microcephaly is a neurological disorder in which the circumference of the head is smaller than average for the age and gender of the infant or child. Microcephaly may be congenital or it may develop in the first few years of life. The disorder may stem from a wide variety of conditions that cause abnormal growth of the brain, or from syndromes associated with chromosomal abnormalities.

Infants with microcephaly are born with either a normal or reduced head size. Subsequently the head fails to grow while the face continues to develop at a normal rate, producing a child with a small head, a large face, a receding forehead, and a loose, often wrinkled scalp. As the child grows older, the smallness of the skull becomes more obvious, although the entire body also is often underweight and dwarfed. Development of motor functions and speech may be delayed. Hyperactivity and cognitive impairment are common occurrences, although the degree of each varies. Convulsions may also occur. Motor ability varies, ranging from clumsiness in some to spastic quadriplegia in others.

Generally there is no specific treatment for microcephaly. Treatment is symptomatic and supportive.

In general, life expectancy for individuals with microcephaly is reduced and the prognosis for normal brain function is poor. The prognosis varies depending on the presence of associated abnormalities.

Porencephaly is an extremely rare disorder of the central nervous system (CNS) involving a cyst or cavity in a cerebral hemisphere. The cysts or cavities are usually the remnants of destructive lesions, but are sometimes the result of abnormal development. The disorder can occur before or after birth.

Porencephaly most likely has a number of different, often unknown causes, including absence of brain development and destruction of brain tissue. The presence of porencephalic cysts can sometimes be detected by transillumination of the skull in infancy. The diagnosis may be confirmed by CT, MRI, or ultrasonography.

More severely affected infants show symptoms of the disorder shortly after birth, and the diagnosis is usually made before age 1. Signs may include delayed growth and development, spastic paresis (slight or incomplete paralysis), hypotonia (decreased muscle tone), seizures (often infantile spasms), and macrocephaly or microcephaly.

Individuals with porencephaly may have poor or absent speech development, epilepsy, hydrocephalus, spastic contractures (shrinkage or shortening of muscles), and cognitive impairment. Treatment may include physical therapy, medication for seizure disorders, and a shunt for hydrocephalus. The prognosis for individuals with porencephaly varies according to the location and extent of the lesion. Some patients with this disorder may develop only minor neurological problems and have normal intelligence, while others may be severely disabled. Others may die before the second decade of life.

Schizencephaly is a rare developmental disorder characterized by abnormal slits, or clefts, in the cerebral hemispheres. Schizencephaly is a form of porencephaly. Individuals with clefts in both hemispheres, or bilateral clefts, are often developmentally delayed and have delayed speech and language skills and corticospinal dysfunction. Individuals with smaller, unilateral clefts (clefts in one hemisphere) may be weak on one side of the body and may have average or near-average intelligence. Patients with schizencephaly may also have varying degrees of microcephaly, delayed development and cognitive impairment, hemiparesis (weakness or paralysis affecting one side of the body), or quadriparesis (weakness or paralysis affecting all four extremities), and may have reduced muscle tone (hypotonia). Most patients have seizures and some may have hydrocephalus.

In schizencephaly, the neurons border the edge of the cleft implying a very early disruption in development. There is now a genetic origin for one type of schizencephaly. Causes of this type may include environmental exposures during pregnancy such as medication taken by the mother, exposure to toxins, or a vascular insult. Often there are associated heterotopias (isolated islands of neurons) which indicate a failure of migration of the neurons to their final position in the brain.

Treatment for individuals with schizencephaly generally consists of physical therapy, treatment for seizures, and, in cases that are complicated by hydrocephalus, a shunt.

The prognosis for individuals with schizencephaly varies depending on the size of the clefts and the degree of neurological deficit.

What Are Other Less Common Cephalies?

Acephaly literally means absence of the head. It is a much rarer condition than anencephaly. The acephalic fetus is a parasitic twin attached to an otherwise intact fetus. The acephalic fetus has a body but lacks a head and a heart; the fetus's neck is attached to the normal twin. The blood circulation of the acephalic fetus is provided by the heart of the twin. The acephalic fetus cannot exist independently of the fetus to which it is attached.

Exencephaly is a condition in which the brain is located outside of the skull. This condition is usually found in embryos as an early stage of anencephaly. As an exencephalic pregnancy progresses, the neural tissue gradually degenerates. It is unusual to find an infant carried to term with this condition because the defect is incompatible with survival.

Macrocephaly is a condition in which the head circumference is larger than average for the age and gender of the infant or child. It is a descriptive rather than a diagnostic term and is a characteristic of a variety of disorders. Macrocephaly also may be inherited. Although one form of macrocephaly may be associated with developmental delays and cognitive impairment, in approximately one-half of cases mental development is normal. Macrocephaly may be caused by an enlarged brain or hydrocephalus. It may be associated with other disorders such as dwarfism, neurofibromatosis, and tuberous sclerosis.

Micrencephaly is a disorder characterized by a small brain and may be caused by a disturbance in the proliferation of nerve cells. Micrencephaly may also be associated with maternal problems such as alcoholism, diabetes, or rubella (German measles). A genetic factor may play a role in causing some cases of micrencephaly. Affected newborns generally have striking neurological defects and seizures.

Severely impaired intellectual development is common, but disturbances in motor functions may not appear until later in life.

Octocephaly is a lethal condition in which the primary feature is
agnathia—a developmental anomaly characterized by total or virtual
absence of the lower jaw. The condition is considered lethal because of
a poorly functioning airway. In octocephaly, agnathia may occur alone
or together with holoprosencephaly.

Another group of less common cephalic disorders are the craniostenoses. Craniostenoses are deformities of the skull caused by the
premature fusion or joining together of the cranial sutures. Cranial
sutures are fibrous joints that join the bones of the skull together. The
nature of these deformities depends on which sutures are affected.

Brachycephaly occurs when the coronal suture fuses prematurely,
causing a shortened front-to-back diameter of the skull. The coronal
suture is the fibrous joint that unites the frontal bone with the two
parietal bones of the skull. The parietal bones form the top and sides
of the skull.

Oxycephaly is a term sometimes used to describe the premature
closure of the coronal suture plus any other suture, or it may be used
to describe the premature fusing of all sutures. Oxycephaly is the most
severe of the craniostenoses.

Plagiocephaly results from the premature unilateral fusion (joining of one side) of the coronal or lambdoid sutures. The lambdoid
suture unites the occipital bone with the parietal bones of the skull.
Plagiocephaly is a condition characterized by an asymmetrical distortion (flattening of one side) of the skull. It is a common finding at birth
and may be the result of brain malformation, a restrictive intrauterine
environment, or torticollis (a spasm or tightening of neck muscles).

Scaphocephaly applies to premature fusion of the sagittal suture.
The sagittal suture joins together the two parietal bones of the skull.
Scaphocephaly is the most common of the craniostenoses and is char-
acterized by a long, narrow head.

Trigonocephaly is the premature fusion of the metopic suture
(part of the frontal suture which joins the two halves of the frontal
bone of the skull) in which a V-shaped abnormality occurs at the front
of the skull. It is characterized by the triangular prominence of the
forehead and closely set eyes.

Chapter 20

Cerebral Palsy

Cerebral palsy (CP) is a group of disorders that affect a person's ability to move and maintain balance and posture. CP is the most common motor disability in childhood. Cerebral means having to do with the brain. Palsy means weakness or problems with using the muscles. CP is caused by abnormal brain development or damage to the developing brain that affects a person's ability to control his or her muscles.

The symptoms of CP vary from person to person. A person with severe CP might need to use special equipment to be able to walk, or might not be able to walk at all and might need lifelong care. A person with mild CP, on the other hand, might walk a little awkwardly, but might not need any special help. CP does not get worse over time, though the exact symptoms can change over a person's lifetime.

All people with CP have problems with movement and posture. Many also have related conditions such as intellectual disability; seizures; problems with vision, hearing, or speech; changes in the spine (such as scoliosis); or joint problems (such as contractures).

Types of Cerebral Palsy (CP)

Doctors classify CP according to the main type of movement disorder involved. Depending on which areas of the brain are affected, one or more of the following movement disorders can occur:

- Stiff muscles (spasticity)

This chapter includes text excerpted from "Facts about Cerebral Palsy," Centers for Disease Control and Prevention (CDC), February 3, 2017.

- Uncontrollable movements (dyskinesia)

- Poor balance and coordination (ataxia)

There are four main types of CP:

Spastic CP

The most common type of CP is spastic CP. Spastic CP affects about 80 percent of people with CP.

People with spastic CP have increased muscle tone. This means their muscles are stiff and, as a result, their movements can be awkward. Spastic CP usually is described by what parts of the body are affected:

- **Spastic diplegia/diparesis.** In this type of CP, muscle stiffness is mainly in the legs, with the arms less affected or not affected at all. People with spastic diplegia might have difficulty walking because tight hip and leg muscles cause their legs to pull together, turn inward, and cross at the knees (also known as scissoring).

- **Spastic hemiplegia/hemiparesis.** This type of CP affects only one side of a person's body; usually the arm is more affected than the leg.

- **Spastic quadriplegia/quadriparesis.** Spastic quadriplegia is the most severe form of spastic CP and affects all four limbs, the trunk, and the face. People with spastic quadriparesis usually cannot walk and often have other developmental disabilities such as intellectual disability; seizures; or problems with vision, hearing, or speech.

Dyskinetic CP (Also Includes Athetoid, Choreoathetoid, and Dystonic CPs)

People with dyskinetic CP have problems controlling the movement of their hands, arms, feet, and legs, making it difficult to sit and walk. The movements are uncontrollable and can be slow and writhing or rapid and jerky. Sometimes the face and tongue are affected and the person has a hard time sucking, swallowing, and talking. A person with dyskinetic CP has muscle tone that can change (varying from too tight to too loose) not only from day to day, but even during a single day.

Ataxic CP

People with ataxic CP have problems with balance and coordination. They might be unsteady when they walk. They might have a hard time with quick movements or movements that need a lot of control, like writing. They might have a hard time controlling their hands or arms when they reach for something.

Mixed CP

Some people have symptoms of more than one type of CP. The most common type of mixed CP is spastic-dyskinetic CP.

Early Signs

The signs of CP vary greatly because there are many different types and levels of disability. The main sign that a child might have CP is a delay reaching motor or movement milestones (such as rolling over, sitting, standing, or walking). Following are some other signs of possible CP. It is important to note that some children without CP also might have some of these signs.

In a baby younger than 6 months of age

- His head lags when you pick him up while he's lying on his back
- He feels stiff
- He feels floppy
- When held cradled in your arms, he seems to overextend his back and neck, constantly acting as if he is pushing away from you
- When you pick him up, his legs get stiff and they cross or scissor

In a baby older than 6 months of age

- She doesn't roll over in either direction
- She cannot bring her hands together
- She has difficulty bringing her hands to her mouth
- She reaches out with only one hand while keeping the other fisted

In a baby older than 10 months of age

- He crawls in a lopsided manner, pushing off with one hand and leg while dragging the opposite hand and leg

- He scoots around on his buttocks or hops on his knees, but does not crawl on all fours

Causes and Risk Factors

CP is caused by abnormal development of the brain or damage to the developing brain that affects a child's ability to control his or her muscles. There are several possible causes of the abnormal development or damage. People used to think that CP was mainly caused by lack of oxygen during the birth process. Now, scientists think that this causes only a small number of CP cases.

The brain damage that leads to CP can happen before birth, during birth, within a month after birth, or during the first years of a child's life, while the brain is still developing. CP related to brain damage that occurred before or during birth is called congenital CP. The majority of CP (85–90%) is congenital. In many cases, the specific cause is not known. A small percentage of CP is caused by brain damage that occurs more than 28 days after birth. This is called acquired CP, and usually is associated with an infection (such as meningitis) or head injury.

Screening and Diagnosis

Diagnosing CP at an early age is important to the well-being of children and their families. Diagnosing CP can take several steps:

Developmental Monitoring

Developmental monitoring (also called surveillance) means tracking a child's growth and development over time. If any concerns about the child's development are raised during monitoring, then a developmental screening test should be given as soon as possible.

Developmental Screening

During developmental screening a short test is given to see if the child has specific developmental delays, such as motor or movement delays. If the results of the screening test are cause for concern, then the doctor will make referrals for developmental and medical evaluations.

Developmental and Medical Evaluations

The goal of a developmental evaluation is to diagnose the specific type of disorder that affects a child.

Treatments and Intervention Services

There is no cure for CP, but treatment can improve the lives of those who have the condition. It is important to begin a treatment program as early as possible.

After a CP diagnosis is made, a team of health professionals works with the child and family to develop a plan to help the child reach his or her full potential. Common treatments include medicines; surgery; braces; and physical, occupational, and speech therapy. No single treatment is the best one for all children with CP. Before deciding on a treatment plan, it is important to talk with the child's doctor to understand all the risks and benefits.

Intervention Services

Both early intervention and school-aged services are available through our nation's special education law—the Individuals with Disabilities Education Act (IDEA). Part C of IDEA deals with early intervention services (birth through 36 months of age), while Part B applies to services for school-aged children (3 through 21 years of age). Even if your child has not been diagnosed with CP, he or she may be eligible for IDEA services.

If You're Concerned

If you think your child is not meeting movement milestones or might have CP, **contact your doctor or nurse and share your concerns.**

If you or your doctor is still concerned, **ask for a referral to a specialist** who can do a more in-depth evaluation of your child and assist in making a diagnosis.

At the same time, call your state's public early childhood system to request a free evaluation to find out if your child qualifies for intervention services. This is sometimes called a Child Find evaluation. You do not need to wait for a doctor's referral or a medical diagnosis to make this call.

Where to call for a free evaluation from the state depends on your child's age:

- If your child is not yet 3 years old, contact your local early intervention system.

  You can find the right contact information for your state by calling the Early Childhood Technical Assistance (ECTA) Center at 919-962-2001 or visit the ECTA Center.

- If your child is 3 years of age or older, contact your local public school system.

  Even if your child is not yet old enough for kindergarten or enrolled in a public school, call your local elementary school or board of education and ask to speak with someone who can help you have your child evaluated.

If you're not sure who to contact, you can call the Early Childhood Technical Assistance (ECTA) Center at 919-962-2001 or visit the ECTA Center.

Chapter 21

Chiari Malformation

What Are Chiari Malformations?

Chiari malformations (CM) are structural defects in the base of the skull and cerebellum, the part of the brain that controls balance. Normally the cerebellum and parts of the brainstem sit above an opening in the skull that allows the spinal cord to pass through it (called the foramen magnum). When part of the cerebellum extends below the foramen magnum and into the upper spinal canal, it is called a CM.

CM may develop when part of the skull is smaller than normal or misshapen, which forces the cerebellum to be pushed down into the foramen magnum and spinal canal. This causes pressure on the cerebellum and brainstem that may affect functions controlled by these areas and block the flow of cerebrospinal fluid (CSF)—the clear liquid that surrounds and cushions the brain and spinal cord. The CSF also circulates nutrients and chemicals filtered from the blood and removes waste products from the brain.

What Are the Causes of CM?

CM has several different causes. Most often it is caused by structural defects in the brain and spinal cord that occur during fetal development. This can be the result of genetic mutations or a maternal diet that lacked certain vitamins or nutrients. This is called primary

This chapter includes text excerpted from "Chiari Malformation Fact Sheet," National Institute of Neurological Disorders and Stroke (NINDS), June 2017.

or congenital CM. It can also be caused later in life if spinal fluid is drained excessively from the lumbar or thoracic areas of the spine either due to traumatic injury, disease, or infection. This is called acquired or secondary CM. Primary CM is much more common than secondary CM.

What Are the Symptoms of a CM?

Headache is the hallmark sign of CM, especially after sudden coughing, sneezing, or straining. Other symptoms may vary among individuals and may include:

- neck pain
- hearing or balance problems
- muscle weakness or numbness
- dizziness
- difficulty swallowing or speaking
- vomiting
- ringing or buzzing in the ears (tinnitus)
- curvature of the spine (scoliosis)
- insomnia
- depression
- problems with hand coordination and fine motor skills

Some individuals with CM may not show any symptoms. Symptoms may change for some individuals, depending on the compression of the tissue and nerves and on the buildup of CSF pressure.

Infants with a CM may have difficulty swallowing, irritability when being fed, excessive drooling, a weak cry, gagging or vomiting, arm weakness, a stiff neck, breathing problems, developmental delays, and an inability to gain weight.

How Are CMs Classified?

CMs are classified by the severity of the disorder and the parts of the brain that protrude into the spinal canal.

CM Type I

Type 1 happens when the lower part of the cerebellum (called the cerebellar tonsils) extends into the foramen magnum. Normally, only the spinal cord passes through this opening. Type 1—which may not cause symptoms—is the most common form of CM. It is usually first noticed in adolescence or adulthood, often by accident during an examination for another condition. Adolescents and adults who have CM but no symptoms initially may develop signs of the disorder later in life.

CM Type II

Individuals with Type II have symptoms that are generally more severe than in Type 1 and usually appear during childhood. This disorder can cause life-threatening complications during infancy or early childhood, and treating it requires surgery.

In Type II, also called classic CM, both the cerebellum and brainstem tissue protrude into the foramen magnum. Also the nerve tissue that connects the two halves of the cerebellum may be missing or only partially formed. Type II is usually accompanied by a myelomeningocele—a form of spina bifida that occurs when the spinal canal and backbone do not close before birth. (Spina bifida is a disorder characterized by the incomplete development of the brain, spinal cord, and/or their protective covering.) A myelomeningocele usually results in partial or complete paralysis of the area below the spinal opening. The term Arnold-Chiari malformation (named after two pioneering researchers) is specific to Type II malformations.

CM Type III

Type III is very rare and the most serious form of CM. In Type III, some of the cerebellum and the brainstem stick out, or herniate, through an abnormal opening in the back of the skull. This can also include the membranes surrounding the brain or spinal cord.

The symptoms of Type III appear in infancy and can cause debilitating and life-threatening complications. Babies with Type III can have many of the same symptoms as those with Type II but can also have additional severe neurological defects such as mental and physical delays, and seizures.

CM Type IV

Type IV involves an incomplete or underdeveloped cerebellum (a condition known as cerebellar hypoplasia). In this rare form of CM, the cerebellum is located in its normal position but parts of it are missing, and portions of the skull and spinal cord may be visible.

What Other Conditions Are Associated with CMs?

- **Hydrocephalus** is an excessive buildup of CSF in the brain. A CM can block the normal flow of this fluid and cause pressure within the head that can result in mental defects and/or an enlarged or misshapen skull. Severe hydrocephalus, if left untreated, can be fatal. The disorder can occur with any type of CM, but is most commonly associated with Type II.

- **Spina bifida** is the incomplete closing of the backbone and membranes around the spinal cord. In babies with spina bifida, the bones around the spinal cord do not form properly, causing defects in the lower spine. While most children with this birth defect have such a mild form that they have no neurological problems, individuals with Type II CM usually have myelomeningocele, and a baby's spinal cord remains open in one area of the back and lower spine. The membranes and spinal cord protrude through the opening in the spine, creating a sac on the baby's back. This can cause a number of neurological impairments such as muscle weakness, paralysis, and scoliosis.

- **Syringomyelia** is a disorder in which a CSF-filled tubular cyst, or syrinx, forms within the spinal cord's central canal. The growing syrinx destroys the center of the spinal cord, resulting in pain, weakness, and stiffness in the back, shoulders, arms, or legs. Other symptoms may include a loss of the ability to feel extremes of hot or cold, especially in the hands. Some individuals also have severe arm and neck pain.

- **Tethered cord syndrome** occurs when a child's spinal cord abnormally attaches to the tissues around the bottom of the spine. This means the spinal cord cannot move freely within the spinal canal. As a child grows, the disorder worsens, and can result in permanent damage to the nerves that control the muscles in the lower body and legs. Children who have a myelomeningocele have an increased risk of developing a tethered cord later in life.

- **Spinal curvature** is common among individuals with syringomyelia or CM Type I. The spine either may bend to the left or right (scoliosis) or may bend forward (kyphosis).

How Common Are CMs?

In the past, it was estimated that the condition occurs in about one in every 1,000 births. However, the increased use of diagnostic imaging has shown that CM may be much more common. Complicating this estimation is the fact that some children who are born with this condition may never develop symptoms or show symptoms only in adolescence or adulthood. CMs occur more often in women than in men and Type II malformations are more prevalent in certain groups, including people of Celtic descent.

How Are CMs Diagnosed?

Currently, no test is available to determine if a baby will be born with a CM. Since CMs are associated with certain birth defects like spina bifida, children born with those defects are often tested for malformations. However, some malformations can be seen on ultrasound images before birth.

Many people with CMs have no symptoms and their malformations are discovered only during the course of diagnosis or treatment for another disorder. The doctor will perform a physical exam and check the person's memory, cognition, balance (functions controlled by the cerebellum), touch, reflexes, sensation, and motor skills (functions controlled by the spinal cord). The physician may also order one of the following diagnostic tests:

- **Magnetic resonance imaging (MRI)** is the imaging procedure most often used to diagnose a CM. It uses radio waves and a powerful magnetic field to painlessly produce either a detailed three-dimensional picture or a two-dimensional "slice" of body structures, including tissues, organs, bones, and nerves.

- **X-rays** use electromagnetic energy to produce images of bones and certain tissues on film. An X-ray of the head and neck cannot reveal a CM but can identify bone abnormalities that are often associated with the disorder.

- **Computed tomography (CT)** uses X-rays and a computer to produce two-dimensional pictures of bone and blood vessels. CT can identify hydrocephalus and bone abnormalities associated with CM.

How Are CMs Treated?

Some CMs do not show symptoms and do not interfere with a person's activities of daily living. In these cases, doctors may only recommend regular monitoring with MRI. When individuals experience pain or headaches, doctors may prescribe medications to help ease symptoms.

Surgery

In many cases, surgery is the only treatment available to ease symptoms or halt the progression of damage to the central nervous system (CNS). Surgery can improve or stabilize symptoms in most individuals. More than one surgery may be needed to treat the condition.

The most common surgery to treat CM is posterior fossa decompression. It creates more space for the cerebellum and relieves pressure on the spinal cord. The surgery involves making an incision at the back of the head and removing a small portion of the bone at the bottom of the skull (craniectomy). In some cases the arched, bony roof of the spinal canal, called the lamina, may also be removed (spinal laminectomy). The surgery should help restore the normal flow of CSF, and in some cases it may be enough to relieve symptoms.

Next, the surgeon may make an incision in the dura, the protective covering of the brain and spinal cord. Some surgeons perform a Doppler ultrasound test during surgery to determine if opening the dura is even necessary. If the brain and spinal cord area is still crowded, the surgeon may use a procedure called electrocautery to remove the cerebellar tonsils, allowing for more free space. These tonsils do not have a recognized function and can be removed without causing any known neurological problems.

The final step is to sew a dura patch to expand the space around the tonsils, similar to letting out the waistband on a pair of pants. This patch can be made of artificial material or tissue harvested from another part of an individual's body.

Infants and children with myelomeningocele may require surgery to reposition the spinal cord and close the opening in the back. Findings from the National Institutes of Health (NIH) show that this surgery is most effective when it is done prenatally (while the baby is still in the womb) instead of after birth. The prenatal surgery reduces the occurrence of hydrocephalus and restores the cerebellum and brainstem to a more normal alignment.

Hydrocephalus may be treated with a shunt (tube) system that drains excess fluid and relieves pressure inside the head. A sturdy tube, surgically inserted into the head, is connected to a flexible tube placed under the skin. These tubes drain the excess fluid into either the chest cavity or the abdomen so it can be absorbed by the body.

An alternative surgical treatment in some individuals with hydrocephalus is third ventriculostomy, a procedure that improves the flow of CSF out of the brain. A small hole is made at the bottom of the third ventricle (brain cavity) and the CSF is diverted there to relieve pressure. Similarly, in cases where surgery was not effective, doctors may open the spinal cord and insert a shunt to drain a syringomyelia or hydromyelia (increased fluid in the central canal of the spinal cord).

Chapter 22

Spina Bifida

Spina bifida is a condition that affects the spine and is usually apparent at birth. It is a type of neural tube defect (NTD).

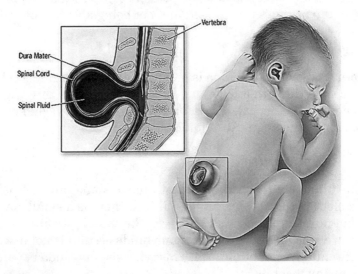

Figure 22.1. *Spina Bifida*

Spina bifida can happen anywhere along the spine if the neural tube does not close all the way. When the neural tube doesn't close all the

---

This chapter includes text excerpted from "Spina Bifida—Basics," Centers for Disease Control and Prevention (CDC), September 11, 2017.

way, the backbone that protects the spinal cord doesn't form and close as it should. This often results in damage to the spinal cord and nerves.

Spina bifida might cause physical and intellectual disabilities that range from mild to severe. The severity depends on:

- The size and location of the opening in the spine.
- Whether part of the spinal cord and nerves are affected.

Types of Spina Bifida

The three most common types of spina bifida are:

Myelomeningocele

When people talk about spina bifida, most often they are referring to myelomeningocele. Myelomeningocele is the most serious type of spina bifida. With this condition, a sac of fluid comes through an opening in the baby's back. Part of the spinal cord and nerves are in this sac and are damaged. This type of spina bifida causes moderate to severe disabilities, such as problems affecting how the person goes to the bathroom, loss of feeling in the person's legs or feet, and not being able to move the legs.

Meningocele

Another type of spina bifida is meningocele. With meningocele a sac of fluid comes through an opening in the baby's back. But, the spinal cord is not in this sac. There is usually little or no nerve damage. This type of spina bifida can cause minor disabilities.

Spina Bifida Occulta

Spina bifida occulta is the mildest type of spina bifida. It is sometimes called "hidden" spina bifida. With it, there is a small gap in the spine, but no opening or sac on the back. The spinal cord and the nerves usually are normal. Many times, spina bifida occulta is not discovered until late childhood or adulthood. This type of spina bifida usually does not cause any disabilities.

Diagnosis

Spina bifida can be diagnosed during pregnancy or after the baby is born. Spina bifida occulta might not be diagnosed until late childhood or adulthood, or might never be diagnosed.

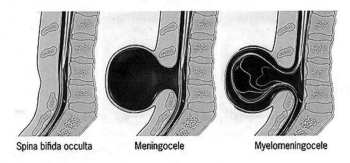

Spina bifida occulta   Meningocele   Myelomeningocele

Figure 22.2. *Spina Bifida Types*

During Pregnancy

During pregnancy there are screening tests (prenatal tests) to check for spina bifida and other birth defects. Talk with your doctor about any questions or concerns you have about this prenatal testing.

- **AFP.** AFP stands for alpha-fetoprotein, a protein the unborn baby produces. This is a simple blood test that measures how much AFP has passed into the mother's bloodstream from the baby. A high level of AFP might mean that the baby has spina bifida. An AFP test might be part of a test called the "triple screen" that looks for neural tube defects and other issues.

- **Ultrasound.** An ultrasound is a type of picture of the baby. In some cases, the doctor can see if the baby has spina bifida or find other reasons that there might be a high level of AFP. Frequently, spina bifida can be seen with this test.

- **Amniocentesis.** For this test, the doctor takes a small sample of the amniotic fluid surrounding the baby in the womb. Higher than average levels of AFP in the fluid might mean that the baby has spina bifida.

After the Baby Is Born

In some cases, spina bifida might not be diagnosed until after the baby is born.

Sometimes there is a hairy patch of skin or a dimple on the baby's back that is first seen after the baby is born. A doctor can use an image scan, such as an, X-ray, magnetic resonance imaging (MRI), or computed tomography (CT), to get a clearer view of the baby's spine and the bones in the back.

Sometimes spina bifida is not diagnosed until after the baby is born because the mother did not receive prenatal care or an ultrasound did not show clear pictures of the affected part of the spine.

Treatment

Not all people born with spina bifida have the same needs, so treatment will be different for each person. Some people have problems that are more serious than others. People with myelomeningocele and meningocele will need more treatments than people with spina bifida occulta.

Causes and Prevention

We do not know all of the causes of spina bifida. The role that genetics and the environment play in causing spina bifida needs to be studied further. However, we do know that there are ways for women to reduce the risk of having a baby with spina bifida both before and during her pregnancy.

If you are pregnant or could get pregnant, use the following tips to help prevent your baby from having spina bifida:

- Take 400 micrograms (mcg) of folic acid every day. If you have already had a pregnancy affected by spina bifida, you may need to take a higher dose of folic acid before pregnancy and during early pregnancy. Talk to your doctor to discuss what's best for you.

- Talk to your doctor or pharmacist about any prescription and over-the-counter (OTC) drugs, vitamins, and dietary or herbal supplements you are taking.

- If you have a medical condition, such as diabetes or obesity, be sure it is under control before you become pregnant.

- Avoid overheating your body, as might happen if you use a hot tub or sauna.

- Treat any fever you have right away with Tylenol® (or store brand acetaminophen).

Remember! Spina bifida happens in the first few weeks of pregnancy, often before a woman knows she's pregnant. Although folic acid is not a guarantee that a woman will have a healthy pregnancy, taking folic acid can help reduce a woman's risk of having a pregnancy affected by spina bifida. Because half of all pregnancies in the United States are unplanned, it is important that all women who can become pregnant take 400 mcg of folic acid daily one month before pregnancy and during early pregnancy.

Living with Spina Bifida

Spina bifida can range from mild to severe. Some people may have little to no disability. Other people may be limited in the way they move or function. Some people may even be paralyzed or unable to walk or move parts of their body.

Even so, with the right care, most people affected by spina bifida lead full, productive lives.

Part Four

Brain Infections

Chapter 23

Acquired Immune Deficiency Syndrome (AIDS): Neurological Complications

What Is AIDS?

Acquired immune deficiency syndrome (AIDS) is a condition that occurs in the most advanced stages of human immunodeficiency virus (HIV) infection. It may take many years for AIDS to develop following the initial HIV infection. Although AIDS is primarily an immune system disorder, it also affects the nervous system and can lead to a wide range of severe neurological disorders.

How Does Aids Affect the Nervous System?

The virus does not appear to directly invade nerve cells but it jeopardizes their health and function. The resulting inflammation may damage the brain and spinal cord and cause symptoms such as confusion and forgetfulness, behavioral changes, headaches, progressive weakness, and loss of sensation in the arms and legs. Cognitive motor impairment or damage to the peripheral nerves is also common.

This chapter includes text excerpted from "Neurological Complications of AIDS Fact Sheet," National Institute of Neurological Disorders and Stroke (NINDS), January 2006. Reviewed February 2018.

Research has shown that the HIV infection can significantly alter the size of certain brain structures involved in learning and information processing.

Other nervous system complications that occur as a result of the disease or the drugs used to treat it include pain, seizures, shingles, spinal cord problems, lack of coordination, difficult or painful swallowing, anxiety disorder, depression, fever, vision loss, gait disorders, destruction of brain tissue, and coma. These symptoms may be mild in the early stages of AIDS but can become progressively severe. In the United States, neurological complications are seen in more than 50 percent of adults with AIDS. Nervous system complications in children may include developmental delays, loss of previously achieved milestones, brain lesions, nerve pain, smaller than normal skull size, slow growth, eye problems, and recurring bacterial infections.

What Are Some of the Neurological Complications That Are Associated with AIDS?

AIDS-related disorders of the nervous system may be caused directly by the HIV virus, by certain cancers and opportunistic infections (illnesses caused by bacteria, fungi, and other viruses that would not otherwise affect people with healthy immune systems), or by toxic effects of the drugs used to treat symptoms. Other neuro-AIDS disorders of unknown origin may be influenced by but are not caused directly by the virus.

AIDS dementia complex (ADC), or HIV-associated dementia (HAD), occurs primarily in persons with more advanced HIV infection. Symptoms include encephalitis (inflammation of the brain), behavioral changes, and a gradual decline in cognitive function, including trouble with concentration, memory, and attention. Persons with ADC also show progressive slowing of motor function and loss of dexterity and coordination. When left untreated, ADC can be fatal. It is rare when antiretroviral therapy is used. Milder cognitive complaints are common and are termed HIV-associated neurocognitive disorder (HAND). Neuropsychologic testing can reveal subtle deficits even in the absence of symptoms.

Central nervous system (CNS) lymphomas are cancerous tumors that either begin in the brain or result from a cancer that has spread from another site in the body. CNS lymphomas are almost always associated with the Epstein-Barr virus (EBV) (a common human virus in the herpes family). Symptoms include headache, seizures, vision problems, dizziness, speech disturbance, paralysis, and mental deterioration. Individuals may develop one or more CNS lymphomas. Prognosis is poor due to advanced and increasing immunodeficiency, but is better with successful HIV therapy.

Cryptococcal meningitis (CM) is seen in about 10 percent of untreated individuals with AIDS and in other persons whose immune systems have been severely suppressed by disease or drugs. It is caused by the fungus *Cryptococcus neoformans,* which is commonly found in dirt and bird droppings. The fungus first invades the lungs and spreads to the covering of the brain and spinal cord, causing inflammation. Symptoms include fatigue, fever, headache, nausea, memory loss, confusion, drowsiness, and vomiting. If left untreated, patients with cryptococcal meningitis may lapse into a coma and die.

Cytomegalovirus (CMV) infections can occur concurrently with other infections. Symptoms of CMV encephalitis include weakness in the arms and legs, problems with hearing and balance, altered mental states, dementia, peripheral neuropathy, coma, and retinal disease that may lead to blindness. CMV infection of the spinal cord and nerves can result in weakness in the lower limbs and some paralysis, severe lower back pain, and loss of bladder function. It can also cause pneumonia and gastrointestinal disease. This is rarely seen in HIV-treated individuals since advanced immunity is required for CMV to emerge.

Herpes virus infections are often seen in people with AIDS. The herpes zoster virus, which causes chickenpox and shingles, can infect the brain and produce encephalitis and myelitis (inflammation of the spinal cord). It commonly produces shingles, which is an eruption of blisters and intense pain along an area of skin supplied by an infected nerve. In people exposed to herpes zoster, the virus can lay dormant in the nerve tissue for years until it is reactivated as shingles. This reactivation is common in persons with AIDS because of their weakened immune systems. Signs of shingles include painful blisters (like those seen in chickenpox), itching, tingling, and pain in the nerves.

People with AIDS may suffer from several different forms of neuropathy, or nerve pain, each strongly associated with a specific stage of active immunodeficiency disease.

Peripheral neuropathy describes damage to the peripheral nerves, the vast communications network that transmits information between the brain and spinal cord to every other part of the body.

Peripheral nerves also send sensory information back to the brain and spinal cord. HIV damages the nerve fibers that help conduct signals and can cause several different forms of neuropathy.

Distal sensory polyneuropathy (DSP) causes either a numbing feeling or a mild to painful burning or tingling sensation that normally begins in the legs and feet. These sensations may be particularly strong at night and may spread to the hands. Affected persons have a heightened sensitivity to pain, touch, or other stimuli. Onset usually occurs in the later stages of the HIV infection and may affect the majority of advanced-stage HIV patients.

Neurosyphilis, the result of an insufficiently treated syphilis infection, seems more frequent and more rapidly progressive in people with HIV infection. It may cause slow degeneration of the nerve cells and nerve fibers that carry sensory information to the brain. Symptoms, which may not appear for some decades after the initial infection and vary from person to person, include weakness, diminished reflexes, unsteady gait, progressive degeneration of the joints, loss of coordination, episodes of intense pain and disturbed sensation, personality changes, dementia, deafness, visual impairment, and impaired response to light. The disease is more frequent in men than in women. Onset is common during midlife.

Progressive multifocal leukoencephalopathy (PML) primarily affects individuals with suppressed immune systems (including nearly 5 percent of people with AIDS). PML is caused by the JC virus, which travels to the brain, infects multiple sites, and destroys the cells that make myelin—the fatty protective covering for many of the body's nerve and brain cells. Symptoms include various types of mental deterioration, vision loss, speech disturbances, ataxia (inability to coordinate movements), paralysis, brain lesions, and, ultimately, coma. Some individuals may also have compromised memory and cognition, and seizures may occur. PML is relentlessly progressive and death usually occurs within 6 months of initial symptoms. However, immune reconstitution with highly active antiretroviral therapy allows survival of more than half of HIV-associated PML cases in the current treatment era.

Psychological and neuropsychiatric disorders can occur in different phases of the HIV infection and AIDS and may take various and complex forms. Some illnesses, such as AIDS dementia complex, are caused directly by HIV infection of the brain, while other conditions may be triggered by the drugs used to combat the infection. Individuals may experience anxiety disorder, depressive disorders, increased thoughts of suicide, paranoia, dementia, delirium, cognitive impairment, confusion, hallucinations, behavioral abnormalities, malaise, and acute mania.

Toxoplasmic encephalitis (TE), also called cerebral toxoplasmosis, occurs in about 10 percent of untreated AIDS patients. It is caused by the parasite *Toxoplasma gondii*, which is carried by cats, birds, and other animals and can be found in soil contaminated by cat feces and sometimes in raw or undercooked meat. Once the parasite invades the immune system, it remains there; however, the immune system in a healthy person can fight off the parasite, preventing disease. Symptoms include encephalitis, fever, severe headache that does not respond to treatment, weakness on one side of the body, seizures, lethargy, increased confusion, vision problems, dizziness, problems with speaking and walking, vomiting, and personality changes. Not all patients show signs of the infection. Antibiotic therapy, if used early, will generally control the complication.

Vacuolar myelopathy (VM) causes the protective myelin sheath to pull away from nerve cells of the spinal cord, forming small holes called vacuoles in nerve fibers. Symptoms include weak and stiff legs and unsteadiness when walking. Walking becomes more difficult as the disease progresses and many patients eventually require a wheelchair. Some people also develop AIDS dementia. Vacuolar myelopathy may affect up to 30 percent of untreated adults with AIDS and its incidence may be even higher in HIV-infected children.

How Are These Disorders Diagnosed?

Based on the results of the individual's medical history and a general physical exam, the physician will conduct a thorough neurological exam to assess various functions: motor and sensory skills, nerve function, hearing and speech, vision, coordination and balance, mental status, and changes in mood or behavior. The physician may order laboratory tests and one or more of the following procedures to help diagnose neurological complications of AIDS.

Brain imaging can reveal signs of brain inflammation, tumors and CNS lymphomas, nerve damage, internal bleeding or hemorrhage, white matter irregularities, and other brain abnormalities. Several painless imaging procedures are used to help diagnose neurological complications of AIDS.

- **Computed tomography** (also called a CT scan) uses X-rays and a computer to produce two-dimensional images of bone and tissue, including inflammation, certain brain tumors and cysts, brain damage from head injury, and other disorders. It provides more details than an X-ray alone.

- **Magnetic resonance imaging** (MRI) uses a computer, radio waves, and a powerful magnetic field to produce either a detailed three-dimensional picture or a two-dimensional "slice" of body structures, including tissues, organs, bones, and nerves. It does not use ionizing radiation (as does an X-ray) and gives physicians a better look at tissue located near bone.

- **Functional MRI** (fMRI) uses the blood's magnetic properties to pinpoint areas of the brain that are active and to note how long they stay active. It can assess brain damage from head injury or degenerative disorders such as Alzheimer disease and can identify and monitor other neurological disorders, including AIDS dementia complex.

- **Magnetic resonance spectroscopy** (MRS) uses a strong magnetic field to study the biochemical composition and concentration of hydrogen-based molecules, some of which are very specific to nerve cells, in various brain regions. MRS is being used experimentally to identify brain lesions in people with AIDS.

Electromyography, or EMG, is used to diagnose nerve and muscle dysfunction (such as neuropathy and nerve fiber damage caused by the HIV virus) and spinal cord disease. It records spontaneous muscle activity and muscle activity driven by the peripheral nerves.

Biopsy is the removal and examination of tissue from the body. A brain biopsy, which involves the surgical removal of a small piece of the brain or tumor, is used to determine intracranial disorders and tumor type. Unlike most other biopsies, it requires hospitalization. Muscle or nerve biopsies can help diagnose neuromuscular problems, while a brain biopsy can help diagnose a tumor, inflammation, or other irregularity.

Cerebrospinal fluid analysis can detect any bleeding or brain hemorrhage, infections of the brain or spinal cord (such as neurosyphilis), and any harmful buildup of fluid. It can also be used to sample viruses that may be affecting the brain. A sample of the fluid is removed by needle, under local anesthesia, and studied to detect any irregularities.

How Are These Disorders Treated?

No single treatment can cure the neurological complications of AIDS. Some disorders require aggressive therapy while others are treated symptomatically.

Neuropathic pain is often difficult to control. Medicines range from analgesics sold over the counter to antiepileptic drugs, opiates, and some classes of antidepressants. Inflamed tissue can press on nerves, causing pain. Inflammatory and autoimmune conditions leading to neuropathy may be treated with corticosteroids, and procedures such as plasmapheresis (or plasma exchange) can clear the blood of harmful substances that cause inflammation.

Treatment options for AIDS- and HIV-related neuropsychiatric or psychotic disorders include antidepressants and anticonvulsants. Psychostimulants may also improve depressive symptoms and combat lethargy. Antidementia drugs may relieve confusion and slow mental decline, and benzodiazepines may be prescribed to treat anxiety. Psychotherapy may also help some individuals.

Aggressive antiretroviral therapy is used to treat AIDS dementia complex, vacuolar myopathy, progressive multifocal leukoencephalopathy (PML), and cytomegalovirus (CMV) encephalitis. Highly active antiretroviral therapy (HAART), or highly active antiretroviral therapy, combines at least three drugs to reduce the amount of virus circulating in the blood and may also delay the start of some infections. Other neuro-AIDS treatment options include physical therapy and rehabilitation, radiation therapy and/or chemotherapy to kill or shrink cancerous brain tumors that may be caused by the HIV virus, antifungal or antimalarial drugs to combat certain bacterial infections associated with the disorder, and penicillin to treat neurosyphilis.

Chapter 24

Brain Abscess

What Is Brain Abscess?

Brain abscess is an accumulation of pus inside the brain that results from a bacterial or fungal infection. The pus can cause swelling, which can affect the brain and spine. It was previously almost always a fatal condition, but progress in research, diagnosis, and treatment have increased the chances for recovery. The effects of a brain abscess can vary depending on where it occurs and its size, but left untreated an abscess can cause serious brain damage and spinal cord dysfunction.

Causes and Risk Factors

Brain abscesses generally result from bacterial, viral, and fungal infections in some part of the brain or elsewhere in the body. Some common causes for brain abscess include:

- **Infection in another part of the skull.** An ear infection, sinus infection, or dental abscess can spread directly to the brain.

- **Infection elsewhere in the body.** An infection that affects other parts of the body can be spread through the bloodstream into the brain. Examples include infections in the lung or chest area.

"Brain Abscess," © 2018 Omnigraphics. Reviewed February 2018.

- **Severe head injury.** An open wound can cause a virus or bacteria to enter the brain directly.

- **Surgery.** Complications from surgery, such as infections, can also cause brain abscess.

Some factors that can increase the risk of brain abscess include:

- weakened immune system due to such conditions as human immunodeficiency virus (HIV) / acquired immunodeficiency syndrome (AIDS)

- congenital heart disease

- chronic sinus or ear infections

- skull fracture or severe head injury

- meningitis

- cancer or chronic illnesses

- immunosuppressant drugs, such as those used in chemotherapy

Signs and Symptoms

Symptoms of brain abscess may develop slowly over a few weeks or can be rapid. Seventy-five percent of patients have a dull, achy headache, along with fever and neurological difficulties. Some other signs and symptoms of the condition include:

- changes in mental processes, such as:

  - confusion

  - drowsiness

  - poor mental focus

  - irritability

  - slow thought process

  - slow responsiveness

- fever

- chills

- neck stiffness or stiffness in the shoulders and back

- vomiting or nausea

- muscle weakness

- speech problems

- paralysis on one side of the body

- blurred or double vision

- seizures

- poor coordination

- changes in personality and behavior

- difficulty walking

Diagnosis

Some of the symptoms of brain abscess are similar to those of other health issues or diseases. However, if a brain abscess is suspected, an assessment is done based on the particular symptoms and medical history of the patient. The doctor evaluates these factors, as well as when the symptoms started and how they progressed. The doctor will ask questions to help determine if, for example, the patient has a weakened immune system or has had an infection recently. Diagnostic tests done to confirm a diagnosis of brain abscess include:

- **Blood tests.** These are done to check for high levels of white blood cells (WBC), which can indicate infection.

- **Computed tomography (CT) and magnetic resonance imaging (MRI).** These scans can help detect the presence of a brain abscess.

- **CT-guided aspiration.** This is a type of needle biopsy through which a pus sample is obtained for analysis.

- **Chest X-ray.** These may be used to help detect a lung infection.

- **Lumbar puncture (also called spinal tap).** This test uses a needle inserted into the spine to remove a small amount of cerebral spinal fluid for laboratory analysis.

Treatment

Brain abscess is a critical medical situation. Swelling inside the brain can cause pressure, which can lead to permanent brain damage. If a brain abscess is suspected, the doctor will usually prescribe antibiotics immediately to treat the underlying infections that can cause an abscess. Several types of antibiotics might be prescribed in order to kill a variety of different bacteria.

Successful treatment for abscess depends on the size of the abscess, the cause, the patient's general health, and the number of abscesses present. If the abscess is less than an inch in size, then the patient might be given antibiotic, antifungal, or antiviral medication intravenously. Abscesses of more than an inch would most likely need to be drained or aspirated.

In some cases, surgery could be necessary to treat a brain abscess. If the pressure keeps building within the brain and antibiotic treatment does not work, and if there is gas in the abscess or a risk of rupture, then surgery is needed. The surgeon performs a procedure known as craniotomy, which helps remove the abscess or drain the pus with the aid of a CT scan. High doses of corticosteroids for a short period can also be effective if there is increased intracranial pressure.

Prognosis

Most people recover from a brain abscess; however, it can prove dangerous or even fatal if not detected and treated early. An abscess is harder to treat when it is deep inside the brain or if there are multiple abscesses present. The sooner the treatment, the higher the chances of survival. Since abscesses can occasionally recur, the patient needs to be monitored on a regular basis.

References

1. "Brain Abscess," Healthline, April 20, 2017.

2. "Brain Abscess," NHS Choices, June 20, 2016.

3. "Brain Abscess," Stanford Children's Health, n.d.

4. Nordqvist, Christian. "What Is a Brain Abscess?" MedicalNews Today, October 5, 2016.

Chapter 25

Cysticercosis

What Is Cysticercosis?

Cysticercosis is an infection caused by the larvae of the parasite *Taenia solium*. This infection occurs after a person swallows tapeworm eggs. The larvae get into tissues such as muscle and brain, and form cysts there (these are called cysticerci). When cysts are found in the brain, the condition is called neurocysticercosis.

How Do Humans Get Cysticercosis?

People get cysticercosis when they swallow *T. solium* eggs that are passed in the feces of a human with a tapeworm. Tapeworm eggs are spread through food, water, or surfaces contaminated with feces. Humans swallow the eggs when they eat contaminated food or put contaminated fingers in their mouth. Importantly, someone with a tapeworm can infect him-or herself with tapeworm eggs (this is called autoinfection), and can infect others in the family. Eating pork cannot give you cysticercosis.

This chapter contains text excerpted from the following sources: Text beginning with the heading "What Is Cysticercosis?" is excerpted from "Cysticercosis FAQs," Centers for Disease Control and Prevention (CDC), April 17, 2014. Reviewed February 2018; Text beginning with the heading "Neurocysticercosis" is excerpted from "Neglected Parasitic Infections in the United States—Neurocysticercosis," Centers for Disease Control and Prevention (CDC), May 5, 2014. Reviewed February 2018.

What Is the Relationship between Human Tapeworm and Porcine (Pig) Cysticercosis?

Humans get the tapeworm infection after eating raw or undercooked pork contaminated with cysts of *T. solium.* When swallowed the cysts pass through the stomach and attach to the lining of the small intestine. In the small intestine the cysts develop into adult tapeworms over about two months.

Where Is Cysticercosis Found?

Cysticercosis is found worldwide. Infection is found most often in rural areas of developing countries where pigs are allowed to roam freely and eat human feces and where hygiene practices are poor. Cysticercosis is rare in people who live in countries where pigs do not have contact with human feces. People can sometimes get cysticercosis even if they have never traveled outside of the United States.

What Are the Signs and Symptoms of Cysticercosis?

Signs and symptoms will depend on the location and number of cysts in your body.

- **Cysts in the muscles:**

  - Cysts in the muscles generally do not cause symptoms. However, you may be able to feel lumps under your skin. The lumps sometimes become tender.

- **Cysts in the eyes:**

  - Although rare, cysts may float in the eye and cause blurry or disturbed vision. Infection in the eyes may cause swelling or detachment of the retina.

- **Neurocysticercosis (cysts in the brain, spinal cord):**

  - Symptoms of neurocysticercosis depend upon where and how many cysts are found in the brain. Seizures and headaches are the most common symptoms. However, confusion, lack of attention to people and surroundings, difficulty with balance, excess fluid around the brain (called hydrocephalus) may also occur. The disease can result in death.

How Long Will I Be Infected before Symptoms Begin?

Symptoms can occur months to years after infection, usually when the cysts start dying. When cysts die, the brain or other tissue around the cyst may swell. The pressure of the swelling is what usually causes the symptoms of the infection. Sometimes symptoms are caused by the pressure of cyst in a small space.

What Should I Do If I Think I Have Cysticercosis?

See your healthcare provider.

How Is Cysticercosis Diagnosed?

Your healthcare provider will ask you about your symptoms, where you have traveled, and the kinds of foods you eat. Diagnosis may require blood tests and/or imaging studies. Diagnosis of neurocysticercosis is usually made by magnetic resonance imaging (MRI) or computed tomography (CT) brain scans. Blood tests are available to help diagnose an infection, but may not always be accurate. If surgery is necessary to remove a cyst, the diagnosis can be made by the pathologist who looks at the cyst.

Is There Treatment for Cysticercosis?

Yes. Infections are generally treated with antiparasitic drugs in combination with anti-inflammatory drugs. Surgery is sometimes necessary to treat cysts in certain locations, when patients are not responsive to drug treatment, or to reduce brain swelling. Not all cases of cysticercosis need treatment. Even if you don't need treatment to kill the parasite, you may need treatment for the symptoms caused by the infection, such as medication to reduce the number of seizures you have.

Can Cysticercosis Be Spread from Person to Person?

No. Someone with cysticercosis cannot spread the disease to other people. However, people with taeniasis (tapeworm infection in the intestine) may spread tapeworm eggs to other people if they do not practice good hygiene (e.g., hand washing after they use the toilet), which may result in cysticercosis if people swallow the eggs.

If I Have Cysticercosis Should I Also Be Tested for an Intestinal Tapeworm Infection?

Yes. Family members may also need to be tested. Because the tapeworm infection can be difficult to diagnose, your healthcare provider may ask you to submit several stool specimens over several days or to examine your stools for evidence of a tapeworm.

How Can I Prevent Cysticercosis and Other Infections Spread through Fecal Contamination?

- Wash your hands with soap and warm water after using the toilet, changing diapers, and before handling food

- Teach children the importance of washing hands to prevent infection

- Wash and peel all raw vegetables and fruits before eating

- Use good food and water safety practices while traveling in developing countries such as:

  - Drink only bottled or boiled (1 minute) water or carbonated (bubbly) drinks in cans or bottles

  - Filter unsafe water through an "absolute 1 micron or less" filter and dissolve iodine tablets in the filtered water; "absolute 1 micron" filters can be found in camping and outdoor supply stores

Neurocysticercosis

Neurocysticercosis is a preventable parasitic infection caused by larval cysts (enclosed sacs containing the immature stage of a parasite) of the pork tapeworm (*Taenia solium*). The larval cysts can infect various parts of the body causing a condition known as cysticercosis. Larval cysts in the brain cause a form of cysticercosis called neurocysticercosis which can lead to seizures. Neurocysticercosis, which affects the brain and is the most severe form of the disease, can be fatal. Neurocysticercosis is considered a Neglected Parasitic Infection (NPI), one of a group of diseases that results in significant illness among those who are infected and is often poorly understood by healthcare providers.

How People Get Neurocysticercosis

A person gets neurocysticercosis by swallowing microscopic eggs passed in the feces of a person who has an intestinal pork tapeworm. For example, a person eats undercooked, infected pork and gets a tapeworm infection in the intestines. She passes tapeworm eggs in her feces. If she doesn't wash her hands properly after using the bathroom, she may contaminate food or surfaces with feces containing these eggs. These eggs may be swallowed by another person if they eat contaminated food. Once inside the body, the eggs hatch and become larvae that find their way to the brain. These larvae cause neurocysticercosis.

Risk Factors for Acquiring Neurocysticercosis

People are at a higher risk for getting neurocysticercosis by swallowing parasite eggs if they:

- Have a pork tapeworm infection (this is called autoinfection)
- Live in a household with someone who has a pork tapeworm
- Eat food made by someone with a pork tapeworm infection

In general, most people in the United States with neurocysticercosis are people who come from regions where the disease is common, including Latin America. Neurocysticercosis is a preventable disease. Good hand washing practices and treating people infected with intestinal tapeworms could drastically reduce the number of new infections.

Why Be Concerned about Neurocysticercosis in the United States?

Neurocysticercosis is a leading cause of adult onset epilepsy worldwide. It is costly to diagnose and treat but entirely preventable. There are an estimated 1,000 new hospitalizations for neurocysticercosis in the United States each year. Cases are most frequently reported in New York, California, Texas, Oregon, and Illinois. Additionally, neurocysticercosis creates a tremendous economic burden. In a study, the average charge of hospitalization due to neurocysticercosis was $37,600, with the most common form of payment being Medicaid (43.9%). Currently, there is little being done to monitor prevent, or identify and treat neurocysticercosis.

Chapter 26

Meningitis and Encephalitis

Infections, and less commonly other causes, in the brain and spinal cord can cause dangerous inflammation. This inflammation can produce a wide range of symptoms, including fever, headache, seizures, change in behavior or confusion and, in extreme cases, can cause brain damage, stroke, or even death.

Infection of the meninges, the membranes that surround the brain and spinal cord, is called meningitis. Inflammation of the brain itself is called encephalitis. Myelitis refers to inflammation of the spinal cord. When both the brain and the spinal cord are involved, the condition is called encephalomyelitis.

What Causes Meningitis and Encephalitis?

Infectious causes of meningitis and encephalitis include bacteria, viruses, fungi, and parasites. Many of these affect healthy people. For others, environmental and exposure history, recent travel or immunocompromised state (such as human immunodeficiency virus (HIV), diabetes, steroids, chemotherapy) are important elements. There are also noninfectious causes such as autoimmune causes and medications.

This chapter includes text excerpted from "Meningitis and Encephalitis Fact Sheet," National Institute of Neurological Disorders and Stroke (NINDS), April 2004. Reviewed February 2018.

Meningitis

Meningitis is most often caused by a bacterial or viral infection. It also may be caused by a fungal infection, parasite, a reaction to certain medications or medical treatments, a rheumatologic disease such as lupus, some types of cancer, or a traumatic injury to the head or spine.

Bacterial meningitis is a rare but potentially fatal disease. It can be caused by several types of bacteria that first cause an upper respiratory tract infection and then travel through the blood-stream to the brain. The disease can also occur when certain bacteria invade the meninges directly. The disease can cause stroke, hearing loss, and permanent brain damage.

Pneumococcal meningitis is the most common form of meningitis and is the most serious form of bacterial meningitis. Some 6,000 cases of pneumococcal meningitis are reported in the United States each year. The disease is caused by the bacterium *Streptococcus pneumoniae*, which also causes pneumonia, blood poisoning (septicemia), and ear and sinus infections. At particular risk are children under age 2 and adults with a weakened or depressed immune system, including the elderly. Persons who have had pneumococcal meningitis often suffer neurological damage ranging from deafness to severe brain damage. There are immunizations available for certain strains of the Pneumococcal bacteria.

Meningococcal meningitis is caused by the bacterium *Neisseria meningitides*. Each year in the United States about 2,600 people get this highly contagious disease. High-risk groups include infants under the age of 1 year, people with suppressed immune systems, travelers to foreign countries where the disease is endemic, and college students (freshmen in particular) who reside in dormitories. Between 10 and 15 percent of cases are fatal, with another 10–15 percent causing brain damage and other serious side effects. If this is diagnosed, people who come in close contact with the affected individual should be given preventative antibiotics.

Haemophilus meningitis was at one time the most common form of bacterial meningitis. Fortunately, the *Haemophilus influenzae b* (Hib) vaccine has greatly reduced the number of cases in the United States. Those most at risk of getting this disease are children in child-care settings and children who do not have access to the vaccine.

Other forms of bacterial meningitis include *Listeria monocytogenes meningitis*. Certain foods such as unpasteurized dairy or deli meats are sometimes implicated. *Escherichia coli meningitis*, which is most common in elderly adults and newborns and may be transmitted to a baby through the birth canal, and *Mycobacterium tuberculosis meningitis*, a rare disease that occurs when the bacterium that causes tuberculosis attacks the meninges.

Viral, or aseptic, meningitis is usually caused by enteroviruses—common viruses that enter the body through the mouth and travel to the brain and surrounding tissues where they multiply. Enteroviruses are present in mucus, saliva, and feces and can be transmitted through direct contact with an infected person or an infected object or surface. Other viruses that cause meningitis include *varicella zoster (the virus that causes chicken pox and can appear decades later as shingles)*, influenza, mumps, HIV, and *herpes simplex type 2* (genital herpes).

Many fungal infections can affect the brain. The most common form of fungal meningitis is caused by the fungus cryptococcus neoformans (found mainly in dirt and bird droppings). Cryptococcal meningitis mostly occurs in immunocompromised individuals such as in AIDS patients but can also occur in healthy people Some of these cases can be indolent and smolder for weeks. Although treatable, fungal meningitis often recurs in nearly half of affected persons.

Parasitic causes include cysticercosis, which is common in other parts of the world as well, and cerebral malaria.

There are rare cases of amoebic meningitis, sometimes related to fresh water swimming, which can be rapidly fatal.

Encephalitis

Encephalitis can be caused by the same infections listed above. However, up to 60 percent of cases remain undiagnosed, so this is an active area of research. Several thousand cases of encephalitis are reported each year, but many more may actually occur since the symptoms may be mild to nonexistent in most patients.

Most diagnosed cases of encephalitis in the United States are caused by enteroviruses, herpes simplex virus types (HSV) 1 and 2, rabies virus (this can occur even without a known animal bite, such as for example due to exposure to bats), or arboviruses such as West Nile virus (WNV), which are transmitted from infected animals to humans through the bite of an infected tick, mosquito, or other blood-sucking insect. Lyme disease, a bacterial infection spread by tick bite, more typically causes meningitis, and rarely encephalitis.

Herpes simplex encephalitis (HSE) is responsible for about 10 percent of all encephalitis cases, with a frequency of about 2 cases per million persons per year. More than half of untreated cases are fatal. About 30 percent of cases result from the initial infection with the herpes simplex virus; the majority of cases are caused by reactivation of an earlier infection. Most people acquire herpes simplex type 1 (the cause of cold sores or fever blisters) in childhood so it is a ubiquitous exposure.

HSE due to herpes simplex virus type 1 can affect any age group but is most often seen in persons under age 20 or over age 40. This rapidly progressing disease is the single most important cause of fatal sporadic encephalitis in the United States Symptoms can include headache and fever for up to 5 days, followed by personality and behavioral changes, seizures, hallucinations, and altered levels of consciousness. Brain damage in adults and in children beyond the neonatal period is usually seen in the frontal (leading to behavioral and personality changes) and temporal lobes (leading to memory and speech problems) and can be severe.

Type 2 virus (genital herpes) is most often transmitted through sexual contact. Many people do not know they are infected and may not have active genital lesions. An infected mother can transmit the disease to her child at birth, and through contact with genital secretions. In newborns, symptoms such as lethargy, irritability, tremors, seizures, and poor feeding generally develop between 4 and 11 days after delivery.

Powassan encephalitis is the only well-documented tick-borne arbovirus in the United States and Canada. Symptoms are noticed 7–10 days following the bite (most people do not notice tick bites) and may include headache, fever, nausea, confusion, partial paralysis, coma, and seizures.

Four common forms of mosquito-transmitted viral encephalitis are seen in the United States:

- **Equine encephalitis** affects horses and humans. Eastern equine encephalitis also infects birds that live in freshwater swamps of the eastern U.S. seaboard and along the Gulf Coast. In humans, symptoms are seen 4–10 days following transmission and include sudden fever, general flu-like muscle pains, and headache of increasing severity, followed by coma and death in severe cases. About half of infected patients die from the disorder. Fewer than 10 human cases are seen annually in the United States. Western equine encephalitis is seen in farming areas in the western and central plains states. Symptoms begin 5–10 days following infection. Children, particularly those under 12 months of age, are affected more severely than adults and may have permanent neurologic damage. Death occurs in about 3 percent of cases. Venezuelan equine encephalitis is very rare in this country. Children are at greatest risk of developing severe complications, while adults generally develop flu-like symptoms. Epidemics in South and Central America have killed thousands of persons and left others with permanent, severe neurologic damage.

• **La Crosse encephalitis** occurs most often in the upper midwestern states (Illinois, Wisconsin, Indiana, Ohio, Minnesota, and Iowa) but also has been reported in the southeastern and mid-Atlantic regions of the country. Most cases are seen in children under age 16. Symptoms such as vomiting, headache, fever, and lethargy appear 5–10 days following infection. Severe complications include seizure, coma, and permanent neurologic damage. About 100 cases of LaCrosse encephalitis are reported each year.

• **St. Louis encephalitis** is most prevalent in temperate regions of the United States but can occur throughout most of the country. The disease is generally milder in children than in adults, with elderly adults at highest risk of severe disease or death. Symptoms typically appear 7–10 days following infection and include headache and fever. In more severe cases, confusion and disorientation, tremors, convulsions (especially in the very young), and coma may occur.

West Nile encephalitis (WNE) was first clinically diagnosed in the United States in 1999; 284 people are known to have died of the virus the following year. There were 9,862 reported cases of human West Nile disease in calendar year 2003, with a total of 560 deaths from this disorder over 5 years. The disease is usually transmitted by a bite from an infected mosquito, but can also occur after transplantation of an infected organ or transfusions of infected blood or blood products. Symptoms are flu-like and include fever, headache, and joint pain. Some patients may develop a skin rash and swollen lymph glands, while others may not show any symptoms. At highest risk are elderly adults and people with weakened immune systems.

Many cases of encephalitis are caused by an autoimmune disorder which may or may not be triggered by an infection.

Who Is at Risk for Encephalitis and Meningitis?

Anyone can get encephalitis or meningitis. People with weakened immune systems, including those persons with HIV or those taking immunosuppressant drugs, are at increased risk.

How Are These Disorders Transmitted?

Some forms of bacterial meningitis and encephalitis are contagious and can be spread through contact with saliva, nasal discharge, feces, or respiratory and throat secretions (often spread through kissing, coughing, or sharing drinking glasses, eating utensils, or such personal items as toothbrushes, lipstick, or cigarettes). For example, people sharing a household, at a day care center, or in a classroom with an infected person can become infected. College students living in dormitories—in particular, college freshmen—have a higher risk of contracting meningococcal meningitis than college students overall. Children who have not been given routine vaccines are at increased risk of developing certain types of bacterial meningitis.

Because these diseases can occur suddenly and progress rapidly, anyone who is suspected of having either meningitis or encephalitis should immediately contact a doctor or go to the hospital.

What Are the Signs and Symptoms?

The hallmark signs of meningitis are sudden fever, severe headache, nausea/vomiting, double vision, drowsiness, sensitivity to bright light, and a stiff neck; encephalitis can be characterized by fever, seizures, change in behavior, confusion and disorientation, and related neurological signs depending on which part of the brain is affected by the encephalitic process, as some of these are quite focal (locally centered) while others are more global.

Meningitis often appears with flu-like symptoms that develop over 1–2 days. Distinctive rashes are typically seen in some forms of the disease. Meningococcal meningitis may be associated with kidney and adrenal gland failure and shock.

Individuals with encephalitis often show mild flu-like symptoms. In more severe cases, patients may experience problems with speech or hearing, double vision, hallucinations, personality changes, loss of consciousness, loss of sensation in some parts of the body, muscle weakness, partial paralysis in the arms and legs, sudden severe dementia, seizures, and memory loss.

Important signs of meningitis or encephalitis to watch for in an infant include fever, lethargy, not waking for feeding, vomiting, body stiffness, unexplained or unusual irritability, and a full or bulging fontanel (the soft spot on the top of the head).

How Are Meningitis and Encephalitis Diagnosed?

Following a physical exam and medical history to review activities of the past several days/weeks (such as recent exposure to insects or animals, any contact with ill persons, recent travel, or preexisting medical conditions and medications list), the doctor may order various diagnostic tests to confirm the presence of infection and inflammation. Early diagnosis is vital, as symptoms can appear suddenly and escalate to brain damage, hearing and/or speech loss, blindness, or even death.

A *neurological examination* involves a series of tests designed to assess motor and sensory function, nerve function, hearing and speech, vision, coordination and balance, mental status, and changes in mood or behavior. Doctors may test the function of the nervous system through tests of strength and sensation, with the aid of items including a tuning fork, small light, reflex hammer, and pins.

Laboratory screening of blood, urine, and body secretions can help detect and identify brain and/or spinal cord infection and determine the presence of antibodies and foreign proteins. Such tests can also rule out metabolic conditions that have similar symptoms. For example, a throat culture may be taken to check for viral or bacterial organisms that cause meningitis or encephalitis. In this procedure, the back of the throat is wiped with a sterile cotton swab, which is then placed on a culture medium. Viruses and bacteria are then allowed to grow on the medium. Samples are usually taken in the physician's office or in a laboratory setting and sent out for analysis to state laboratories or to the U.S. Centers for Disease Control and Prevention (CDC). Results are usually available in 2–3 days.

Analysis of the cerebrospinal fluid that surrounds and protects the brain and spinal cord can detect infections in the brain and/or spinal cord, acute and chronic inflammation, and other diseases. In a procedure known as a spinal tap (or lumbar puncture), a small amount of cerebrospinal fluid is removed by a special needle that is inserted into the lower back. The skin is anesthetized with a local anesthetic prior to the sampling. The fluid, which is completely clear in healthy people, is tested to detect the presence of bacteria or blood, as well as to measure glucose levels (a low glucose level can be seen in bacterial or fungal meningitis) and white blood cells (elevated white blood cell counts are also a sign of infection). The procedure is done in a hospital and takes about 45 minutes. The individual will most often be placed on antibiotics and an antiviral drug while awaiting the final microbiology results as delay in treatment can be life-threatening.

Brain imaging can reveal signs of brain inflammation, internal bleeding or hemorrhage, or other brain abnormalities. Two painless, noninvasive imaging procedures are routinely used to diagnose meningitis and encephalitis.

- *Computed tomography*, also known as a CT scan, combines X-rays and computer technology to produce rapid, clear, two-dimensional images of organs, bones, and tissues. Occasionally a contrast dye is injected into the bloodstream to highlight the different tissues in the brain and to detect signs of encephalitis or inflammation of the meninges. CT scans can also detect bone and blood vessel irregularities, certain brain tumors and cysts, herniated discs, spinal stenosis (narrowing of the spinal canal), blood clots or intracranial bleeding in patients with stroke, brain damage from a head injury, and other disorders. If the individual has abnormal results on a neurological examination, often a CT scan is performed to look for brain swelling, hemorrhage, or abscess which if present, could make a spinal tap unsafe.

- *Magnetic resonance imaging (MRI)* uses computer-generated radio waves and a strong magnet to produce detailed images of body structures, including tissues, organs, bones, and nerves. There is no radiation involved in this test and it gives a much better picture of the actual brain tissue. this may not be available in the emergency setting so a CT scan is usually performed first in very ill individuals. The pictures, which are clearer than those produced by CT, can help identify brain and spinal cord inflammation, infection, tumors, eye disease, and blood vessel irregularities that may lead to stroke. A contrast dye may be injected prior to the test to reveal more detail.

Electroencephalography, or EEG, can identify abnormal brainwaves by monitoring electrical activity in the brain through the skull. Among its many functions, EEG is used to help diagnose seizures or patterns that may suggest specific viral infections such as herpes virus, and to detect subclinical seizures which may contribute to abnormalities in level of consciousness in critically ill individuals.

How Are These Infections Treated?

Persons who are suspected of having meningitis or encephalitis should receive immediate, aggressive medical treatment. Both diseases can progress quickly and have the potential to cause severe, irreversible neurological damage.

Meningitis

Early treatment of bacterial meningitis is important to its outcome, with antibiotics that can cross the protective blood-brain lining. Appropriate antibiotic treatment for most types of meningitis can reduce the risk of dying from the disease to below 15 percent.

Infected sinuses may need to be drained. Corticosteroids such as prednisone may be ordered to relieve brain pressure and swelling and to prevent hearing loss that is common in patients with Haemophilus influenza meningitis. Lyme disease is treated with intravenous antibiotics.

Unlike bacteria, viruses cannot be killed by antibiotics; generally there is no specific treatment for viruses except for the herpes virus, which can be treated with the antiviral drug acyclovir. The physician may prescribe anticonvulsants such as dilantin or phenytoin to prevent seizures and corticosteroids to reduce brain inflammation. If inflammation is severe, pain medicine and sedatives may be prescribed to make the person more comfortable.

Acute disseminated encephalomyelitis is treated with steroids. Fungal meningitis is treated with intravenous antifungal medications.

Encephalitis

Antiviral drugs used to treat viral encephalitis include acyclovir and ganciclovir.

Anticonvulsants may be prescribed to stop or prevent seizures. Corticosteroids can reduce brain swelling. Individuals with breathing difficulties may require artificial respiration.

Autoimmune causes of encephalitis are treated with additional immunosuppressant drugs and screening for tumors when appropriate.

Individuals should receive evaluation for comprehensive rehabilitation that might include cognitive rehabilitation, physical, speech, and occupational therapy once the acute illness is under control.

Can Meningitis and Encephalitis Be Prevented?

Avoid sharing food, utensils, glasses, and other objects with a person who may be exposed to or have the infection. Wash hands often with soap and rinse under running water.

Effective vaccines are available to prevent pneumonia, H. influenza, pneumococcal meningitis, and infection with other bacteria that can cause meningococcal meningitis.

People who live, work, or go to school with someone who has been diagnosed with bacterial meningitis may be asked to take antibiotics for a few days as a preventive measure.

To lessen the risk of being bitten by an infected mosquito or other insect, people should limit outdoor activities at night, wear long-sleeved clothing when outdoors, use insect repellents that are most effective for that particular region of the country, and rid lawn and outdoor areas of free-standing pools of water, in which mosquitoes breed. Do not over-apply repellants, particularly on young children and especially infants, as chemicals such as DEET may be absorbed through the skin.

What Is the Prognosis for These Infections?

Outcome generally depends on the particular infectious agent involved, the severity of the illness, and how quickly treatment is given. In most cases, people with very mild encephalitis or meningitis can make a full recovery, although the process may be slow.

Individuals who experience only headache, fever, and stiff neck may recover in 2–4 weeks. Those with bacterial meningitis typically show some relief 48–72 hours following initial treatment but are more likely to experience complications caused by the disease. In more serious cases, these diseases can cause hearing and/or speech loss, blindness, permanent brain and nerve damage, behavioral changes, cognitive disabilities, lack of muscle control, seizures, and memory loss. These patients may need long-term therapy, medication, and supportive care. The recovery from encephalitis is variable depending on the cause and extent of brain inflammation.

What Research Is Being Done?

The National Institute of Neurological Disorders and Stroke (NINDS), a component of the National Institutes of Health (NIH) within the U.S. Department of Health and Human Services (HHS), conducts and supports a wide range of research on neurological disorders, including meningitis and encephalitis. Current research efforts include gaining a better understanding of how the central nervous system responds to inflammation and to better understand the molecular mechanisms involved in the protection and disruption of the blood-brain barrier, which could lead to the development of new treatments for several neuroinflammatory diseases such as meningitis and encephalitis. A possible therapeutic approach under investigation involves testing neuroprotective compounds that block the damage that accumulates after the infection, and how the inflammation of meningitis and encephalitis can lead to potential complications including loss of cognitive function and dementia.

Chapter 27

Progressive Multifocal Leukoencephalopathy (PML)

Progressive multifocal leukoencephalopathy (PML) is a disease of the white matter of the brain, caused by a virus infection that targets cells that make myelin—the material that insulates nerve cells (neurons). Polyomavirus JC (often called JC virus) is carried by a majority of people and is harmless except among those with lowered immune defenses. The disease is rare and occurs in patients undergoing chronic corticosteroid or immunosuppressive therapy for organ transplant, or individuals with cancer (such as Hodgkin disease or lymphoma). Individuals with autoimmune conditions such as multiple sclerosis, rheumatoid arthritis, and systemic lupus erythematosis—some of whom are treated with biological therapies that allow JC virus reactivation—are at risk for PML as well.

PML is most common among individuals with human immunodeficiency virus (HIV)-1 infection/acquired immune deficiency syndrome (AIDS). Studies estimate that prior to effective antiretroviral therapy, as many as 5 percent of persons infected with HIV-1 eventually develop PML that is an AIDS-defining illness. However, current HIV therapy using antiretroviral drugs (ART), which effectively restores immune system function, allows as many as half of all HIV-PML patients to

---

This chapter includes text excerpted from "Progressive Multifocal Leukoencephalopathy Information Page," National Institute of Neurological Disorders and Stroke (NINDS), May 24, 2017.

survive, although they may sometimes have an inflammatory reaction in the regions of the brain affected by PML.

Symptoms

The symptoms of PML are diverse, since they are related to the location and amount of damage in the brain, and may evolve over the course of several weeks to months The most prominent symptoms are clumsiness; progressive weakness; and visual, speech, and sometimes personality changes. The progression of deficits leads to life-threatening disability and (frequently) death. A diagnosis of PML can be made following brain biopsy or by combining observations of a progressive course of the disease, consistent white matter lesions visible on a magnetic resonance imaging (MRI) scan, and the detection of the JC virus in spinal fluid.

Treatment

Currently, the best available therapy is reversal of the immune-deficient state, since there are no effective drugs that block virus infection without toxicity. Reversal may be achieved by using plasma exchange to accelerate the removal of the therapeutic agents that put patients at risk for PML. In the case of HIV-associated PML, immediately beginning antiretroviral therapy will benefit most individuals. Several new drugs that laboratory tests found effective against infection are being used in PML patients with special permission of the U.S. Food and Drug Administration (FDA). Hexadecyloxypropyl-cidofovir (CMX001) is currently being studied as a treatment option for JVC because of its ability to suppress JVC by inhibiting viral deoxyribonucleic acid (DNA) replication.

Prognosis

In general, PML has a mortality rate of 30–50 percent in the first few months following diagnosis but depends on the severity of the underlying disease and treatment received. Those who survive PML can be left with severe neurological disabilities.

Chapter 28

Rabies

Rabies is a preventable viral disease of mammals most often transmitted through the bite of a rabid animal. The vast majority of rabies cases reported to the Centers for Disease Control and Prevention (CDC) each year occur in wild animals like raccoons, skunks, bats, and foxes. The rabies virus infects the central nervous system, ultimately causing disease in the brain and death. The early symptoms of rabies in people are similar to that of many other illnesses, including fever, headache, and general weakness or discomfort. As the disease progresses, more specific symptoms appear and may include insomnia, anxiety, confusion, slight or partial paralysis, excitation, hallucinations, agitation, hypersalivation (increase in saliva), difficulty swallowing, and hydrophobia (fear of water). Death usually occurs within days of the onset of these symptoms.

How Is Rabies Transmitted?

All species of mammals are susceptible to rabies virus infection, but only a few species are important as reservoirs for the disease. In the United States, distinct strains of rabies virus have been identified in raccoons, skunks, foxes, and coyotes. Several species of insectivorous bats are also reservoirs for strains of the rabies virus.

This chapter contains text excerpted from the following sources: Text in this chapter begins with excerpts "Rabies," Centers for Disease Control and Prevention (CDC), September 28, 2017; Text under the heading "Side Effects of Rabies Vaccine" is excerpted from "Rabies," Vaccines.gov, U.S. Department of Health and Human Services (HHS), January 18, 2018.

Transmission of rabies virus usually begins when infected saliva of a host is passed to an uninfected animal. The most common mode of rabies virus transmission is through the bite and virus-containing saliva of an infected host. Though transmission has been rarely documented via other routes such as contamination of mucous membranes (i.e., eyes, nose, mouth), aerosol transmission, and corneal and organ transplantations.

What Are the Signs and Symptoms of Rabies?

The first symptoms of rabies may be very similar to those of the flu including general weakness or discomfort, fever, or headache. These symptoms may last for days.

There may be also discomfort or a prickling or itching sensation at the site of bite, progressing within days to symptoms of cerebral dysfunction, anxiety, confusion, and agitation. As the disease progresses, the person may experience delirium, abnormal behavior, hallucinations, and insomnia. The acute period of disease typically ends after 2–10 days. Once clinical signs of rabies appear, the disease is nearly always fatal, and treatment is typically supportive. Disease prevention includes administration of both passive antibody, through an injection of human immune globulin and a round of injections with rabies vaccine. Once a person begins to exhibit signs of the disease, survival is rare. To date less than 10 documented cases of human survival from clinical rabies have been reported and only two have not had a history of pre- or post-exposure prophylaxis.

What Is the Risk for My Pet?

Any animal bitten or scratched by either a wild, carnivorous mammal or a bat that is not available for testing should be regarded as having been exposed to rabies. Unvaccinated dogs, cats, and ferrets exposed to a rabid animal should be euthanized immediately. If the owner is unwilling to have this done, the animal should be placed in strict isolation for 6 months and vaccinated 1 month before being released.

Animals with expired vaccinations need to be evaluated on a case-by-case basis. Dogs and cats that are currently vaccinated are kept under observation for 45 days. Small mammals such as squirrels, rats, mice, hamsters, guinea pigs, gerbils, chipmunks, rabbits, and hares are almost never found to be infected with rabies and have not been known to cause rabies among humans in the United States. Bites by these animals are usually not considered a risk of rabies unless the animal was sick or behaving in any unusual manner and rabies is widespread in your area.

However, from 1985 through 1994, woodchucks accounted for 86 percent of the 368 cases of rabies among rodents reported to CDC. Woodchucks or groundhogs (Marmota monax) are the only rodents that may be frequently submitted to state health department because of a suspicion of rabies. In all cases involving rodents, the state or local health department should be consulted before a decision is made to initiate postexposure prophylaxis (PEP).

How Is Rabies Diagnosed?

In animals, rabies is diagnosed using the direct fluorescent antibody (DFA) test, which looks for the presence of rabies virus antigens in brain tissue. In humans, several tests are required. Rapid and accurate laboratory diagnosis of rabies in humans and other animals is essential for timely administration of postexposure prophylaxis. Within a few hours, a diagnostic laboratory can determine whether or not an animal is rabid and inform the responsible medical personnel. The laboratory results may save a patient from unnecessary physical and psychological trauma, and financial burdens, if the animal is not rabid.

In addition, laboratory identification of positive rabies cases may aid in defining current epidemiologic patterns of disease and provide appropriate information for the development of rabies control programs. The nature of rabies disease dictates that laboratory tests be standardized, rapid, sensitive, specific, economical, and reliable.

When Should I Seek Medical Attention?

The rabies virus is transmitted through saliva or brain/nervous system tissue. You can only get rabies by coming in contact with these specific bodily excretions and tissues. It's important to remember that rabies is a medical urgency but not an emergency. Decisions should not be delayed. Wash any wounds immediately. One of the most effective ways to decrease the chance for infection is to wash the wound thoroughly with soap and water. See your doctor for attention for any trauma due to an animal attack before considering the need for rabies vaccination. Your doctor, possibly in consultation with your state or local health department, will decide if you need a rabies vaccination. Decisions to start vaccination, known as postexposure prophylaxis (PEP), will be based on your type of exposure and the animal you were exposed to, as well as laboratory and surveillance information for the geographic area where the exposure occurred.

In the United States, postexposure prophylaxis consists of a regimen of one dose of immune globulin and four doses of rabies vaccine over a 14-day period. Rabies immune globulin and the first dose of rabies vaccine should be given by your healthcare provider as soon as possible after exposure. Additional doses or rabies vaccine should be given on days 3, 7, and 14 after the first vaccination. Current vaccines are relatively painless and are given in your arm, like a flu or tetanus vaccine.

What Care Will I Receive?

Wound Care

Regardless of the risk of rabies, bite wounds can cause serious injury such as nerve or tendon laceration and local and system infection. Your doctor will determine the best way to care for your wound, and will also consider how to treat the wound for the best possible cosmetic results. For many types of bite wounds, immediate gentle irrigation with water or a dilute water Povidone-iodine solution has been shown to markedly decrease the risk of bacterial infection.

Wound cleansing is especially important in rabies prevention since, in animal studies, thorough wound cleansing alone without other postexposure prophylaxis has been shown to markedly reduce the likelihood of rabies. You should receive a tetanus shot if you have not been immunized in ten years. Decisions regarding the use of antibiotics, and primary wound closure should be decided together with your doctor.

Rabies Postexposure Vaccinations

For people who have never been vaccinated against rabies previously, postexposure anti-rabies vaccination should always include administration of both passive antibody and vaccine. The combination of human rabies immune globulin (HRIG) and vaccine is recommended for both bite and nonbite exposures, regardless of the interval between exposure and initiation of treatment. People who have been previously vaccinated or are receiving pre-exposure vaccination for rabies should receive only vaccine.

Adverse reactions to rabies vaccine and immune globulin are not common. Newer vaccines in use today cause fewer adverse reactions than previously available vaccines. Mild, local reactions to the rabies vaccine, such as pain, redness, swelling, or itching at the injection site, have been reported. Rarely, symptoms such as headache, nausea, abdominal pain, muscle aches, and dizziness have been reported. Local pain and low-grade fever may follow injection of rabies immune globulin.

The vaccine should be given at recommended intervals for best results. Talk to your doctor or state or local public health officials if you will not be able to have shot at the recommended interval. Rabies prevention is a serious matter and changes should not be made in the schedule of doses. People cannot transmit rabies to other people unless they themselves are sick with rabies. The prophylaxis you are receiving will protect you from developing rabies, and therefore you cannot expose other people to rabies. You should continue to participate in your normal activities.

Table 28.1. Rabies Vaccines and Immunoglobulin Available in the United States

Type	Name	Route	Indications
Human Diploid Cell Vaccine (HDCV)	Imovax® Rabies	Intramuscular	Preexposure or Postexposure
Purified Chick Embryo Cell Vaccine (PCEC)	RabAvert®	Intramuscular	Preexposure or Postexposure
Human Rabies Immune Globulin	Imogam® Rabies-HT	Local infusion at wound site, with additional amount intramuscular at site distant from vaccine	Postexposure
Human Rabies Immune Globulin	HyperRab TM S/D	Local infusion at wound site, with additional amount intramuscular at site distant from vaccine	Postexposure

Side Effects of Rabies Vaccine

Side effects are usually mild and go away in a few days. They include pain, swelling, or redness where the shot was given, headache, upset stomach, stomach pain, muscle aches, and dizziness. Less common side effects of the rabies vaccine include hives (itchy spots on the skin), joint pain, and fever.

Table 28.2. Rabies Postexposure Prophylaxis (PEP) Schedule

Vaccination status	Intervention	Regimen*
Not previously vaccinated	Wound cleansing	All PEP should begin with immediate thorough cleansing of all wounds with soap and water. If available, a virucidal agent (e.g., povidine-iodine solution) should be used to irrigate the wounds.
	Human rabies immune globulin (HRIG)	Administer 20 IU/kg body weight. If anatomically feasible, the full dose should be infiltrated around and into the wound(s), and any remaining volume should be administered at an anatomical site (intramuscular [IM]) distant from vaccine administration. Also, HRIG should not be administered in the same syringe as vaccine. Because RIG might partially suppress active production of rabies virus antibody, no more than the recommended dose should be administered.
	Vaccine	Human diploid cell vaccine (HDCV) or purified chick embryo cell vaccine (PCECV) 1.0 mL, IM (deltoid area†), 1 each on days 0,§ 3, 7 and 14.
Previously vaccinated**	Wound cleansing	All PEP should begin with immediate thorough cleansing of all wounds with soap and water. If available, a virucidal agent such as povidine-iodine solution should be used to irrigate the wounds.
	HRIG	HRIG should not be administered.
	Vaccine	HDCV or PCECV 1.0 mL, IM (deltoid area†), 1 each on days 0§ and 3.

*These regimens are applicable for persons in all age groups, including children.
§Day 0 is the day dose 1 of vaccine is administered.
**Any person with a history of pre-exposure vaccination with HDCV, PCECV, or rabies vaccine adsorbed (RVA); prior PEP with HDCV, PCECV or RVA; or previous vaccination with any other type of rabies vaccine and a documented history of antibody response to the prior vaccination.
†The deltoid area is the only acceptable site of vaccination for adults and older children. For younger children, the outer aspect of the thigh may be used. Vaccine should never be administered in the gluteal area.

Chapter 29

West Nile Virus

West Nile is a virus most commonly spread to people by mosquito bites. In North America, cases of West Nile virus (WNV) occur during mosquito season, which starts in the summer and continues through fall. WNV cases have been reported in all of the continental United States. There are no vaccines to prevent or medications to treat WNV. Fortunately, most people infected with WNV do not have symptoms. About 1 in 5 people who are infected develop a fever and other symptoms. About 1 out of 150 infected people develop a serious, sometimes fatal, illness. You can reduce your risk of WNV by using insect repellent and wearing protective clothing to prevent mosquito bites.

Symptoms

No symptoms in most people. Most people (8 out of 10) infected with West Nile virus do not develop any symptoms.

Febrile illness (fever) in some people. About 1 in 5 people who are infected develop a fever with other symptoms such as headache, body aches, joint pains, vomiting, diarrhea, or rash. Most people with this type of WNV disease recover completely, but fatigue and weakness can last for weeks or months.

This chapter includes text excerpted from "West Nile Virus," Centers for Disease Control and Prevention (CDC), February 21, 2018.

Serious symptoms in a few people. About 1 in 150 people who are infected develop a severe illness affecting the central nervous system such as encephalitis (inflammation of the brain) or meningitis (inflammation of the membranes that surround the brain and spinal cord).

- Symptoms of severe illness include high fever, headache, neck stiffness, stupor, disorientation, coma, tremors, convulsions, muscle weakness, vision loss, numbness, and paralysis.

- Severe illness can occur in people of any age; however, people over 60 years of age are at greater risk. People with certain medical conditions, such as cancer, diabetes, hypertension, kidney disease, and people who have received organ transplants, are also at greater risk.

- Recovery from severe illness might take several weeks or months. Some effects to the central nervous system might be permanent.

- About 1 out of 10 people who develop severe illness affecting the central nervous system die.

Diagnosis

- See your healthcare provider if you develop the symptoms described above.

- Your healthcare provider can order tests to look for WNV infection.

Treatment

- No vaccine or specific antiviral treatments for WNV infection are available.

- Over-the-counter (OTC) pain relievers can be used to reduce fever and relieve some symptoms.

- In severe cases, patients often need to be hospitalized to receive supportive treatment, such as intravenous fluids, pain medication, and nursing care.

- If you think you or a family member might have WNV disease, talk with your healthcare provider.

Transmission

WNV is most commonly spread to people by the bite of an infected mosquito. Mosquitoes become infected when they feed on infected birds. Infected mosquitoes then spread WNV to people and other animals by biting them.

In a very small number of cases, WNV has been spread through:

- Exposure in a laboratory setting.

- Blood transfusion and organ donation.

- Mother to baby, during pregnancy, delivery, or breastfeeding.

West Nile virus is not spread:

- Through coughing, sneezing, or touching.

- By touching live animals.

- From handling live or dead infected birds. Avoid bare-handed contact when handling any dead animal. If you are disposing of a dead bird, use gloves or double plastic bags to place the carcass in a garbage can.

- Through eating infected birds or animals. Always follow instructions for fully cooking meat from either birds or mammals.

Prevention

The most effective way to avoid WNV disease is to prevent mosquito bites. Be aware of the WNV activity in your area and take action to protect yourself and your family.

Prevent Mosquito Bites

Use Insect Repellent

Use U.S. Environmental Protection Agency (EPA)-registered insect repellents with one of the active ingredients below. When used as directed, EPA-registered insect repellents are proven safe and effective, even for pregnant and breastfeeding women.

Tips for Everyone

- Always follow the product label instructions.

- Reapply insect repellent as directed.

  - Do not spray repellent on the skin under clothing.

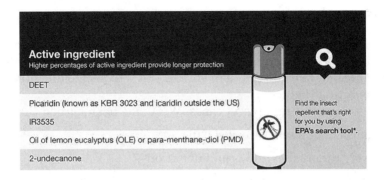

Figure 29.1. *Insect-Repellent*

- If you are also using sunscreen, apply sunscreen first and insect repellent second.

Tips for Babies and Children

- Always follow instructions when applying insect repellent to children.

- Do not use insect repellent on babies younger than 2 months old.

- Do not apply insect repellent onto a child's hands, eyes, mouth, and cut or irritated skin.

  - Adults: Spray insect repellent onto your hands and then apply to a child's face.

- Do not use products containing oil of lemon eucalyptus (OLE) or para-menthane-diol (PMD) on children under 3 years old.

Natural Insect Repellents (Repellents Not Registered with EPA)

- We do not know the effectiveness of non-EPA registered insect repellents, including some natural repellents.

- To protect yourself against diseases spread by mosquitoes, Centers for Disease Control and Prevention (CDC) and EPA recommend using an EPA-registered insect repellent.

- Choosing an EPA-registered repellent ensures the EPA has evaluated the product for effectiveness.

Protect Your Baby or Child

- Dress your child in clothing that covers arms and legs.

- Cover crib, stroller, and baby carrier with mosquito netting.

Wear Long-Sleeved Shirts and Long Pants

- Treat items, such as boots, pants, socks, and tents, with permethrin* or buy permethrin-treated clothing and gear.

  - Permethrin-treated clothing will protect you after multiple washings. See product information to find out how long the protection will last.

  - If treating items yourself, follow the product instructions.

  - Do not use permethrin products directly on skin.

In some places, such as Puerto Rico, where permethrin products have been used for years in mosquito control efforts, mosquitoes have become resistant to it. In areas with high levels of resistance, use of permethrin is not likely to be effective.

Take Steps to Control Mosquitoes Inside and Outside Your Home

- Use screens on windows and doors. Repair holes in screens to keep mosquitoes outside.

- Use air conditioning when available.

  - Sleep under a mosquito bed net if air-conditioned or screened rooms are not available or if sleeping outdoors.

- Once a week, empty and scrub, turn over, cover, or throw out items that hold water, such as tires, buckets, planters, toys, pools, birdbaths, flowerpots, or trash containers. Check inside and outside your home. Mosquitoes lay eggs near water.

Part Five

Traumatic and Acquired Brain Injuries

Chapter 30

Concussion (Mild Traumatic Brain Injury)

What Is a Concussion?

A concussion is a type of traumatic brain injury—or TBI—caused by a bump, blow, or jolt to the head or by a hit to the body that causes the head and brain to move rapidly back and forth. This sudden movement can cause the brain to bounce around or twist in the skull, creating chemical changes in the brain and sometimes stretching and damaging brain cells.

Concussions Are Serious

Medical providers may describe a concussion as a "mild" brain injury because concussions are usually not life-threatening. Even so, the effects of a concussion can be serious.

Concussion: Signs and Symptoms

Children and teens who show or report one or more of the signs and symptoms listed below, or simply say they just "don't feel right" after a bump, blow, or jolt to the head or body, may have a concussion or more serious brain injury.

This chapter includes text excerpted from "Heads Up—Brain Injury Basics," Centers for Disease Control and Prevention (CDC), January 31, 2017.

Concussion Signs Observed

- Can't recall events *prior to* or *after* a hit or fall.
- Appears dazed or stunned.
- Forgets an instruction, is confused about an assignment or position, or is unsure of the game, score, or opponent.
- Moves clumsily.
- Answers questions slowly.
- Loses consciousness (even briefly).
- Shows mood, behavior, or personality changes.

Concussion Symptoms Reported

- Headache or "pressure" in head.
- Nausea or vomiting.
- Balance problems or dizziness, or double or blurry vision.
- Bothered by light or noise.
- Feeling sluggish, hazy, foggy, or groggy.
- Confusion, or concentration or memory problems.
- Just not "feeling right," or "feeling down."

Signs and symptoms generally show up soon after the injury. However, you may not know how serious the injury is at first and some symptoms may not show up for hours or days. For example, in the first few minutes your child or teen might be a little confused or a bit dazed, but an hour later your child might not be able to remember how he or she got hurt.

You should continue to check for signs of concussion right after the injury and a few days after the injury. If your child or teen's concussion signs or symptoms get worse, you should take him or her to the emergency department right away.

Concussion Danger Signs

In rare cases, a dangerous collection of blood (hematoma) may form on the brain after a bump, blow, or jolt to the head or body that may squeeze the brain against the skull. Call 9-1-1 right away, or take your child or teen to the emergency department if he or she has one or more of the following danger signs after a bump, blow, or jolt to the head or body:

Dangerous Signs and Symptoms of a Concussion

- One pupil larger than the other.
- Drowsiness or inability to wake up.
- A headache that gets worse and does not go away.
- Slurred speech, weakness, numbness, or decreased coordination.
- Repeated vomiting or nausea, convulsions or seizures (shaking or twitching).
- Unusual behavior, increased confusion, restlessness, or agitation.
- Loss of consciousness (passed out/knocked out). Even a brief loss of consciousness should be taken seriously.

Dangerous Signs and Symptoms of a Concussion for Toddlers and Infants

Any of the signs and symptoms listed above and:

- Will not stop crying and cannot be consoled.
- Will not nurse or eat.

Severe Brain Injury

Long-Term Effects

A person with a severe brain injury will need to be hospitalized and may have long-term problems affecting things such as:

- Thinking
- Memory
- Learning
- Coordination and balance
- Speech, hearing or vision
- Emotions

A severe brain injury can affect all aspects of people's lives, including relationships with family and friends, as well as their ability to work or be employed, do household chores, drive, and/or do other normal daily activities.

Recovery from Concussion

Most children with a concussion feel better within a couple of weeks. However for some, symptoms will last for a month or longer. Concussion symptoms may appear during the normal healing process or as your child gets back to their regular activities. If there are any symptoms that concern you or are getting worse, be sure to seek medical care as soon as possible.

What Steps Should My Child Take to Feel Better?

Making short-term changes to your child's daily activities can help him or her get back to a regular routine more quickly. As your child begins to feel better, you can slowly remove these changes. Use your child's symptoms to guide return to normal activities. If your child's symptoms do not worsen during an activity then this activity is OK for them. If symptoms worsen, your child should cut back on how much he or she can do that activity without experiencing symptoms. It is important to remember that each concussion and each child is unique, so your child's recovery should be customized based on his or her symptoms.

Rest

Your child should take it easy the first few days after the injury when symptoms are more severe.

- Early on, limit physical and thinking/remembering activities to avoid symptoms getting worse.

- Avoid activities that put your child at risk for another injury to the head and brain.

- Get a good night's sleep and take naps during the day as needed.

Light Activity

As your child starts to feel better, gradually return to regular (nonstrenuous) activities.

- Find relaxing activities at home. Avoid activities that put your child at risk for another injury to the head and brain.

- Return to school gradually. If symptoms do not worsen during an activity, then this activity is OK for your child. If symptoms worsen, cut back on that activity until it is tolerated.

- Get maximum nighttime sleep. (Avoid screen time and loud music before bed, sleep in a dark room, and keep to a fixed bedtime and wake up schedule.)

- Reduce daytime naps or return to a regular daytime nap schedule (as appropriate for their age).

Moderate Activity

When symptoms are mild and nearly gone, your child can return to most regular activities.

- Help your child take breaks only if concussion symptoms worsen.

- Return to a regular school schedule.

Back to Regular Activity

Recovery from a concussion is when your child is able to do all of their regular activities without experiencing any symptoms.
Also, be sure to:

- Schedule a follow-up appointment for your child's doctor or nurse.

- Ask your child's doctor or nurse about safe over-the-counter (OTC) or prescription medications to help with symptoms (e.g., Ibuprofen or acetaminophen for headache).

- Limit the number of soft drinks or caffeinated items to help your child rest.

Postconcussive Syndrome

While most children and teens with a concussion feel better within a couple of weeks, some will have symptoms for months or longer. Talk with your children' or teens' healthcare provider if their concussion symptoms do not go away or if they get worse after they return to their regular activities.

If your child or teen has concussion symptoms that last weeks to months after the injury, their medical provider may talk to you about postconcussive syndrome. While rare after only one concussion, postconcussive syndrome is believed to occur most commonly in patients with a history of multiple concussions.

There are many people who can help you and your family as your child or teen recovers. You do not have to do it alone. Keep talking with your medical provider, family members, and loved ones about how your child or teen is feeling. If you do not think he or she is getting better, tell your medical provider.

Chapter 31

Traumatic Brain Injury (TBI)

Chapter Contents

Section 31.1

What Is Traumatic Brain Injury (TBI)?

This section includes text excerpted from "TBI: Get the
Facts—Traumatic Brain Injury and Concussion," Centers for
Disease Control and Prevention (CDC), April 27, 2017.

Traumatic Brain Injury: Facts

Traumatic brain injury (TBI) is a major cause of death and disability in the United States. TBIs contribute to about 30 percent of all injury deaths. Every day, 153 people in the United States die from injuries that include TBI. Those who survive a TBI can face effects that last a few days, or the rest of their lives. Effects of TBI can include impaired thinking or memory, movement, sensation (e.g., vision or hearing), or emotional functioning (e.g., personality changes, depression). These issues not only affect individuals but can have lasting effects on families and communities.

What Is TBI?

A TBI is caused by a bump, blow, or jolt to the head that disrupts the normal function of the brain. Not all blows or jolts to the head result in a TBI. The severity of a TBI may range from "mild" (i.e., a brief change in mental status or consciousness) to "severe" (i.e., an extended period of unconsciousness or memory loss after the injury). Most TBIs that occur each year are mild, commonly called concussions.

How Big Is the Problem?

- In 2013, about 2.8 million TBI-related U.S. Emergency Department (ED) visits, hospitalizations, and deaths occurred in the United States.

  - TBI contributed to the deaths of nearly 50,000 people.

  - TBI was a diagnosis in more than 282,000 hospitalizations and 2.5 million ED visits. These consisted of TBI alone or TBI in combination with other injuries.

- Over the span of six years (2007–2013), while rates of TBI-related ED visits increased by 47 percent, hospitalization rates decreased by 2.5 percent and death rates decreased by 5 percent.

- In 2012, an estimated 329,290 children (age 19 or younger) were treated in U.S. EDs for sports and recreation-related injuries that included a diagnosis of concussion or TBI.

  - From 2001–2012, the rate of ED visits for sports and recreation-related injuries with a diagnosis of concussion or TBI, alone or in combination with other injuries, more than doubled among children (age 19 or younger).

What Are the Leading Causes of TBI?

- In 2013, falls were the leading cause of TBI. Falls accounted for 47 percent of all TBI-related ED visits, hospitalizations, and deaths in the United States. Falls disproportionately affect the youngest and oldest age groups:

  - More than half (54%) of TBI-related ED visits hospitalizations, and deaths among children 0–14 years were caused by falls.

  - Nearly 4 in 5 (79%) TBI-related ED visits, hospitalizations, and deaths in adults aged 65 and older were caused by falls.

- Being struck by or against an object was the second leading cause of TBI, accounting for about 15 percent of TBI-related ED visits, hospitalizations, and deaths in the United States in 2013.

  - Over 1 in 5 (22%) TBI-related ED visits, hospitalizations, and deaths in children less than 15 years of age were caused by being struck by or against an object.

- Among all age groups, motor vehicle crashes were the third overall leading cause of TBI-related ED visits, hospitalizations, and deaths (14%). When looking at just TBI-related deaths, motor vehicle crashes were the third leading cause (19%) in 2013.

- Intentional self-harm was the second leading cause of TBI-related deaths (33%) in 2013.

Risk Factors for TBI

Among TBI-related deaths in 2013:

- Rates were highest for persons 75 years of age and older.

- The leading cause of TBI-related death varied by age.

  - Falls were the leading cause of death for persons 65 years of age or older.

  - Intentional self-harm was the leading cause of death for persons 25–64 years of age.

  - Motor vehicle crashes were the leading cause of death for persons 5–24 years of age.

  - Assaults were the leading cause of death for children ages 0–4 years.
  Among nonfatal TBI-related injuries in 2013:

- Hospitalization rates were highest among persons 75 years of age and older.

- Rates of ED visits were highest for persons 75 years of age and older and children 0–4 years of age.

- Falls were the leading cause of TBI-related ED visits for all but one age group.

  - Being struck by or against an object was the leading cause of TBI-related ED visits for persons 15–24 years of age.

- The leading cause of TBI-related hospitalizations varied by age:

  - Falls were the leading cause among children 0–14 years of age and adults 45 years of age and older.

  - Motor vehicle crashes were the leading cause of hospitalizations for adolescents and persons 15–44 years of age.

Signs and Symptoms

What Are the Signs and Symptoms of Concussion?

Most people with a concussion recover well from symptoms experienced at the time of the injury. But for some people, symptoms can last for days, weeks, or longer. In general, recovery may be slower among older adults, young children, and teens. Those who have had a concussion in the past are also at risk of having another one. Some people may also find that it takes longer to recover if they have another concussion.

Symptoms of concussion usually fall into four categories:

Table 31.1. Symptoms of Concussion

Thinking/ Remembering	Physical	Emotional/ Mood	Sleep
Difficulty thinking clearly	Headache Fuzzy or blurry vision	Irritability	Sleeping more than usual
Feeling slowed down	Nausea or vomiting (early on) Dizziness	Sadness	Sleep less than usual
Difficulty concentrating	Sensitivity to noise or light Balance problems	More emotional	Trouble falling asleep
Difficulty remembering new information	Feeling tired, having no energy	Nervousness or anxiety	

Some of these symptoms may appear right away. Others may not be noticed for days or months after the injury, or until the person resumes their everyday life. Sometimes, people do not recognize or admit that they are having problems. Others may not understand their problems and how the symptoms they are experiencing impact their daily activities.

The signs and symptoms of a concussion can be difficult to sort out. Early on, problems may be overlooked by the person with the concussion, family members, or doctors. People may look fine even though they are acting or feeling differently.

When to Seek Immediate Medical Attention

Danger Signs in Adults

In rare cases, a person with a concussion may form a dangerous blood clot that crowds the brain against the skull. Contact your healthcare professional or emergency department right away if you experience these danger signs after a bump, blow, or jolt to your head or body:

- Headache that gets worse and does not go away.

- Weakness, numbness or decreased coordination.

- Repeated vomiting or nausea.

- Slurred speech.

The people checking on you should take you to an emergency department right away if you:

- Look very drowsy or cannot wake up.

- Have one pupil (the black part in the middle of the eye) larger than the other.

- Have convulsions or seizures.

- Cannot recognize people or places.

- Are getting more and more confused, restless, or agitated.

- Have unusual behavior.

- Lose consciousness.

Danger Signs in Children

Take your child to the emergency department right away if they received a bump, blow, or jolt to the head or body, and:

- Have any of the danger signs for adults listed above.

- Will not stop crying and are inconsolable.

- Will not nurse or eat.

Response

What Should I Do If a Concussion Occurs?

People with a concussion need to be seen by a healthcare professional. If you think you or someone you know has a concussion, contact your healthcare professional. Your healthcare professional can evaluate your concussion and determine if you need to be referred to a neurologist, neuropsychologist, neurosurgeon, or specialist in rehabilitation (such as a speech pathologist) for specialized care. Getting help soon after the injury by trained specialists may improve recovery.

What to Expect When You See a Healthcare Professional

While most people are seen in an emergency department or medical office, some people must stay in the hospital overnight. Your healthcare professional may do a scan of your brain (such as a computed tomography (CT) scan) or other tests. Additional tests might be necessary, such as tests of your learning, memory concentration, and problem solving. These tests are called "neuropsychological" or "neurocognitive" tests and can help your healthcare professional identify the effects of a concussion. Even if the concussion doesn't show up on these tests, you may still have a concussion.

Your healthcare professional will send you home with important instructions to follow. Be sure to follow all of your healthcare professional's instructions carefully.

If you are taking medications—prescription, over-the-counter (OTC) medicines, or "natural remedies"—or if you drink alcohol or take illicit drugs, tell your healthcare professional. Also, tell your healthcare professional if you are taking blood thinners (anticoagulant drugs), such as Coumadin and aspirin, because they can increase the chance of complications.

Recovery

What Can I Do to Help Feel Better after a Mild TBI?

Although most people recover after a concussion, how quickly they improve depends on many factors. These factors include how severe their concussion was, their age, how healthy they were before the concussion, and how they take care of themselves after the injury.

Some people who have had a concussion find that at first it is hard to do their daily activities, their job, to get along with everyone at home, or to relax.

Rest is very important after a concussion because it helps the brain to heal. Ignoring your symptoms and trying to "tough it out" often makes symptoms worse. Be patient because healing takes time. Only when your symptoms have reduced significantly, in consultation with your healthcare professional, should you slowly and gradually return to your daily activities, such as work or school. If your symptoms come back or you get new symptoms as you become more active, this is a sign that you are pushing yourself too hard. Stop these activities and take more time to rest and recover. As the days go by, you can expect to gradually feel better.

Getting Better: Tips for Adults

- Get plenty of sleep at night, and rest during the day.

- Avoid activities that are physically demanding (e.g., heavy house cleaning, weightlifting/working-out) or require a lot of concentration (e.g., balancing your checkbook). They can make your symptoms worse and slow your recovery.

• Avoid activities, such as contact or recreational sports, that could lead to another concussion. (It is best to avoid roller coasters or other high speed rides that can make your symptoms worse or even cause a concussion.)

• When your healthcare professional says you are well enough, return to your normal activities gradually, not all at once.

• Because your ability to react may be slower after a concussion, ask your healthcare professional when you can safely drive a car, ride a bike, or operate heavy equipment.

• Talk with your healthcare professional about when you can return to work. Ask about how you can help your employer understand what has happened to you.

• Consider talking with your employer about returning to work gradually and about changing your work activities or schedule until you recover (e.g., work half-days).

• Take only those drugs that your healthcare professional has approved.

• Do not drink alcoholic beverages until your healthcare professional says you are well enough. Alcohol and other drugs may slow your recovery and put you at risk of further injury.

• Write down the things that may be harder than usual for you to remember.

• If you're easily distracted, try to do one thing at a time. For example, don't try to watch TV while fixing dinner.

• Consult with family members or close friends when making important decisions.

• Do not neglect your basic needs, such as eating well and getting enough rest.

• Avoid sustained computer use, including computer/video games early in the recovery process.

• Some people report that flying in airplanes makes their symptoms worse shortly after a concussion.

Getting Better: Tips for Children

Parents and caregivers of children who have had a concussion can help them recover by taking an active role in their recovery:

- Having the child get plenty of rest. Keep a regular sleep schedule, including no late nights and no sleepovers.

- Making sure the child avoids high-risk/high-speed activities such as riding a bicycle, playing sports, or climbing playground equipment, roller coasters or rides that could result in another bump, blow, or jolt to the head or body. Children should not return to these types of activities until their healthcare professional says they are well enough.

- Giving the child only those drugs that are approved by the pediatrician or family physician.

- Talking with their healthcare professional about when the child should return to school and other activities and how the parent or caregiver can help the child deal with the challenges that the child may face. For example, your child may need to spend fewer hours at school, rest often, or require more time to take tests.

- Sharing information about concussion with parents, siblings, teachers, counselors, babysitters, coaches, and others who interact with the child helps them understand what has happened and how to meet the child's needs.

Help Prevent Long-Term Problems

If you already had a medical condition at the time of your concussion (such as chronic headaches), it may take longer for you to recover from the concussion. Anxiety and depression may also make it harder to adjust to the symptoms of a concussion. While you are healing, you should be very careful to avoid doing anything that could cause a bump, blow, or jolt to the head or body. On rare occasions, receiving another concussion before the brain has healed can result in brain swelling, permanent brain damage, and even death, particularly among children and teens.

After you have recovered from your concussion, you should protect yourself from having another one. People who have had repeated concussions may have serious long-term problems, including chronic difficulty with concentration, memory, headache, and occasionally, physical skills, such as keeping one's balance.

Potential Effects

What Are the Potential Effects of TBI?

The severity of a TBI may range from "mild" (i.e., a brief change in mental status or consciousness) to "severe" (i.e., an extended period of unconsciousness or amnesia after the injury).

A TBI can cause a wide range of functional short- or long-term changes affecting:

- **Thinking** (i.e., memory and reasoning);

- **Sensation** (i.e., sight and balance);

- **Language** (i.e., communication, expression, and understanding); and

- **Emotion** (i.e., depression, anxiety, personality changes, aggression, acting out, and social inappropriateness).

A TBI can also cause epilepsy and increase the risk for conditions such as Alzheimer disease, Parkinson disease, and other brain disorders.

About 75 percent of TBIs that occur each year are concussions or other forms of mild TBI.

Repeated mild TBIs occurring over an extended period of time can result in cumulative neurological and cognitive deficits. Repeated mild TBIs occurring within a short period of time (i.e., hours, days, or weeks) can be catastrophic or fatal.

Prevention

What Can I Do to Help Prevent TBI?

There are many ways to reduce the chances of sustaining a traumatic brain injury, including:

1. Buckling your child in the car using a child safety seat, booster seat, or seat belt (according to the child's height, weight, and age).

2. Wearing a seat belt every time you drive or ride in a motor vehicle.

3. Never driving while under the influence of alcohol or drugs.

4. Wearing a helmet and making sure your children wear helmets when:

    -   Riding a bike, motorcycle, snowmobile, scooter, or all-terrain vehicle;

    -   Playing a contact sport, such as football, ice hockey, or boxing;

    -   Using in-line skates or riding a skateboard;

    -   Batting and running bases in baseball or softball;

    -   Riding a horse; or

    -   Skiing or snowboarding.

5. Making living areas safer for seniors, by:

    -   Removing tripping hazards such as throw rugs and clutter in walkways;

    -   Using nonslip mats in the bathtub and on shower floors; Installing grab bars next to the toilet and in the tub or shower;

    -   Installing handrails on both sides of stairways;

    -   Improving lighting throughout the home; and

    -   Maintaining a regular physical activity program, if your doctor agrees, to improve lower body strength and balance.

6. Making living areas safer for children, by:

    -   Installing window guards to keep young children from falling out of open windows; and

    -   Using safety gates at the top and bottom of stairs when young children are around.

7. Making sure the surface on your child's playground is made of shock-absorbing material, such as hardwood mulch or sand.

Know the Stages

Birth up to Age 2

Rear-facing car seat. For the best possible protection, infants and children should be kept in a rear-facing car seat, in the back seat buckled with the seat's harness, until they reach the upper weight or height limits of their particular seat. Check the seat owner's manual for weight and height limits.

Age 2 up to at least Age 5

Forward-facing car seat. When children outgrow their rear-facing seats they should ride in forward-facing car seats, in the back seat buckled with the seat's harness, until they reach the upper weight or height limit of their particular seat. Check the seat owner's manual for weight and height limits.

Age 5 up to at least Age 9

Booster seat. Once children outgrow their forward-facing seats (by reaching the upper height and weight limits of their seat), they should ride in belt positioning booster seats. Remember to keep children in the back seat for the best possible protection.

Once Seat Belts Fit Properly

Children should use booster seats until adult seat belts fit them properly. Seat belts fit properly when the lap belt lays across the upper thighs (not the stomach) and the shoulder belt fits across the chest (not the neck). The recommended height for proper seat belt fit is 57 inches tall. For the best possible protection keep children in the back seat and use lap-and-shoulder belts.

Severe TBI

Each year, TBIs contribute to a substantial number of deaths and cases of permanent disability. In fact, TBI is a contributing factor to a third (30%) of all injury-related deaths in the United States. In 2010, approximately 2.5 million people sustained a traumatic brain injury. Individuals with more severe injuries are more likely to require hospitalization.

Changes in the rates of TBI-related hospitalizations vary depending on age. For persons 44 years of age and younger, TBI-related hospitalizations decreased between the periods of 2001–2002 and 2009–2010. However, rates for age groups 45–64 years of age and 65 years and older increased between these time periods. Rates in persons 45–64 years of age increased almost 25 percent from 60.1–79.4 per 100,000. Rates of TBI-related hospitalizations in persons 65 years of age and older increased more than 50 percent, from 191.5–294.0 per 100,000 during the same period, largely due to a substantial increase (39%) between 2007–2008 and 2009–2010. In contrast, rates of TBI-related hospitalizations in youth 5–14 years of age fell from 54.5–23.1 per 100,000, decreasing by more than 50 percent during this period.

A severe TBI not only impacts the life of an individual and their family, but it also has a large societal and economic toll. The estimated economic cost of TBI in 2010, including direct and indirect medical costs, is estimated to be approximately $76.5 billion. Additionally, the cost of fatal TBIs and TBIs requiring hospitalization, many of which are severe, account for approximately 90 percent of the total TBI medical costs.

TBI Classification Systems

TBI injury severity can be described using several different tools.

The Glasgow Coma Scale (GCS), a clinical tool designed to assess coma and impaired consciousness, is one of the most commonly used severity scoring systems. Persons with GCS scores of 3–8 are classified with a severe TBI, those with scores of 9–12 are classified with a moderate TBI, and those with scores of 13–15 are classified with a mild TBI.

Other classification systems include the Abbreviated Injury Scale (AIS), the Trauma Score, and the Abbreviated Trauma Score. Despite their limitations, these systems are crucial to understanding the clinical management and the likely outcomes of this injury as the prognosis for milder forms of TBIs is better than for moderate or severe TBIs.

Potential Effects of Severe TBI

A nonfatal severe TBI may result in an extended period of unconsciousness (coma) or amnesia after the injury. For individuals hospitalized after a TBI, almost half (43%) have a related disability one year after the injury. A TBI may lead to a wide range of short- or long-term issues affecting:

- **Cognitive function** (e.g., attention and memory)

- **Motor function** (e.g., extremity weakness, impaired coordination and balance)

- **Sensation** (e.g., hearing, vision, impaired perception and touch)

- **Emotion** (e.g., depression, anxiety, aggression, impulse control, personality changes)

Approximately 5.3 million Americans are living with a TBI-related disability and the consequences of severe TBI can affect all aspects of an individual's life. This can include relationships with family and friends, as well as their ability to work or be employed, do household tasks, drive, and/or participate in other activities of daily living.

Meeting the Challenge of Severe TBI

While there is no one size fits all solution, there are interventions that can be effective to help limit the impact of this injury. These measures include primary prevention, early management, and treatment of severe TBI.

Section 31.2

Diagnosis and Treatment for TBI

This section includes text excerpted from "Traumatic Brain Injury: Hope through Research," National Institute of Neurological Disorders and Stroke (NINDS), September 2015.

How Is Traumatic Brain Injury (TBI) Diagnosed?

Although the majority of TBIs are mild they can still have serious health implications. Of greatest concern are injuries that can quickly grow worse. All TBIs require immediate assessment by a professional who has experience evaluating head injuries. A neurological exam will assess motor and sensory skills and the functioning of one or more cranial nerves. It will also test hearing and speech, coordination and balance, mental status, and changes in mood or behavior, among other abilities. Screening tools for coaches and athletic trainers can identify the most concerning concussions for medical evaluation.

Initial assessments may rely on standardized instruments such as the **Acute Concussion Evaluation (ACE)** form from the Centers for Disease Control and Prevention (CDC) or the **Sport Concussion Assessment Tool 2,** which provide a systematic way to assess a person who has suffered a mild TBI. Reviewers collect information about the characteristics of the injury, the presence of amnesia (loss of memory) and/or seizures, as well as the presence of physical, cognitive, emotional, and sleep-related symptoms. The ACE is also used to track symptom recovery over time. It also takes into account risk factors (including concussion, headache, and psychiatric history) that can impact how long it takes to recover from a TBI.

When necessary, medical providers will use brain scans to evaluate the extent of the primary brain injuries and determine if surgery will be needed to help repair any damage to the brain. The need for imaging is based on a physical examination by a doctor and a person's symptoms.

Computed tomography (CT) is the most common imaging technology used to assess people with suspected moderate to severe TBI. CT scans create a series of cross-sectional X-ray images of the skull and brain and can show fractures, hemorrhage, hematomas, hydrocephalus, contusions, and brain tissue swelling. CT scans are often used to assess the damage of a TBI in emergency room settings.

Magnetic resonance imaging (MRI) may be used after the initial assessment and treatment as it is a more sensitive test and picks up subtle changes in the brain that the CT scan might have missed.

Unlike moderate or severe TBI, mild TBI may not involve obvious signs of damage (hematomas, skull fracture, or contusion) that can be identified with current neuroimaging. Instead, much of what is believed to occur to the brain following mild TBI happens at the cellular level. Significant advances have been made in the last decade to image milder TBI damage. For example, diffusion tensor imaging (DTI) can image white matter tracts, more sensitive tests like fluid-attenuated inversion recovery (FLAIR) can detect small areas of damage, and susceptibility-weighted imaging very sensitively identifies bleeding. Despite these improvements, currently available imaging technologies, blood tests, and other measures remain inadequate for detecting these changes in a way that is helpful for diagnosing the mild concussive injuries.

Neuropsychological tests to gauge brain functioning are often used in conjunction with imaging in people who have suffered mild TBI. Such tests involve performing specific cognitive tasks that help assess memory, concentration, information processing, executive functioning, reaction time, and problem solving. The Glasgow Coma Scale (GCS) is the most widely used tool for assessing the level of consciousness after TBI. The standardized 15-point test measures a person's ability to open his or her eyes and respond to spoken questions or physical prompts for movement. A total score of 3–8 indicates a severe head injury; 9–12 indicates moderate injury; and 13–15 is classified as mild injury.

Many athletic organizations recommend establishing a baseline picture of an athlete's brain function at the beginning of each season, ideally before any head injuries have occurred. Baseline testing should begin as soon as a child begins a competitive sport. Brain function tests yield information about an individual's memory, attention, and ability to concentrate and solve problems. Brain function tests can be repeated at regular intervals (every 1–2 years) and also after a suspected concussion. The results may help healthcare providers identify any effects from an injury and allow them make more informed decisions about whether a person is ready to return to their normal activities.

How Is TBI Treated?

Many factors, including the size, severity, and location of the brain injury, influence how a TBI is treated and how quickly a person might recover. One of the critical elements to a person's prognosis is the severity of the injury. Although brain injury often occurs at the moment of head impact, much of the damage related to severe TBI develops from secondary injuries which happen days or weeks after the initial trauma. For this reason, people who receive immediate medical attention at a certified trauma center tend to have the best health outcomes.

Treating Mild TBI

Individuals with mild TBI, such as concussion, should focus on symptom relief and "brain rest." In these cases, headaches can often be treated with over-the-counter (OTC) pain relievers. People with mild TBI are also encouraged to wait to resume normal activities until given permission by a doctor. People with a mild TBI should:

- Make an appointment for a follow-up visit with their healthcare provider to confirm the progress of their recovery.

- Inquire about new or persistent symptoms and how to treat them.

- Pay attention to any new signs or symptoms even if they seem unrelated to the injury (for example, mood swings, unusual feelings of irritability). These symptoms may be related even if they occurred several weeks after the injury.

Even after symptoms resolve entirely, people should return to their daily activities gradually. Brain functionality may still be limited despite an absence of outward symptoms. Very little is known about the long-term effects of concussions on brain function. There is no clear timeline for a safe return to normal activities although there are guidelines such as those from the American Academy of Neurology (AAN) and the American Medical Society for Sports Medicine (AMSSM) to help determine when athletes can return to practice or competition. Further research is needed to better understand the effects of mild TBI on the brain and to determine when it is safe to resume normal activities.

Preventing future concussions is critical. While most people recover fully from a first concussion within a few weeks, the rate of recovery from a second or third concussion is generally slower.

In the days or weeks after a concussion, a minority of individuals may develop postconcussion syndrome (PCS). People can develop this syndrome even if they never lost consciousness. The symptoms include headache, fatigue, cognitive impairment, depression, irritability, dizziness and balance trouble, and apathy. These symptoms usually improve without medical treatment within one to a few weeks but some people can have longer lasting symptoms.

In some cases of moderate to severe TBI, persistent symptoms may be related to conditions triggered by imbalances in the production of hormones required for the brain to function normally. Hormone imbalances can occur when certain glands in the body, such as the pituitary gland, are damaged over time as result of the brain injury. Symptoms of these hormonal imbalances include weight loss or gain, fatigue, dry skin, impotence, menstrual cycle changes, depression, difficulty concentrating, hair loss, or cold intolerance. When these symptoms persist 3 months after their initial injury or when they occur up to 3 years after the initial TBI, people should speak with a healthcare provider about their condition.

Treating Severe TBI

Immediate treatment for the person who has suffered a severe TBI focuses on preventing death; stabilizing the person's spinal cord, heart, lung, and other vital organ functions; and preventing further brain damage. Persons with severe TBI generally require a breathing machine to ensure proper oxygen delivery and breathing.

During the acute management period, healthcare providers monitor the person's blood pressure, flow of blood to the brain, brain temperature, pressure inside the skull, and the brain's oxygen supply. A common practice called intracranial pressure (ICP) monitoring involves inserting a special catheter through a hole drilled into the skull. Doctors frequently rely on ICP monitoring as a way to determine if and when medications or surgery are needed in order to prevent secondary brain injury from swelling. People with severe head injury may require surgery to relieve pressure inside the skull, get rid of damaged or dead brain tissue (especially for penetrating TBI), or remove hematomas.

In-hospital strategies for managing people with severe TBI aim to prevent conditions including:

- Infection, particularly pneumonia

- Deep vein thrombosis (DVT) (blood clots that occur deep within a vein; risk increases during long periods of inactivity)

People with TBIs may need nutritional supplements to minimize the effects that vitamin, mineral, and other dietary deficiencies may cause over time. Some individuals may even require tube feeding to maintain the proper balance of nutrients.

Following the acute care period, people with severe TBI are often transferred to a rehabilitation center where a multidisciplinary team of healthcare providers help with recovery. The rehabilitation team includes neurologists, nurses, psychologists, nutritionists, as well as physical, occupational, vocational, speech, and respiratory therapists.

Cognitive rehabilitation therapy (CRT) is a strategy aimed at helping individuals regain their normal brain function through an individualized training program. Using this strategy, people may also learn compensatory strategies for coping with persistent deficiencies involving memory, problem solving, and the thinking skills to get things done. CRT programs tend to be highly individualized and their success varies. A 2011 Institute of Medicine (IOM) report concluded that cognitive rehabilitation interventions need to be developed and assessed more thoroughly.

Other Factors That Influence Recovery

Genes

Evidence suggests that genetics play a role in how quickly and completely a person recovers from a TBI. For example, researchers have found that apolipoprotein E ε4 (ApoE4)—a genetic variant associated with higher risks for Alzheimer disease (AD)—is associated with worse health outcomes following a TBI. Much work remains to be done to understand how genetic factors, as well as how specific types of head injuries in particular locations, affect recovery processes. It is hoped that this research will lead to new treatment strategies and improved outcomes for people with TBI.

Age

Studies suggest that age and the number of head injuries a person has suffered over his or her lifetime are two critical factors that impact recovery. For example, TBI-related brain swelling in children can be very different from the same condition in adults, even when the primary injuries are similar. Brain swelling in newborns, young infants, and teenagers often occurs much more quickly than it does in older individuals. Evidence from very limited chronic traumatic encephalopathy (CTE) studies suggest that younger people (ages 20–40) tend to have behavioral and mood changes associated with CTE, while those who are older (ages 50+) have more cognitive difficulties.

Compared with younger adults with the same TBI severity, older adults are likely to have less complete recovery. Older people also have more medical issues and are often taking multiple medications that may complicate treatment (e.g., blood-thinning agents when there is a risk of bleeding into the head). Further research is needed to determine if and how treatment strategies may need to be adjusted based on a person's age.

Researchers are continuing to look for additional factors that may help predict a person's course of recovery.

Section 31.3

Epilepsy Can Follow Traumatic Brain Injury

This section includes text excerpted from "Epilepsy Can Follow
Traumatic Brain Injury," Centers for Disease Control and
Prevention (CDC), March 27, 2017.

A traumatic brain injury (TBI) can happen to anyone, especially
young children and older adults. TBIs can range from mild TBIs (such
as concussions) to severe, life-threatening injuries. They can cause
problems such as changes in:

- Thinking and memory;

- Sensations and balance;

- Language, such as talking and understanding; and

- Emotions, such as depression, anxiety, or aggression.

TBI Can Cause Epilepsy

Epilepsy is a broad term used for a brain disorder that causes reoc-
curing seizures. There are many types of epilepsy and there are also
many different kinds of seizures. TBIs can cause a seizure right after
the injury happens or even months or years later. Researchers agree
that the more severe the TBI, the greater the chance the person may
develop epilepsy. Factors such as age and other medical conditions
also influence the chance a person may develop epilepsy after a TBI.

The terms post-traumatic epilepsy (PTE) and post-traumatic seizures (PTS) are both used to describe seizures that happen because
of a TBI. In 2013 there were over 280,000 hospitalizations for TBI
in the United States. A Centers for Disease Control and Prevention
(CDC)-funded study found that among people aged 15 years and older,
about 1 out of 10 developed epilepsy in the 3 years following a TBI that
required hospitalization.

Everyone should:

- Learn the signs and symptoms of TBI and when to seek medical
care.

- Take the CDC's HEADS UP training to learn how to recognize,
respond to, and minimize the risk of concussion or TBI if you're
a parent, coach, child care provider, or school professional.

If you or someone you care for has a head injury, here's what you need to know:

- Seek medical attention and share information about TBI signs and symptoms.

- Talk to the doctor about the risk for having seizures or developing epilepsy after a TBI.

- Learn to recognize the signs of a seizure. Sometimes it can be hard to tell. Some seizures cause a person to fall, cry out, shake or jerk, and become unaware of what's going on around them. Other seizures can make a person appear confused, make it hard for them to answer questions, twitch, or cause the person to feel like they taste, see or smell something unusual.

- Learn first aid so you are prepared if someone has a seizure.

To prevent TBIs that may cause epilepsy, protect your brain from injury. For example:

- Use seat belts and properly installed car safety seats every time you drive or ride in a motor vehicle.

- Never drive while under the influence of alcohol or drugs.

- Wear a helmet when playing certain sports and riding bikes, horses, motorcycles, or all-terrain vehicles.

- Prevent falls, especially in older adults and young children.

Section 31.4

Life after TBI

This section includes text excerpted from "Moderate to Severe Traumatic Brain Injury Is a Lifelong Condition," Centers for Disease Control and Prevention (CDC), September 15, 2016.

Moderate and severe traumatic brain injury (TBI) can lead to a lifetime of physical, cognitive, emotional, and behavioral changes. These changes may affect a person's ability to function in their everyday life. Despite initial hospitalization and inpatient rehabilitation services, about 50 percent of people with TBI will experience further decline in their daily lives or die within 5 years of their injury. Some of the health consequences of TBI can be prevented or reduced. Attending to these lifelong issues also known as chronic disease management, is crucial for improving the lives of persons with TBI. This section outlines the estimated burden of moderate and severe TBI on public health, and highlights key policy strategies to address the long-term consequences of TBI. The national estimates are based on data from the TBI Model Systems (TBIMS) National Database. It contains data from the largest study of people with moderate or severe TBI who receive inpatient rehabilitation, and includes information from the time of injury to the end of life. Those requiring inpatient rehabilitation are among the most severely injured and constitute less than 10 percent of all persons hospitalized with a TBI.

Long-Term Negative Effects of TBI Are Significant

Even after surviving a moderate or severe TBI and receiving inpatient rehabilitation services, a person's life expectancy is 9 years shorter. TBI increases the risk of dying from several causes. Compared to people without TBI, people with TBI are more likely to die from:

- Seizures (50x more likely)

- Accidental Drug Poisoning (11x more likely)

- Infections (9x more likely)

- Pneumonia (6x more likely)

After inpatient rehabilitation for TBI, the following groups are more likely to die sooner:

- Older adults

- Men

- Unemployed

- People who are not married

- People with fewer years of education

- People with more severe TBI

- People with fall-related TBI

In addition, people with moderate to severe TBI typically face a variety of chronic health problems. These issues add costs and burden to people with TBI, their families, and society. Among those still alive 5 years after injury:

- 57 percent are moderately or severely disabled.

- 55 percent do not have a job (but were employed at the time of their injury).

- 50 percent return to a hospital at least once.

- 33 percent rely on others for help with everyday activities.

- 29 percent are not satisfied with life.

- 29 percent use illicit drugs or misuse alcohol.

- 12 percent reside in nursing homes or other institutions.

Policy Implications: Proactive Management of TBI

With proper healthcare and community services, some causes of TBI-related problems can be prevented or treated, and the impact can be reduced. Because the problems faced by people with TBI are lasting, they require long-term solutions. While coordinated approaches to acute care and rehabilitation after TBI are available, only a few promote long-term health and well-being. At the federal level, decision-makers can:

- Recognize TBI as a chronic health condition.

- Review policies that affect access to rehabilitation services over the lifespan.

- Further research that addresses the future management of TBI.

- Enhance surveillance to monitor the national burden of TBI.

At the state level, decision-makers can:

- Identify the prevalence of disabilities due to TBI among their residents.

- Screen for TBI history among persons who receive state-funded health and social services.

- Train health and social service professionals to recognize and minimize the effects of TBI on behavior.

- Make home and community services more accessible to people with TBI.

  Healthcare providers can:

- Determine if their patients have experienced TBI and understand the impact of TBI

- on the current health status of patients.

- Screen for and treat common, late-developing problems, such as depression, substance misuse, and weight gain.

- Encourage lifestyles that promote brain health.

- Educate patients and their families to prevent or reduce late-occurring problems.

Section 31.5

After Effects of TBI

This section includes text excerpted from "Traumatic Brain Injury:
A Guide For Patients," U.S. Department of Veterans Affairs (VA),
January 18, 2009. Reviewed February 2018.

Poor Concentration

The main cause of poor concentration is tiredness. When it becomes difficult to concentrate on what you're doing, take a break and relax. Between 15 and 30 minutes a day should be enough. If you still continue to have problems, your work day, class schedule, or daily routine should be temporarily shortened. Trying to "stick to it" won't help, and usually makes things worse.

Reducing distractions can help. Turn down the radio or try to work where it's quiet. At first, avoiding noisy environments may be helpful, then return to them gradually. Don't try to do too many things at once. Writing while you talk on the phone or taking notes as you listen to someone are examples of doing two things at the same time. It may be difficult for you to concentrate on more than one thing at first. You will be able to concentrate when you've had enough rest. So, if you really need to concentrate on something important, do so when you're feeling fresh.

Fatigue

It is normal to be more tired after a head injury. Most people experience some degree of fatigue during their recovery. The only sensible treatment for being tired is rest. Avoid wearing yourself out. Gradually increase your activity level. You may find that you need to sleep more than usual, in which case it is a good idea to get the extra sleep that you need. Most patients have more energy in the morning than later in the day. An afternoon nap can help if you find that it is harder to do things at the end of the day. Physical and mental fatigue usually diminishes over time; it should be greatly improved within 6 months after a brain injury.

It may seem counterintuitive, but a well-designed exercise program can help your physical and mental endurance. Adding activity gradually is the key. For instance, an hour of morning activity may be all that you can handle. From there, you slowly and incrementally add activity followed by rest breaks. Closely monitor your fatigue levels until you reach an acceptable level that you can tolerate, and be careful to avoid extreme fatigue.

Sleep Difficulties

You might expect that the fatigue you experience during recovery would cause you to sleep more soundly. However, sleep disturbance is actually quite common following a brain injury. Studies have shown that individuals who suffer a brain injury often have difficulty getting to sleep and maintaining uninterrupted sleep at night, and thus experience excessive daytime sleepiness. When they do sleep, their sleep is lighter and less restful, and they frequently awaken. Getting adequate sleep is very important in the healing process. If you don't sleep well at night, you'll be more tired during the day. When you're tired during the day, you'll find it difficult to concentrate, and may become irritable and angry more easily. Thus, lack of sleep can exacerbate your other symptoms.

Irritability and Emotional Changes

Some people show emotions more easily after a brain injury. They may yell at people or say things they wouldn't normally say, or get annoyed easily by things that normally would not upset them. Some may even get violent. You may also find that you get more emotional in other ways, getting frustrated or tearful when you normally wouldn't. This behavior does not necessarily mean that you are feeling a deep emotion, but can occur because the brain is not regulating emotions to the same extent as before the injury. If any of these episodes happen, it is usually a sign that it is time to take a rest from what you are doing and get away from it. There are a variety of different techniques to deal with irritability. Some people find that leaving the frustrating situation temporarily is helpful. Others employ relaxation techniques or attempt to use up emotional energy through exercise. One frequent cause of irritability and emotionality is fatigue. People lose their tempers more easily when they are tired or overworked. Adjust your schedule and get more rest if you notice yourself becoming irritable or emotional.

Everyone gets angry from time to time, often with good reason. Being irritable only becomes a problem when it interferes with your ability to get along with people from day to day. If you find yourself getting into arguments that cause trouble at home or work, try to change the way you think about things. Thoughts often make us more angry than what actually happened. You can see this yourself by imagining an irritating situation and why it would make you angry.

There is usually a reason that irritating things happen. When something makes you angry, ask yourself what caused it. Family, friends, or coworkers can do things that bother us at times. Try to think of why they did whatever it was that irritated you. What would they say the reason was? Thinking about what caused a problem is the first step toward solving it. Problems can usually be solved better if you stay calm and explain your point of view. The steps you need to take to solve a problem will be the same when you are calm as they would be if you were irritated. Try to remind yourself of this when you find yourself becoming irritable.

You can usually come up with several ways to solve a problem. Try to think of at least five different ways, and then decide on which is best. Just realizing that there are several things you can do to solve a problem will make it a lot less irritating.

Depression

For reasons we do not fully understand, depression seems to occur more often after a brain injury. More than one-third of people with recent traumatic brain injury become depressed, especially during the first year after injury. One reason for this increase in depression may be because brain injury causes an imbalance in certain chemicals in the brain and disrupts brain networks critical for mood regulation.

Another cause of depression in TBI may be psychological and social changes such as losing friends, losing abilities, and not being able to return to work or other meaningful activities after injury. Simply put, people become depressed when unpleasant things happen to them, and a head injury is unpleasant. We feel good when good things happen to us. Thus, an effective way to treat depression is to make sure that good things happen. One way to do this is to plan to do something enjoyable for yourself each day. Make your plan specific, and then be sure to stick to it. Decide on an activity you like and exactly when you are going to do it. That way you can look forward to it. Anticipating and doing enjoyable things each day will improve your mood.

Chances are that if you are depressed, you are telling yourself things that are depressing. Thinking that the situation is terrible, that there is no end to it in sight, that you aren't able to do anything about it, and that it is your fault are all depressing things to tell yourself. Thinking this way can become a habit if you do it enough. Usually, when people tell themselves unpleasant things all the time it is out of habit, not because those things are really true. If you find yourself thinking depressing thoughts, stop. Simply stopping a depressing thought can make you feel better. See if what you are telling yourself is really true.

Memory Problems

Memory difficulties have several causes. The part of our brain that stores memories is called the temporal lobe. This is the part of the brain that is most likely to be bruised in a head injury. Some memory difficulties can be caused by the bruises, which is why you may not remember the accident very well. Like a black and blue mark on your arm or leg, these bruises will recover with time. Your memory will most likely improve as this happens. Most of the memory problems that patients notice after a head injury are not caused by bruising.

They usually come from poor concentration and being tired. For you to remember something, you have to pay attention to it first. If you don't concentrate long enough, the information is never stored in your memory. Concentration problems are a normal part of recovering from a head injury and some memory trouble is a normal side effect of this. You will probably be able to concentrate and remember better when you get enough rest. Memory problems can be a sign that you are pushing yourself too hard. Writing important things down, using a pocket tape recorder, and asking for reminders are other excellent ways of coping with temporary memory difficulties. They will help recovery and not slow it down.

Of course, nobody's memory is perfect anyway. After a head injury, it can be easy to forget that we sometimes had trouble remembering things even before the accident. Some of the symptoms you notice may actually have nothing to do with your head injury. A list of common memory "problems" is shown below along with the percentage of people who experience each "symptom" even though they didn't have a head injury.

Worrying about remembering things that you would normally forget can make your memory seem worse to you. If you can remember your memory problems, you probably don't have much of a memory problem! People with serious memory difficulties are usually not upset by their symptoms. They don't remember that they have any memory trouble.

Headaches

Headaches are part of the normal recovery process, but that doesn't make them any less bothersome. Not only are they painful to experience, but frequent headaches can take a toll on you mentally and emotionally, and are a common cause of irritability and concentration problems following a head injury. This guide cannot replace the medical advice that you should get if you are bothered by headaches. Headaches can have many causes, and your doctor will want to diagnose the problem and prescribe medication that can help if you need it.

One of the most common causes of headaches after a head injury is stress or tension. This is usually the cause when the headaches start for the first time several weeks after the injury.

These headaches mean that you are trying to do too much. They will probably disappear if you take a break and relax. Your workday, class schedule, or daily routine should be temporarily shortened if you continue to have headaches. Stress or worry cause tension headaches by increasing muscle tension in your neck or forehead. These muscles become tense and can stay tight without you realizing it, out of habit. They can become even tighter once a headache starts, because muscles automatically tense in reaction to pain. This muscle tension makes the headaches worse.

If you have tension headaches, relaxing your muscles can help. One way to do this is with a method called progressive muscle relaxation. Start by clenching your hand into a fist, as hard as you can. Notice how the muscle tension feels. Now relax your hand completely and notice the difference. Now clench both your hands as hard as you can and hold them that way for a moment or two before letting them relax completely. Notice the difference. Now continue to tense and relax more muscles groups by adding a different set each time: hands, arms, face, chest, stomach, buttocks, legs, feet. This method works best if you are lying on your back. Finally, tense all the muscles in your body at once as hard as you can, and then let them relax.

At this point all your muscles will be very, very relaxed. Progressive muscle relaxation can help prevent tension headaches by relaxing your muscles. This works best if you practice it each day at about the same time for 5 minutes or so. But, be sure that you DO NOT use this technique while you are having a headache.

Anxiety

Worry about symptoms and problems at work is the main cause of anxiety for many patients. Anxiety should not be a problem for you if you understand that your symptoms are a normal part of recovery, get enough rest, and gradually increase your responsibilities at work. If you are anxious, chances are that you are telling yourself things that are making you that way. Usually, when people worry all the time it is out of habit, not because the things that they are telling themselves are really true. The steps you need to take to solve a problem will be the same when you are calm as they would be if you were anxious. If you find yourself thinking anxious thoughts, stop. Simply stopping an anxious thought can make you feel better. See if what you are telling yourself is really true.

Confusion and Trouble Thinking

Many people feel uncertain, perplexed, or confused after a head injury. They find that their mind and feelings don't react in the ways they used to. They may fear that they are "going crazy." This is a normal reaction to a head injury. If you have these feelings, it is good to talk about them with someone you trust.

Trouble thinking is often a side effect of other symptoms. Concentration problems, being tired, headaches, and anxiety can all make it hard to think clearly. Like these other symptoms, trouble thinking is probably a sign that you are doing too much too soon. Dizziness, visual difficulties, and light sensitivity Dizziness and visual difficulties should be checked by your doctor. These symptoms usually go away

353

by themselves in 3–6 months or less in most patients. If you find these symptoms troublesome, your doctor may want to prescribe medication for motion sickness, or eyeglasses. Some motion sickness medications are very effective for dizziness, but can make you drowsy or reduce your attention span as side effects.

You may notice some increased sensitivity to bright light or loud noise, particularly if you have headaches. Some increased sensitivity is normal after a head injury. But, scientific studies by neurosurgeons and neuropsychologists in New Zealand show that a person's actual sensitivity to light and noise has nothing to do with how much light and noise bother them. Paying attention to these symptoms makes them seem worse, because paying attention to a feeling seems to magnify or increase it. The less you think and worry about your symptoms, the faster they will usually go away.

Chapter 32

Abusive Head Trauma (Shaken Baby Syndrome)

What Is Shaken Baby Syndrome?

Shaken baby syndrome (SBS) is a severe form of physical child abuse. SBS may be caused from vigorously shaking an infant by the shoulders, arms, or legs. The "whiplash" effect can cause intracranial (within the brain) or intraocular (within the eyes) bleeding. Often there is no obvious external head trauma. Still, children with SBS may display some outward signs:

- Change in sleeping pattern or inability to be awakened

- Confused, restless, or agitated state

- Convulsions or seizures

- Loss of energy or motivation

- Slurred speech

- Uncontrollable crying

This chapter contains text excerpted from the following sources: Text beginning with the heading "What Is Shaken Baby Syndrome?" is excerpted from "Gateway to Health Communication—Shaken Baby Syndrome," Centers for Disease Control and Prevention (CDC), September 15, 2017; Text beginning with the heading "Is There Any Treatment?" is excerpted from "Shaken Baby Syndrome," National Institute of Neurological Disorders and Stroke (NINDS), December 21, 2016.

355

- Inability to be consoled

- Inability to nurse or eat

SBS can result in death, mental retardation or developmental delays, paralysis, severe motor dysfunction, spasticity, blindness, and seizures.

Who's at Risk?

Small children are especially vulnerable to this type of abuse. Their heads are large in comparison to their bodies, and their neck muscles are weak. Children under one year of age are at highest risk, but SBS has been reported in children up to five years of age. Shaking often occurs in response to a baby crying or having a toilet-training accident. The perpetrator tends to be male and is primarily the biological father or the mother's boyfriend or partner. Caregivers are responsible for about 9–21 percent of cases. The explanation typically provided by the caregiver—"I was playing with the baby"—does not begin to account for the severity of trauma. Many times there is also a history of child abuse.

Can It Be Prevented?

SBS is completely preventable. However, it is not known whether educational efforts will effectively prevent this type of abuse. Home visitation programs are shown to prevent child abuse in general. Because the child's father or the mother's partner often causes SBS, they should be included in home visitation programs. Home visits bring community resources to families in their homes. Health professionals provide information, healthcare, psychological support, and other services that can help people to be more effective parents and caregivers.

SBS is completely preventable. However, it is not known whether educational efforts will effectively prevent this type of abuse. Home visitation programs are shown to prevent child abuse in general. Because the child's father or the mother's partner often causes SBS, they should be included in home visitation programs. Home visits bring community resources to families in their homes. Health professionals provide information, healthcare, psychological support, and other services that can help people to be more effective parents and caregivers.

Is There Any Treatment?

Emergency treatment for a shaken baby often includes life support measures such as breathing support and surgery to stop internal bleeding and brain hemorrhage. Doctors can make diagnostic images of the brain, using magnetic resonance imaging (MRI) or computed tomography (CT), to make the definitive diagnosis.

What Is the Prognosis?

Compared with accidental brain trauma in babies, shaken baby injuries have a worse prognosis. Damage to the retina can cause blindness. Most babies who survive severe shaking will have some form of neurological or mental disability, such as cerebral palsy (CP), or mental retardation, which may not be apparent until they are 6 years old. Children who suffer shaken baby syndrome may need medical care for the rest of their lives.

Chapter 33

Preventing Traumatic Brain Injuries

General Prevention

Car and Booster Seats

- Motor vehicle injuries are a leading cause of death among children in the United States. But many of these deaths can be prevented. Buckling children in age- and size-appropriate car seats, booster seats, and seat belts reduces serious and fatal injuries by more than half.

Helmets

Making sure your child always wears the right helmet for their activity and that it fits correctly. Wearing a helmet is a must to help reduce the risk of a serious brain injury or skull fracture. However, helmets are not designed to prevent concussions. There is no "concussion proof" helmet.

Your child's helmet should fit properly and be:

- Well maintained

- Age appropriate

This chapter includes text excerpted from "Brain Injury Safety Tips and Prevention," Centers for Disease Control and Prevention (CDC), March 14, 2017.

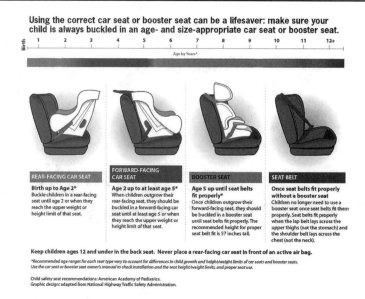

Using the correct car seat or booster seat can be a lifesaver: make sure your child is always buckled in an age- and size-appropriate car seat or booster seat.

REAR-FACING CAR SEAT

Birth up to Age 2*
Buckle children in a rear-facing seat until age 2 or when they reach the upper weight or height limit of that seat.

FORWARD-FACING CAR SEAT

Age 2 up to at least age 5*
When children outgrow their rear-facing seat, they should be buckled in a forward-facing car seat until at least age 5 or when they reach the upper weight or height limit of that seat.

BOOSTER SEAT

Age 5 up until seat belts fit properly*
Once children outgrow their forward-facing seat, they should be buckled in a booster seat until seat belts fit properly. The recommended height for proper seat belt fit is 57 inches tall.

SEAT BELT

Once seat belts fit properly without a booster seat
Children no longer need to use a booster seat once seat belts fit them properly. Seat belts fit properly when the lap belt lays across the upper thighs (not the stomach) and the shoulder belt lays across the chest (not the neck).

Keep children ages 12 and under in the back seat. Never place a rear-facing car seat in front of an active air bag.

*Recommended age ranges for each seat type vary to account for differences in child growth and height/weight limits of car seats and booster seats. Use the car seat or booster seat owner's manual to check installation and the seat height/weight limits, and proper seat use.

Child safety seat recommendations: American Academy of Pediatrics.
Graphic design: adapted from National Highway Traffic Safety Administration.

Figure 33.1. *Rear Facing Car Seat Positions*

- Worn consistently and correctly
- Appropriately certified for use

While there is no concussion-proof helmet, a helmet can help protect your child or teen from a serious brain or head injury. Even with a helmet, it is important for your child or teen to avoid hits to the head.

Stair Gates

Using gates at the top and bottom of stairs to prevent serious falls in infants and toddlers. We all want to keep our children safe and secure and help them live to their full potential. Knowing how to prevent leading causes of child injury, like falls, is a step toward this goal.

Falls are the leading cause of nonfatal injuries for all children ages 0–19. Every day, approximately 8,000 children are treated in U.S. emergency rooms for fall-related injuries. This adds up to almost 2.8 million children each year. Thankfully, many falls can be prevented, and parents and caregivers can play a key role in protecting children.

Soft Surfaces

Using playgrounds with soft material under them like mulch or sand, not grass or dirt.

Preventing Brain Injuries in Sports

Create a Safe Sport Culture

Young athletes deserve to play sports in a culture that celebrates their hard work, dedication, and teamwork, and in programs that seek to create a safe environment—especially when it comes to concussion. As a youth sports coach or parent, your actions can create a safe sport culture and can lower an athlete's chance of getting a concussion or other serious injury.

Athletes thrive when they:

- Have fun playing their sport.

- Receive positive messages and praise from their coaches for concussion symptom reporting.

- Have parents who talk with them about concussion and model and expect safe play.

- Get written instructions from a healthcare provider on when to return to school and play.

- Support their teammates sitting out of play if they have concussion.

- Feel comfortable reporting symptoms of a possible concussion to coaches.

Enforce the Rules

Enforce the rules of the sport for fair play, safety, and sportsmanship. Ensure athletes avoid unsafe actions such as:

- Striking another athlete in the head;

- Using their head or helmet to contact another athlete;

- Making illegal contacts or checking, tackling, or colliding with an unprotected opponent; and/or

- Trying to injure or put another athlete at risk for injury.

Tell athletes you expect good sportsmanship at all times, both on and off the playing field.

Talk about Concussion Reporting

Talk with athletes about the importance of reporting a concussion.

Some athletes may not report a concussion because they don't think a concussion is serious. They may also worry about:

- Losing their position on the team or during the game.

- Jeopardizing their future sports career.

- Looking weak.

- Letting their teammates down.

- What their coach or teammates might think of them.

Get a Concussion Action Plan in Place

Create an action plan that includes information on how to teach athletes ways to lower their chances of getting a concussion. If you think an athlete may have a concussion, you should:

1. **Remove the athlete from play.**

2. **Keep an athlete with a possible concussion out of play on the same day of the injury and until cleared by a healthcare provider.** Do not try to judge the severity of the injury yourself. Only a healthcare provider should assess an athlete for a possible concussion.

3. **Record and share information about the injury,** such as how it happened and the athlete's symptoms, to help a healthcare provider assess the athlete.

4. **Inform the athlete's parent(s) or guardian(s)** about a possible concussion.

5. **Ask for written instructions from the athlete's healthcare provider** about the steps you should take to help the athlete safely return to play. Before returning to play an athlete should:

   - Be back to doing their regular school activities.

   - Not have any symptoms from the injury when doing normal activities.

   - Have the green light from their healthcare provider to begin the return to play process.

Why This Is Important

Athletes May Try to Hide Concussion Symptoms

- As many as 7 in 10 young athletes with a possible concussion report playing with concussion symptoms.

- Out of those, 4 in 10 said their coaches were unaware that they had a possible concussion.

Enforce Safe Play. You Set the Tone for Safety

- As many as 25 percent of the concussions reported among high school athletes result from aggressive or illegal play.

Young Athletes Are More Likely to Play with a Concussion during a Big Game

- In almost all sports, concussion rates are higher during competitions than in practice.
- Athletes may be less likely to tell their coach or athletic trainer about a possible concussion during a championship game or other important event.

Most Sports Related Concussions Are Caused by Player to Player Contact

- Over two-thirds (70%) of concussions among young athletes result from contact with another athlete.
- This is followed by player to surface contact (17%), such as hitting the ground or other obstacle.

Headache Is Most Commonly Reported Concussion Symptom

- Almost all (94%) high school athletes with a concussion reported having a headache.
- Other commonly reported symptoms include:
  - Dizziness (76%)
  - Trouble concentrating (55%)
  - Confusion (45%)
  - Bothered by light (36%)
  - Nausea (31%)

Chapter 34

Agnosia

Agnosia is characterized by an inability to recognize and identify objects and/or persons. Symptoms may vary, according to the area of the brain that is affected. It can be limited to one sensory modality such as vision or hearing; for example, a person may have difficulty in recognizing an object as a cup or identifying a sound as a cough.

Agnosia can result from strokes, traumatic brain injury (TBI), dementia, a tumor, developmental disorders, overexposure to environmental toxins (e.g., carbon monoxide poisoning), or other neurological conditions. **Visual agnosia** may also occur in association with other underlying disorders.

Symptoms

People with **primary visual agnosia** may have one or several impairments in visual recognition without impairment of intelligence, motivation, and/or attention. Vision is almost always intact and the mind is clear. Some affected individuals do not have the ability to recognize familiar objects. They can see objects, but are unable to identify them by sight. However, objects may be identified by touch, sound, and/or smell. For example, affected individuals may not be able to identify a set of keys by sight, but can identify them upon holding them in their hands.

This chapter includes text excerpted from "Agnosia," Genetic and Rare Diseases Information Center (GARD), National Center for Advancing Translational Sciences (NCATS), April 22, 2011. Reviewed February 2018.

Some researchers separate visual agnosia into two broad categories: apperceptive agnosia and associative agnosia. **Apperceptive agnosia** refers to individuals who cannot properly process what they see, meaning they have difficult identifying shapes or differentiating between different objects (visual stimuli). Affected individuals may not be able to recognize that pictures of the same object from different angles are of the same object. Affected individuals may be unable to copy (e.g., draw a picture) of an object. **Associative agnosia** refers to people who cannot match an object with their memory. They can accurately describe an object and even draw a picture of the object, but are unable to state what the object is or is used for. However, if told verbally what the object is, an affected individual will be able to describe what it is used for.

In some cases, individuals with primary visual agnosia cannot identify familiar people **(prosopagnosia)**. They can see the person clearly and can describe the person (e.g., hair and eye color), but cannot identify the person by name. People with prosopagnosia may identify people by touch, smell, speech, or the way that they walk (gait). In some rare cases, affected individuals cannot recognize their own face.

Some people have a form of **primary visual agnosia** associated with the loss of the ability to identify their surroundings (loss of environmental familiarity agnosia). Symptoms include the inability to recognize familiar places or buildings. Affected individuals may be able to describe a familiar environment from memory and point to it on a map.

Simultanagnosia is characterized by the inability to read and the inability to view one's surroundings as a whole. The affected individual can see parts of the surrounding scene, but not the whole. There is an inability to comprehend more than one part of a visual scene at a time or to coordinate the parts.

In rare cases, people with primary visual agnosia may not be able to recognize or point to various parts of the body **(autotopagnosia)**. Symptoms may also include loss of the ability to distinguish left from right.

Cause

Primary visual agnosia occurs as a result of damage to the brain. Symptoms develop due to the inability to retrieve information from those damaged areas that are associated with visual memory. Lesions may occur as a result of traumatic brain injury, stroke, tumor, or overexposure to dangerous environmental toxins (e.g., carbon monoxide poisoning). In some cases, the cause of the brain damage may not be known. Symptoms may vary, according to the area of the brain that is affected.

Visual agnosia may also occur in association with other underlying disorders (secondary visual agnosia) such as Alzheimer disease (AD), agenesis of the corpus callosum, Mitochondrial encephalomyopathy, lactic acidosis, and stroke-like episodes (MELAS), and other diseases that result in progressive dementia. Disorders that may precede the development of primary visual agnosia (and may be useful in identifying an underlying cause of some forms of this disorder) include AD, Pick disease, and a rare disorder called Balint syndrome.

Diagnosis

A variety of psychophysical tests can be conducted to pinpoint the nature of the visual process that is disrupted in an individual. Brain damage that causes visual agnosia may be identified through imaging techniques, including computed tomography (CT scan) and magnetic resonance imaging (MRI).

Treatment

People with agnosia may retain their cognitive abilities in other areas. Treatment of primary agnosia is symptomatic and supportive; when it is caused by an underlying disorder, treatment of the disorder may reduce symptoms and help prevent further brain damage.

Chapter 35

Cerebral Aneurysm

What Is a Cerebral Aneurysm?

A cerebral aneurysm (also known as an intracranial or intracerebral aneurysm) is a weak or thin spot in a cerebral blood vessel that sticks out like a balloon and fills with blood. The outgoing aneurysm can put pressure on a nerve or surrounding brain tissue. They can also lose or break, spilling blood into the surrounding tissue (called hemorrhage). Some brain aneurysms, particularly very small ones, do not bleed or cause other problems. Brain aneurysms can occur anywhere in the brain, but most are located next to the loop of arteries that pass between the lower part of the brain and the base of the skull.

What Causes a Cerebral Aneurysm?

Most cerebral aneurysms are congenital, due to an inborn abnormality of an arterial wall. Cerebral aneurysms are more common in people with certain genetic diseases, such as connective tissue disorders (CTD) and polycystic kidney disease (PKD), and certain circulatory disorders, such as arteriovenous malformations.*

Other causes can be trauma or head injury, high blood pressure (BP), infection, tumors, atherosclerosis (a disease of the blood vessels where fats accumulate inside the arterial walls) and other diseases

---

This chapter includes text excerpted from "Cerebral Aneurysms Fact Sheet," National Institute of Neurological Disorders and Stroke (NINDS), December 20, 2016.

369

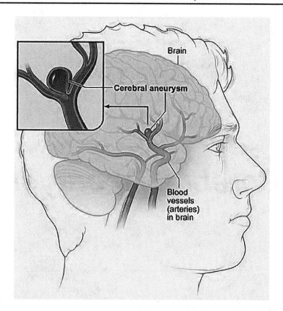

Figure 35.1. *Brain Aneurysm*

The illustration shows a typical location of a brain aneurysm in the arteries that supply blood to the brain. The inset image shows a closeup view of the sac-like aneurysm. (Source: "Aneurysm," National Heart, Lung, and Blood Institute (NHLBI).)

of the vascular system, cigarette smoking, and drug abuse. Some researchers have speculated that oral contraceptives may increase the risk of developing aneurysms.

The aneurysms that result from an infection in the arterial wall are called fungal aneurysms. Aneurysms related to cancer are often associated with primary or metastatic tumors of the head and neck. Drug abuse, particularly habitual cocaine use, can inflame blood vessels and lead to the development of cerebral aneurysms.

A congenital malformation where a tangle of cerebral arteries and veins interrupts the blood flow.

How Are Aneurysms Classified?

There are three types of cerebral aneurysm. The saccular aneurysm is a sack of blood that is rounded or resembles a sachet that is attached by the neck or peduncle to an artery or branch of a blood vessel. Also known as "berry" aneurysm (because it looks like a berry hanging from a vine), this common form of cerebral aneurysm is typically found in arteries at the base of the brain. Saccular aneurysms appear more frequently in adults. A lateral aneurysm appears as a lump on a wall of the blood vessel, while a fusiform aneurysm is formed by the widening of all the walls of the vessel.

Aneurysms are also classified by size. Small aneurysms are less than 11 millimeters in diameter (about the size of a standard pencil eraser), larger aneurysms are 11–25 millimeters (about the width of a dime), and giant aneurysms have more than 25 millimeters in diameter (more than the width of a 25 cents coin).

Who Is at Risk?

Brain aneurysms can occur in anyone, at any age. They are more common in adults than in children and slightly more common in women than men. People with certain inherited disorders are also at higher risk.

All brain aneurysms have the potential to rupture and cause bleeding within the brain. The reported incidence of ruptured aneurysm is about 10 out of every 100,000 people per year (about 27,000 patients per year in the United States), commonly in people between 30–60 years old. The possible risk factors for rupture are hypertension, alcohol abuse, drug abuse (particularly cocaine), and smoking. In addition, the state and size of the aneurysm affect the risk of rupture.

What Are the Dangers?

Aneurysms can burst and bleed inside the brain, causing serious complications such as hemorrhagic stroke, permanent nerve damage, or both. Once it bursts, the aneurysm may burst again and bleed back into the brain, and additional aneurysms may occur. Commonly, rupture can cause a subarachnoid hemorrhage, bleeding in the space between the skull and the brain. A delayed but serious complication of subarachnoid hemorrhage is hydrocephalus, where the excessive accumulation of cerebrospinal fluid in the skull dilates the fluid pathways called ventricles that can swell and compress brain tissue. Another delayed complication after rupture is vasospasm, where other cerebral blood vessels contract and limit blood flow to vital areas of the brain. This reduced blood flow can cause a stroke or tissue damage.

What Are the Symptoms?

Most brain aneurysms show no symptoms until they are very large or burst. Small aneurysms that do not change usually will not have symptoms, while a larger aneurysm that grows constantly can compress nerves and tissues. Symptoms may include pain above and behind the eyes; numbness, weakness, or paralysis on one side of the face; dilated pupils and changes in vision. When an aneurysm bleeds, the individual may have severe sudden headache, double vision, nausea, vomiting, stiff neck, or loss of consciousness. Patients generally describe headache as "the worst of their life" and are generally different in intensity and severity from other headaches they have had. Warning headaches or "sentinels" They may be due to an aneurysm that you lose from days to weeks before breaking up. Only a minority of patients have a sentinel headache before the rupture of the aneurysm.

Other signs that a brain aneurysm has burst are nausea and vomiting associated with severe headache, a drooping eyelid, sensitivity to light and changes in mental status or level of consciousness. Some individuals may have seizures, others may briefly lose consciousness or enter a prolonged coma. People who have the "worst headache," especially when combined with other symptoms should seek immediate medical attention.

How Are Brain Aneurysms Diagnosed?

Most brain aneurysms go unnoticed until it is broken or detected by brain images that may have been obtained from another condition. Various diagnostic methods are available to provide information about the aneurysm and the best form of treatment. The tests are usually obtained after a subarachnoid hemorrhage to confirm the diagnosis of an aneurysm.

Angiography is a test with dye used to analyze the arteries or veins. An intracerebral angiography can detect the degree of narrowing or obstruction of an artery or blood vessel in the brain, head or neck, and can identify changes in an artery or vein such as a weak spot, such as an aneurysm. It is used to diagnose stroke and to accurately determine the location, size, and shape of a brain tumor, aneurysm, or blood vessel that has bled. This test is usually done in the angiography room of a hospital. After the injection of a local anesthetic, a flexible catheter is inserted into an artery and advanced through the body to the affected artery. A small amount of contrast dye (which is highlighted on X-rays) is released into the bloodstream and allowed to travel to the head and neck.

The computed tomography (CT) of the head is a tool quick, painless and noninvasive diagnosis may reveal cerebral aneurysm and determine, for those aneurysms bursting, if liquid has passed the brain.

Often, this is the first diagnostic procedure indicated by a doctor after the suspected rupture. X-rays of the head are processed in a computer as two-dimensional transverse images, or "slices," of the brain and skull. Occasionally a contrast dye is injected into the bloodstream before the test. This process, called CT angiography, produces sharper and more detailed images of blood flow and cerebral arteries. CT is usually done in a testing center or outpatient hospital setting.

The magnetic resonance imaging (MRI) using radio waves computer and a powerful magnetic field to produce detailed images of the brain and other body structures generated. The magnetic resonance angiography (MRA) produces more detailed images of blood vessels. The images can be viewed as three-dimensional or two-dimensional cross sections of the brain and vessels. These painless and noninvasive procedures can show the size and shape of an unruptured aneurysm and can detect bleeding in the brain.

A cerebrospinal fluid (CSF) test may be ordered if a ruptured aneurysm is suspected. After the application of a local anesthetic, a small amount of this fluid (which protects the brain and spinal cord) is removed from the subarachnoid space, located between the spinal cord and the surrounding membranes, with a surgical needle and examined to detect any bleeding or cerebral hemorrhage. In patients with suspected subarachnoid hemorrhage, this procedure is usually done in a hospital.

How Are Cerebral Aneurysms Treated?

Not all brain aneurysms burst. Some patients with very small aneurysms can be monitored for growth or onset of symptoms and to ensure aggressive treatment of coexisting medical problems and risk factors. Each case is unique, and the considerations for treating an unruptured aneurysm are the type, size and location of the aneurysm; the risk of rupture; the patient's age, health, personal and family medical history and the risk of treatment.

Two surgical options are available to treat cerebral aneurysms, where both carry some risk to the patient (such as possible damage to other blood vessels, the potential for recurrence of the aneurysm and new bleeding, and the risk of a postoperative stroke).

Microvascular clipping involves cutting the blood flow to the aneurysm. Under anesthesia, a section of the skull is removed and the aneurysm is located. The neurosurgeon uses a microscope to isolate the blood vessel that feeds the aneurysm and places a small, metal, brooch like clip around his neck, stopping the blood supply. The clip remains in the patient and avoids the risk of future bleeding. Then the piece of skull is replaced and the scalp is closed. It has been shown that clipping is highly effective, depending on the location, shape and size of the aneurysm. In general, aneurysms that close completely do not return.

A related procedure is occlusion, in which the surgeon closes (occludes) the entire artery leading to the aneurysm. This procedure is often done when the aneurysm has damaged the artery. Sometimes an occlusion is accompanied by a bypass, in which a small blood vessel is surgically grafted to the cerebral artery, recanalizing the blood flow out of the section of the damaged artery.

Endovascular embolization is an alternative to surgery. Once the patient has been anesthetized, the doctor inserts a hollow plastic tube (a catheter) into an artery (usually in the groin) and advances it, using angiography, through the body to the site of the aneurysm. Using a guidewire, removable spirals (platinum wire coils) or small latex balloons are passed through the catheter and released into the aneurysm. Spirals or balloons fill the aneurysm, block it from circulation, and cause the blood to clot, effectively destroying the aneurysm. It is possible that the procedure should be performed more than once in the patient's life.

Patients who are treated for an aneurysm should stay in bed until the bleeding stops. Underlying conditions, such as high blood pressure, should be treated. Another treatment of cerebral aneurysm is symptomatic and may include anticonvulsants to prevent seizures and analgesics to treat headaches. Vasospasm can be treated with calcium channel blockers, and sedatives may be indicated if the patient is restless. A shunt can be surgically inserted into a ventricle several months after the rupture if the accumulation of cerebrospinal fluid is causing harmful pressure on the surrounding tissue. Patients who have suffered a subarachnoid hemorrhage often need rehabilitation therapy.

Can Cerebral Aneurysms Be Prevented?

There are no known ways to prevent a brain aneurysm from forming. People with a diagnosed brain aneurysm should carefully monitor high blood pressure, stop smoking, and avoid the use of cocaine or other stimulant drugs. They should also consult with a doctor about the benefits and risks of taking aspirin or other blood thinning medications. Women should consult with their doctors about the use of oral contraceptives.

What Is the Prognosis?

An unruptured aneurysm can go unnoticed throughout the person's life. However, a ruptured aneurysm can be fatal or lead to a hemorrhagic stroke, a vasospasm (the leading cause of disability or death after the bursting of an aneurysm), hydrocephalus, coma, or short-term or permanent brain damage.

The prognosis for people whose aneurysm has burst depends greatly on the age and general health of the individual, other pre-existing neurological conditions, the location of the aneurysm, the extent of bleeding (and the new bleeding), and the time between rupture and medical care. It is estimated that about 40 percent of patients whose aneurysm has ruptured do not survive the first 24 hours; Up to 25 percent die of complications within 6 months. Patients who have subarachnoid hemorrhage can have permanent neurological damage. Other individuals can recover with little or no neurological deficit. Delayed complications from the bursting of an aneurysm can be hydrocephalus and vasospasm. Early diagnosis and treatment are important.

Individuals receiving treatment for an unruptured aneurysm usually require less rehabilitation therapy and recover more quickly than people whose aneurysm flared. Recovery from treatment or rupture can take weeks to months.

Chapter 36

Cerebral Cavernous Malformations (Cavernous Angioma)

Cerebral cavernous malformations (CCMs) are collections of small blood vessels (capillaries) in the brain that are enlarged and irregular in structure which lead to altered blood flow. CCMs can occur anywhere in the body, but usually produce serious signs and symptoms only when they occur in the central nervous system (CNS) (the brain and spinal cord). Cavernous malformations in the brain and/or spinal cord are called CCMs. Approximately 25 percent of individuals with cerebral cavernous malformations never experience any related medical problems. Other people with CCMs may experience serious symptoms such as headaches, seizures, paralysis, hearing, or vision deficiencies, and bleeding in the brain (cerebral hemorrhage). These malformations can change in size and number over time, but they do not become cancerous. This condition can be sporadic or it can be inherited in an autosomal dominant pattern. Mutations in the *KRIT1* (CCM1), *CCM2*, and *PDCD10* (CCM3) genes cause CCMs. Treatment depends upon the symptoms. Seizures are usually treated with antiepileptic medications or surgery.

This chapter includes text excerpted from "Cerebral Cavernous Malformation," Genetic and Rare Diseases Information Center (GARD), National Center for Advancing Translational Sciences (NCATS), December 15, 2015.

Symptoms

Approximately 25 percent of individuals with CCMs never experience any related medical problems. Other people with this condition may experience serious symptoms including headaches, seizures, muscle weakness, loss of sensation, paralysis, hearing or vision deficiencies, and bleeding in the brain (cerebral hemorrhage). Severe brain hemorrhages can result in death. Although CCMs have been reported in infants and children, the majority of individuals present with symptoms between the second and fifth decades.

Cause

CCMs are collections of small blood vessels (capillaries) in the brain that are enlarged and irregular in structure. These capillaries have abnormally thin walls that are prone to leak. They also lack other support tissues, such as elastic fibers, which normally make them stretchy. As a result, when the capillaries fill with blood, they stretch out and create "caverns." They may not return to their normal size when the blood vessels empty.

CCMs may be familial or sporadic. Familial cases are caused by a mutation in one of at least three particular genes (*KRIT1, CCM2, and PDCD10*). While the precise functions of these genes are not fully understood, they are believed to interact with each other as part of a complex that strengthens the interactions between cells and limits leakage from the blood vessels. The underlying cause of sporadic CCMs in unknown and the primary focus of many researchers.

Inheritance

CCMs occur in about 0.5 percent of the general population. There are two forms: familial and sporadic.

Familial CCMs, which account for at least 20 percent of all cases, can be passed from parent to child. Individuals with familial CCMs typically have multiple lesions. Familial CCMs are passed through families in an autosomal dominant manner, which means one copy of the altered gene in each cell is sufficient to cause the disorder. Each child of an individual with familial CCM has a 50 percent chance of inheriting the mutation.

Sporadic CCMs occur in people with no family history of the disorder. These individuals tend to have only one CCM. Those with sporadic

CCM do not have a greater chance of having a child with a CCM than anyone else in the general population.

Treatment

Seizures are usually treated with antiepileptic medications. If seizures don't respond to medication, there is recurring bleeding in the brain, or the lesions are in a surgically accessible location, surgical removal of the lesion(s) using microsurgical techniques may be recommended. Headaches are managed symptomatically and/or prophylactically. Other neurological symptoms may be managed through rehabilitation.

Prognosis

Some people with CCMs will never know they have the disorder because they will never experience symptoms. Individuals who have increases in size and number of lesions, or an acute brain hemorrhage, may be directed to consider surgical removal. Symptomatic lesions are likely to remain symptomatic or progress. If treated surgically, many of these individuals will experience remission or reduction of symptoms. Overall, the prognosis for CCMs is variable, as the location, size and number of lesions determine the severity of the disorder. In some cases, CCMs can be fatal, in particular if they cause severe brain hemorrhage.

Chapter 37

Hydrocephalus

What Is Hydrocephalus?

The term hydrocephalus is derived from the Greek words "hydro" meaning water and "cephalous" meaning head. As its name suggests, it is a condition in which the main characteristic is the excessive accumulation of fluid in the brain. Although hydrocephalus was formerly known as "water in the brain," "water" is actually cerebrospinal fluid (CSF)—a clear fluid that surrounds the brain and spinal cord. Excessive accumulation of CSF results in abnormal dilation of spaces in the brain called ventricles. This dilation causes a potentially damaging pressure on the tissues of the brain.

The ventricular system consists of four ventricles connected by narrow pathways. Normally, CSF flows through the ventricles, exits to cisterns (closed spaces that serve as reservoirs) at the base of the brain, bathes the surface of the brain and spinal cord, and is then absorbed into the bloodstream.

CSF has three important vital functions:

1. Keeping brain tissue floating, acting as a cushion or cushion;

2. Serve as a vehicle to transport nutrients to the brain and eliminate waste; and

3. Flow between the skull and the spine to compensate for changes in intracranial blood volume (the amount of blood within the brain).

This chapter includes text excerpted from "Hydrocephalus," National Institute of Neurological Disorders and Stroke (NINDS), December 21, 2016.

The balance between the production and the absorption of CSF is of vital importance. Under ideal conditions, the fluid is almost completely absorbed into the bloodstream as it circulates. However, there are circumstances that, when present, will impede or disrupt the production of CSF or inhibit its normal flow. When this balance is disturbed, hydrocephalus results.

What Are the Different Types of Hydrocephalus?

Hydrocephalus can be congenital or acquired. **Congenital hydrocephalus** is present at birth and may be caused by environmental influences during the development of the fetus or by genetic predisposition. **Acquired hydrocephalus** develops at the time of birth or at a later point. This type of hydrocephalus can affect people of all ages and can be caused by an injury or illness.

Hydrocephalus can also be communicating or noncommunicating. **Communicating hydrocephalus** occurs when the flow of CSF is blocked after leaving the ventricles. This form is called communicating because the CSF can still flow between the ventricles, which remain open. **Noncommunicating hydrocephalus**—also called "obstructive" hydrocephalus occurs when the flow of CSF is blocked along one or more of the narrow pathways that connect the ventricles. One of the most common causes of hydrocephalus is "aqueductal stenosis." In this case, hydrocephalus results from a narrowing of the aqueduct of Silvio, a small conduit between the third and fourth ventricle in the middle of the brain.

There are two other forms of hydrocephalus that do not clearly fit into the categories described above and that primarily affect adults: *ex-vacuo hydrocephalus* and *normal pressure hydrocephalus*.

Ex vacated hydrocephalus occurs when there is damage to the brain caused by a stroke or a traumatic injury. In these cases, there may be a true contraction (atrophy or wasting) of brain tissue. **Normal pressure hydrocephalus** commonly occurs in the elderly and is characterized by many of the same symptoms associated with other conditions that occur more often in the elderly, such as memory loss, dementia, pathological walking disorder (PWD), urinary incontinence (UI), and general reduction of the normal activity of the daily life.

Who Gets Hydrocephalus?

Data on incidence and prevalence are difficult to establish since there is no national registry or database of people who have hydrocephalus and disorders closely associated with this disease; however, it is believed that hydrocephalus affects one in 500 children. Currently, most of these cases are diagnosed prenatally, at the time of birth or in the first years of childhood. Advances in diagnostic imaging technology allow for more accurate diagnoses in people who have atypical presentations, including adults with conditions such as normal pressure hydrocephalus.

What Causes Hydrocephalus?

The causes of hydrocephalus are not all well understood. Hydrocephalus can result from genetic inheritance (aqueductal stenosis) or from developmental disorders such as those associated with neural tube defects, including spina bifida and encephalocele. Other possible causes are complications of premature birth, such as intraventricular hemorrhage (IVH), diseases such as meningitis, tumors, traumatic head injury (TBI), or subarachnoid hemorrhage (SAH) that blocks the exit of the ventricles to the cisterns and eliminates the cisterns themselves.

What Are the Symptoms?

The symptoms of hydrocephalus vary with age, the progression of the disease and individual differences in the tolerance of the disease. For example, a child's ability to tolerate CSF pressure differs from that of an adult. The child's skull can expand to accommodate the increase in CSF because the sutures (the fibrous joints that connect the bones of the skull) have not yet closed.

In childhood, the most obvious indication of hydrocephalus is typically the rapid increase in head circumference or an extraordinarily large head size. Other symptoms may include vomiting, sleepiness, irritability, deviation of the eyes down (also called "sunset"), and seizures.

Older children and adults may experience different symptoms because their skull cannot expand to accommodate the increase in CSF. Symptoms may include headaches followed by vomiting, nausea, blurred, or double vision, deviation of the eyes down, problems with balance, poor coordination, gait disturbances, UI, reduction or loss of evolution in development, lethargy, drowsiness, irritability, or other changes in personality or knowledge, including loss of memory.

The symptoms described in this chapter are related to the most typical forms in which progressive hydrocephalus manifests; however, it is important to remember that the symptoms vary greatly from one person to another.

How Is Hydrocephalus Diagnosed?

Hydrocephalus is diagnosed by clinical neurological evaluation and by the use of cranial imaging techniques such as ultrasonography, computed tomography (CT), magnetic resonance imaging (MRI) or pressure monitoring techniques. A physician selects the appropriate diagnostic tool based on age, the clinical presentation of the patient, and the presence of other known or suspected abnormalities of the brain or spinal cord.

How Is Hydrocephalus Treated?

Hydrocephalus is treated more frequently by surgical placement of a shunt system. This system diverts the flow of CSF from one place within the CNS to another area of the body where it can be absorbed as part of the circulatory process.

A bypass is a flexible but robust silastic tube. A bypass system consists of the tube, a catheter and a valve. One end of the catheter is placed in the CNS—most often within the ventricle inside the brain, but it can also be placed inside a cyst or near the spinal cord. The other end of the catheter is normally placed inside the perito-neal (abdominal) cavity, but it can also be placed in other places inside the body, such as in a heart chamber or in a cavity in the lung where the CSF can drain and be absorbed. A valve located along the catheter maintains flow in one direction and regulates the amount of CSF flow.

A limited number of patients can be treated with a different proce-dure called third ventriculostomy. With this procedure, a neuroendo-scope a small camera designed to visualize small surgical areas that are difficult to access, allows a doctor to see the ventricular surface using fiber optic technology. The neuroendoscope is guided in position so that a small hole can be made in the base of the third ventricle, allowing the CSF to pass the obstruction and flow to the place of resorp-tion around the surface of the brain.

What Are the Possible Complications of a Referral System?

Bypass systems are imperfect devices. Complications can include mechanical failure, infections, obstructions and the need to prolong or replace the catheter. In general, referral systems require regular medical monitoring and follow-up.

When complications occur, subsequent surgery may be necessary to replace the defective part or the entire bypass system. Some complications can lead to other problems such as excessive drainage or insufficient drainage. Excessive drainage occurs when the bypass allows the CSF to drain from the ventricles more rapidly than the one from which it is produced. This excessive drainage can cause the ventricles to collapse, breaking blood vessels and causing headache, hemorrhage (subdural hematoma) or cleft ventricles (cloven ventricular syndrome). Insufficient drainage occurs when the CSF does not withdraw quickly enough and the symptoms of hydrocephalus reappear. Excessive drainage and insufficient CSF drainage are treated by adjusting the drain pressure of the bypass valve; If the bypass has an adjustable pressure valve these changes can be made by placing a special magnet on the scalp over the valve.

In addition to the common symptoms of hydrocephalus, shunt infections can also produce symptoms such as low grade fever, pain in the muscles of the neck or shoulders, and redness or tenderness along the shunt. When there is reason to suspect that a referral system is not working properly (for example, if the symptoms of hydrocephalus reappear), medical attention should be sought immediately. pain in the muscles of the neck or shoulders and redness or tenderness along the bypass duct.

What Is the Prognosis of Hydrocephalus?

The prognosis for patients who have been diagnosed with hydrocephalus is difficult to predict, although there is some correlation between the specific cause of hydrocephalus and the outcome of the condition. The prognosis is further complicated due to the presence of associated disorders, the opportunity of diagnosis and treatment success. The extent to which decompression (relief of pressure or increased CSF) after bypass surgery can reduce or reverse brain damage is not well understood.

Affected individuals and their families should be aware that hydrocephalus presents risks for both cognitive and physical development. However, many children who have been diagnosed with the disorder benefit from rehabilitation therapies and educational interventions that help them lead a normal life with few limitations. The treatment by an interdisciplinary team of medical professionals, rehabilitation specialists and educational experts is vital for a positive outcome.

The treatment of patients with hydrocephalus saves and sustains the life of the patient. If left untreated, progressive hydrocephalus, with rare exceptions, is fatal.

Chapter 38

Stroke

Chapter Contents

Section 38.1

Stroke Basics

This section includes text excerpted from "Stroke Information—About Stroke," Centers for Disease Control and Prevention (CDC), November 13, 2017.

A stroke, sometimes called a brain attack, occurs when something blocks blood supply to part of the brain or when a blood vessel in the brain bursts. In either case, parts of the brain become damaged or die. A stroke can cause lasting brain damage, long-term disability, or even death.

Understanding Stroke

To understand stroke, it helps to understand the brain. The brain controls our movements, stores our memories, and is the source of our thoughts, emotions, and language. The brain also controls many functions of the body, like breathing and digestion.

To work properly, your brain needs oxygen. Although your brain makes up only 2 percent of your body weight, it uses 20 percent of the oxygen you breathe. Your arteries deliver oxygen-rich blood to all parts of your brain.

What Happens during a Stroke

If something happens to block the flow of blood, brain cells start to die within minutes because they can't get oxygen. This causes a stroke. There are two types of stroke:

- An **ischemic stroke** occurs when blood clots or other particles block the blood vessels to the brain. Fatty deposits called plaque can also cause blockages by building up in the blood vessels.

- A **hemorrhagic stroke** occurs when a blood vessel bursts in the brain. Blood builds up and damages surrounding brain tissue.

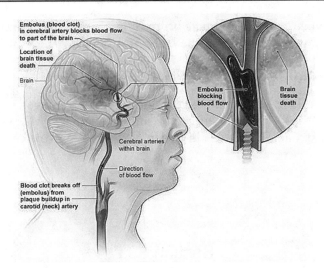

Figure 38.1. *Ischemic Stroke*

The illustration shows how an ischemic stroke can occur in the brain. If a blood clot breaks away from plaque buildup in a carotid (neck) artery, it can travel to and lodge in an artery in the brain. The clot can block blood flow to part of the brain, causing brain tissue death.

(Source: "Stroke," National Heart, Lung, and Blood Institute (NHLBI).)

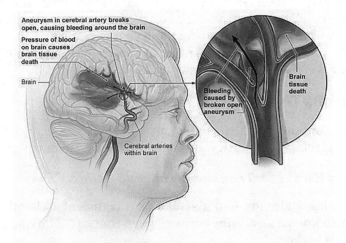

Figure 38.2. *Hemorrhagic Stroke*

The illustration shows how a hemorrhagic stroke can occur in the brain. An aneurysm in a cerebral artery breaks open, which causes bleeding in the brain. The pressure of the blood causes brain tissue death.

(Source: "Stroke," National Heart, Lung, and Blood Institute (NHLBI).)

Both types of stroke damage brain cells. Symptoms of that damage start to show in the parts of the body controlled by those brain cells.

Quick Treatment Is Critical for Stroke

A stroke is a serious medical condition that requires emergency care. Call 9-1-1 right away if you or someone you are with shows any signs of a stroke. **Time lost is brain lost. Every minute counts.**

Section 38.2

Stroke Risk

This section includes text excerpted from "Stroke Information—Stroke Risk," Centers for Disease Control and Prevention (CDC), January 17, 2017.

Anyone can have a stroke at any age. But certain things can increase your chances of having a stroke. The best way to protect yourself and your loved ones from a stroke is to understand your risk and how to control it.

While you can't control your age or family history, you can take steps to lower your chances of having a stroke.

Conditions That Increase Risk for Stroke

Many common medical conditions can increase your chances of having a stroke. Work with your healthcare team to control your risk.

Previous Stroke or Transient Ischemic Attack (TIA)

If you have already had a stroke or a transient ischemic attack (TIA), also known as a "mini-stroke," your chances of having another stroke are higher.

High Blood Pressure

High blood pressure is a leading cause of stroke. It occurs when the pressure of the blood in your arteries and other blood vessels is too high.

There are often no symptoms of high blood pressure. Get your blood pressure checked often. If you have high blood pressure, lowering your blood pressure through lifestyle changes or medicine can also lower your risk for stroke.

High Cholesterol

Cholesterol is a waxy, fat-like substance made by the liver or found in certain foods. Your liver makes enough for your body's needs, but we often get more cholesterol from the foods we eat. If we take in more cholesterol than the body can use, the extra cholesterol can build-up in the arteries, including those of the brain. This can lead to narrowing of the arteries, stroke, and other problems.

A blood test can tell your doctor if you have high levels of cholesterol and triglycerides (a related kind of fat) in your blood.

Heart Disease

Common heart disorders can increase your risk for stroke. For example, coronary artery disease increases your risk for stroke, because plaque builds up in the arteries and blocks the flow of oxygen-rich blood to the brain. Other heart conditions, such as heart valve defects, irregular heartbeat (including atrial fibrillation), and enlarged heart chambers, can cause blood clots that may break loose and cause a stroke.

Diabetes

Diabetes increases your risk for stroke. Your body needs glucose (sugar) for energy. Insulin is a hormone made in the pancreas that helps move glucose from the food you eat to your body's cells. If you have diabetes, your body doesn't make enough insulin, can't use its own insulin as well as it should, or both.

Diabetes causes sugars to build-up in the blood and prevent oxygen and nutrients from getting to the various parts of your body, including your brain. High blood pressure is also common in people with diabetes. High blood pressure is the leading cause of stroke and is the main cause for increased risk of stroke among people with diabetes.

Talk to your doctor about ways to keep diabetes under control.

Sickle Cell Disease

Sickle cell disease is a blood disorder linked to ischemic stroke that affects mainly black and Hispanic children. The disease causes some red blood cells to form an abnormal sickle shape. A stroke can happen if sickle cells get stuck in a blood vessel and block the flow of blood to the brain.

Behaviors That Increase Risk for Stroke

Your lifestyle choices can affect your chances of having a stroke. To lower your risk, your doctor may suggest changes to your lifestyle. that healthy behaviors can lower your risk for stroke.

Unhealthy Diet

Diets high in saturated fats, trans fat, and cholesterol have been linked to stroke and related conditions, such as heart disease. Also, getting too much salt (sodium) in the diet can raise blood pressure levels.

Physical Inactivity

Not getting enough physical activity can lead to other health conditions that can raise the risk for stroke. These health conditions include obesity, high blood pressure, high cholesterol, and diabetes. Regular physical activity can lower your chances for stroke.

Obesity

Obesity is excess body fat. Obesity is linked to higher "bad" cholesterol and triglyceride levels and to lower "good" cholesterol levels. Obesity can also lead to high blood pressure and diabetes.

Too Much Alcohol

Drinking too much alcohol can raise blood pressure levels and the risk for stroke. It also increases levels of triglycerides, a form of fat in your blood that can harden your arteries.

- Women should have no more than one drink a day.

- Men should have no more than two drinks a day.

Tobacco Use

Tobacco use increases the risk for stroke. Cigarette smoking can damage the heart and blood vessels, increasing your risk for stroke. The nicotine in cigarettes raises blood pressure, and the carbon monoxide from cigarette smoke reduces the amount of oxygen that your blood can carry. Even if you don't smoke, breathing in other people's secondhand smoke can make you more likely to have a stroke.

Family History and Other Characteristics That Increase Risk for Stroke

Family members share genes, behaviors, lifestyles, and environments that can influence their health and their risk for disease. Stroke risk can be higher in some families than in others, and your chances of having a stroke can go up or down depending on your age, sex, and race or ethnicity.

The good news is you can take steps to prevent stroke. Work with your healthcare team to lower your risk for stroke.

Genetics and Family History

When members of a family pass traits from one generation to another through genes, that process is called heredity.

Genetic factors likely play some role in high blood pressure, stroke, and other related conditions. Several genetic disorders can cause a stroke, including sickle cell disease. People with a family history of stroke are also likely to share common environments and other potential factors that increase their risk.

The chances for stroke can increase even more when heredity combines with unhealthy lifestyle choices, such as smoking cigarettes and eating an unhealthy diet.

Age

The older you are, the more likely you are to have a stroke. The chance of having a stroke doubles every 10 years after age 55. Although stroke is common among older adults, many people younger than 65 years also have strokes.

In fact, about one in seven strokes occur in adolescents and young adults ages 15–49. Experts think younger people are having more strokes because more young people are obese and have high blood pressure and diabetes.

Sex

Stroke is more common in women than men, and women of all ages are more likely than men to die from stroke. Pregnancy and use of birth control pills pose special stroke risks for women.

Race or Ethnicity

Blacks, Hispanics, American Indians, and Alaska Natives may be more likely to have a stroke than non-Hispanic whites or Asians. The risk of having a first stroke is nearly twice as high for blacks as for whites. Blacks are also more likely to die from stroke than whites are.

Section 38.3

Preventing Stroke

This section includes text excerpted from "Stroke—Preventing Stroke: What You Can Do," Centers for Disease Control and Prevention (CDC), January 17, 2017.

You can help prevent stroke by making healthy choices and controlling any health conditions you may have.

Preventing Stroke: Healthy Living Habits

You can help prevent stroke by making healthy lifestyle choices.

Healthy Diet

Choosing healthy meal and snack options can help you prevent stroke. Be sure to eat plenty of fresh fruits and vegetables.

Eating foods low in saturated fats, *trans* fat, and cholesterol and high in fiber, can help prevent high cholesterol. Limiting salt (sodium) in your diet can also lower your blood pressure. High cholesterol and high blood pressure increase your chances of having a stroke.

Healthy Weight

Being overweight or obese increases your risk for stroke. To determine whether your weight is in a healthy range, doctors often calculate your body mass index (BMI). Doctors sometimes also use waist and hip measurements to measure excess body fat.

Physical Activity

Physical activity can help you stay at a healthy weight and lower your cholesterol and blood pressure levels. For adults, the Surgeon General recommends 2 hours and 30 minutes of moderate-intensity aerobic physical activity, such as a brisk walk, each week. Children and teens should get 1 hour of physical activity every day.

No Smoking

Cigarette smoking greatly increases your chances of having a stroke. If you don't smoke, don't start. If you do smoke, quitting will lower your risk for stroke. Your doctor can suggest ways to help you quit.

Limited Alcohol

Avoid drinking too much alcohol, which can raise your blood pressure. Men should have no more than two drinks per day, and women only one.

Preventing Stroke: Control Medical Conditions

If you have heart disease, high cholesterol, high blood pressure, or diabetes you can take steps to lower your risk for stroke.

Check Cholesterol

Your doctor should test your cholesterol levels at least once every 5 years. Talk with your healthcare team about this simple blood test. If you have high cholesterol, medicine and lifestyle changes can help lower your risk for stroke.

Control Blood Pressure

High blood pressure usually has no symptoms, so be sure to have it checked on a regular basis. Talk to your healthcare team about how often you should check your levels. You can check your blood pressure at home, at a doctor's office, or at a pharmacy.

If you have high blood pressure, your doctor might prescribe medicine, suggest some changes in your lifestyle, or recommend you to choose foods with lower sodium (salt).

Control Diabetes

If your doctor thinks you have symptoms of diabetes, he or she may recommend that you get tested. If you have diabetes, check your blood sugar levels regularly. Talk with your healthcare team about treatment options. Your doctor may recommend certain lifestyle changes, such as getting more physical activity or choosing healthier foods. These actions will help keep your blood sugar under good control and help lower your risk for stroke.

Treat Heart Disease

If you have certain heart conditions, such as coronary artery disease atrial fibrillation (irregular heartbeat), your healthcare team may recommend medical treatment or surgery. Taking care of heart problems can help prevent stroke.

Take Your Medicine

If you take medicine to treat heart disease, high cholesterol, high blood pressure, or diabetes, follow your doctor's instructions carefully. Always ask questions if you don't understand something. Never stop taking your medicine without first talking to your doctor or pharmacist.

Work with Your Healthcare Team

You and your healthcare team can work together to prevent or treat the medical conditions that lead to stroke. Discuss your treatment plan regularly, and bring a list of questions to your appointments.

If you've already had a stroke or transient ischemic attack (TIA) your healthcare team will work with you to prevent further strokes. Your treatment plan will include medicine or surgery and lifestyle changes to lower your risk for another stroke. Be sure to take your medicine as directed and follow your doctor's instructions.

Part Six

Brain Tumors

Chapter 39

Brain Tumor: Overview

Understanding Brain Tumor

A tumor in the brain isn't like tumors in other parts of your body. It has limited room for growth because of the skull. This means that a growing tumor can squeeze vital parts of the brain and lead to serious health problems. Learning about the possible symptoms of brain tumors can help you know when to tell a doctor about them.

A tumor is an abnormal mass of cells. When most normal cells grow old or get damaged, they die, and new cells take their place. Sometimes, this process goes wrong. New cells form when the body doesn't need them, and old or damaged cells don't die as they should. The extra cells can form a tumor.

A tumor that starts in the brain is called a primary brain tumor. People of all ages can develop this type of tumor, even children. And there are many different ways they can form.

"There are over 130 different types of primary brain tumors," says Dr. Mark R. Gilbert, National Institutes of Health (NIH) brain tumor expert. About 80,000 people in the United States are diagnosed with a primary brain tumor each year.

Cancer that has spread to the brain from another part of the body is called a metastatic brain tumor. Metastatic brain tumors are far more common than primary tumors. Both primary and metastatic

This chapter includes text excerpted from "Spotlight on Brain Tumors," *NIH News in Health,* National Institutes of Health (NIH), October 2017.

brain tumors can cause similar symptoms. Symptoms depend mainly on where the tumor is in the brain.

"The symptoms of brain tumors can be either dramatic or subtle," Gilbert says. A seizure is an example of a dramatic symptom. About 3 of every 10 patients with a brain tumor are diagnosed after having a seizure, he explains.

Possible Symptoms of a Brain Tumor

The symptoms of a brain tumor depend on its size, type, and location. The most common ones are listed below. These do not mean you have a brain tumor. But talk with your doctor if you experience any of the following:

- Severe headaches
- Muscle jerking or twitching (seizures or convulsions)
- Nausea and vomiting
- Changes in speech, vision, or hearing
- Problems balancing or walking
- Changes in your mood, personality, or ability to concentrate
- Problems with memory
- Numbness, tingling, or weakness in the arms or legs

Other symptoms are less obvious. For example, you might notice memory problems or weakness on one side of your body.

Diagnosis of Brain Tumor

Until symptoms develop, you may not know you have a brain tumor. If you have symptoms that suggest a brain tumor, tell your doctor. Your doctor will give you a physical exam and ask about your personal and family health history. You may need to have additional tests. Tumors can be detected by imaging methods such as magnetic resonance imaging (MRI) or computed tomography (CT) scans.

"Brain imaging technology has really changed the way we are able to visualize abnormalities," Gilbert explains. It allows brain surgeons to learn as much as possible about the tumor and remove it more safely.

Treatment for Brain Tumor

Treatments differ depending on the type and location of the tumor. Treatment can involve surgery, radiation (beams of high energy rays aimed at the tumor), or drugs that kill or block the growth of cancer cells.

Usually, brain tumor treatment requires a team of healthcare professionals. This may include surgeons, cancer specialists, nutritionists, nurses, and mental health providers. The team does more than treat the tumor. They also try to minimize its impact on a patient's quality of life.

"There is a definite advantage to being cared for by people who do this on a routine basis," Gilbert says. A person who has been diagnosed with a brain tumor may want to seek treatment at a nearby cancer center, if possible.

Chapter 40

Adult Central Nervous System (CNS) Tumors

The Human Brain

The brain controls many important body functions. It has three major parts:

- The **cerebrum** is the largest part of the brain. It is at the top of the head. The cerebrum controls thinking, learning, problem solving, emotions, speech, reading, writing, and voluntary movement.

- The **cerebellum** is in the lower back of the brain (near the middle of the back of the head). It controls movement, balance, and posture.

- The **brainstem** connects the brain to the spinal cord. It is in the lowest part of the brain (just above the back of the neck). The brainstem controls breathing, heart rate, and the nerves and muscles used to see, hear, walk, talk, and eat.

This chapter includes text excerpted from "Adult Central Nervous System Tumors Treatment (PDQ®)—Patient Version," National Cancer Institute (NCI), January 12, 2018.

Spinal Cord and Its Function

The spinal cord connects the brain to nerves in most parts of the body. It is a column of nerve tissue that runs from the brainstem down the center of the back. It is covered by three thin layers of tissue called membranes. These membranes are surrounded by the vertebrae (back bones). Spinal cord nerves carry messages between the brain and the rest of the body, such as a message from the brain to cause muscles to move or a message from the skin to the brain to feel touch.

An adult central nervous system tumor is a disease in which abnormal cells form in the tissues of the brain and/or spinal cord.

Types of Brain and Spinal Cord Tumors

There are many types of brain and spinal cord tumors. The tumors are formed by the abnormal growth of cells and may begin in different parts of the brain or spinal cord. Together, the brain and spinal cord make up the central nervous system (CNS).

The tumors may be either benign (not cancer) or malignant (cancer):

- **Benign brain and spinal cord tumors** grow and press on nearby areas of the brain. They rarely spread into other tissues and may recur (come back).

- **Malignant brain and spinal cord tumors** are likely to grow quickly and spread into other brain tissue.

When a tumor grows into or presses on an area of the brain, it may stop that part of the brain from working the way it should. Both benign and malignant brain tumors cause signs and symptoms and need treatment.

Brain and spinal cord tumors can occur in both adults and children. However, treatment for children may be different than treatment for adults.

Tumors that start in the brain are called primary brain tumors. Primary brain tumors may spread to other parts of the brain or to the spine. They rarely spread to other parts of the body.

Often, tumors found in the brain have started somewhere else in the body and spread to one or more parts of the brain. These are called metastatic brain tumors (or brain metastases). Metastatic brain tumors are more common than primary brain tumors.

Up to half of metastatic brain tumors are from lung cancer. Other types of cancer that commonly spread to the brain include:

- Melanoma
- Breast cancer
- Colon cancer
- Kidney cancer
- Nasopharyngeal cancer
- Cancer of unknown primary site

Cancer may spread to the leptomeninges (the two innermost membranes covering the brain and spinal cord). This is called leptomeningeal carcinomatosis. The most common cancers that spread to the leptomeninges include:

- Breast cancer
- Lung cancer
- Leukemia
- Lymphoma

Brain and spinal cord tumors are named based on the type of cell they formed in and where the tumor first formed in the CNS. The grade of a tumor may be used to tell the difference between slow-growing and fast-growing types of the tumor. The World Health Organization (WHO) tumor grades are based on how abnormal the cancer cells look under a microscope and how quickly the tumor is likely to grow and spread.

WHO Tumor Grading System

- **Grade I (low-grade).** The tumor cells look more like normal cells under a microscope and grow and spread more slowly than grade II, III, and IV tumor cells. They rarely spread into nearby tissues. Grade I brain tumors may be cured if they are completely removed by surgery.

- **Grade II.** The tumor cells grow and spread more slowly than grade III and IV tumor cells. They may spread into nearby tissue and may recur (come back). Some tumors may become a higher-grade tumor.

- **Grade III.** The tumor cells look very different from normal cells under a microscope and grow more quickly than grade I and II tumor cells. They are likely to spread into nearby tissue.

- **Grade IV (high-grade).** The tumor cells do not look like normal cells under a microscope and grow and spread very quickly. There may be areas of dead cells in the tumor. Grade IV tumors usually cannot be cured.

Types of Primary Tumors in the Brain or Spinal Cord

The following types of primary tumors can form in the brain or spinal cord:

Astrocytic tumors. An astrocytic tumor begins in star-shaped brain cells called astrocytes, which help keep nerve cells healthy. An astrocyte is a type of glial cell. Glial cells sometimes form tumors called gliomas. Astrocytic tumors include the following:

- **Brainstem glioma (usually high grade).** A brainstem glioma forms in the brainstem, which is the part of the brain connected to the spinal cord. It is often a high-grade tumor, which spreads widely through the brainstem and is hard to cure. Brainstem gliomas are rare in adults.

- **Pineal astrocytic tumor (any grade).** A pineal astrocytic tumor forms in tissue around the pineal gland and may be any grade. The pineal gland is a tiny organ in the brain that makes melatonin, a hormone that helps control the sleeping and waking cycle.

- **Pilocytic astrocytoma (grade I).** A pilocytic astrocytoma grows slowly in the brain or spinal cord. It may be in the form of a cyst and rarely spreads into nearby tissues. Pilocytic astrocytomas can often be cured.

- **Diffuse astrocytoma (grade II).** A diffuse astrocytoma grows slowly, but often spreads into nearby tissues. The tumor cells look something like normal cells. In some cases, a diffuse astrocytoma can be cured. It is also called a low-grade diffuse astrocytoma.

- **Anaplastic astrocytoma (grade III).** An anaplastic astrocytoma grows quickly and spreads into nearby tissues. The tumor cells look different from normal cells. This type of tumor usually cannot be cured. An anaplastic astrocytoma is also called a malignant astrocytoma or high-grade astrocytoma.

- **Glioblastoma (grade IV).** A glioblastoma grows and spreads very quickly. The tumor cells look very different from normal cells. This type of tumor usually cannot be cured. It is also called glioblastoma multiforme.

Oligodendroglial tumors. An oligodendroglial tumor begins in brain cells called oligodendrocytes, which help keep nerve cells healthy. An oligodendrocyte is a type of glial cell. Oligodendrocytes sometimes form tumors called oligodendrogliomas. Grades of oligodendroglial tumors include the following:

- **Oligodendroglioma (grade II).** An oligodendroglioma grows slowly, but often spreads into nearby tissues. The tumor cells look something like normal cells. In some cases, an oligodendroglioma can be cured.

- **Anaplastic oligodendroglioma (grade III).** An anaplastic oligodendroglioma grows quickly and spreads into nearby tissues. The tumor cells look different from normal cells. This type of tumor usually cannot be cured.

Mixed gliomas. A mixed glioma is a brain tumor that has two types of tumor cells in it—oligodendrocytes and astrocytes. This type of mixed tumor is called an oligoastrocytoma.

- **Oligoastrocytoma (grade II).** An oligoastrocytoma is a slow-growing tumor. The tumor cells look something like normal cells. In some cases, an oligoastrocytoma can be cured.

- **Anaplastic oligoastrocytoma (grade III).** An anaplastic oligoastrocytoma grows quickly and spreads into nearby tissues. The tumor cells look different from normal cells. This type of tumor has a worse prognosis than oligoastrocytoma (grade II).

Ependymal tumors. An ependymal tumor usually begins in cells that line the fluid-filled spaces in the brain and around the spinal cord. An ependymal tumor may also be called an ependymoma. Grades of ependymomas include the following:

- **Ependymoma (grade I or II).** A grade I or II ependymoma grows slowly and has cells that look something like normal cells. There are two types of grade I ependymoma—myxopapillary ependymoma and subependymoma. A grade II ependymoma grows in a ventricle (fluid-filled space in the brain) and its connecting paths or in the spinal cord. In some cases, a grade I or II ependymoma can be cured.

- **Anaplastic ependymoma (grade III).** An anaplastic ependymoma grows quickly and spreads into nearby tissues. The tumor cells look different from normal cells. This type of tumor usually has a worse prognosis than a grade I or II ependymoma.

Medulloblastomas. A medulloblastoma is a type of embryonal tumor. Medulloblastomas are most common in children or young adults.

Pineal parenchymal tumors. A pineal parenchymal tumor forms in parenchymal cells or pinelocytes, which are the cells that make up most of the pineal gland. These tumors are different from pineal astrocytic tumors. Grades of pineal parenchymal tumors include the following:

- Pineocytoma (grade II). A pineocytoma is a slow-growing pineal tumor.
- Pineoblastoma (grade IV). A pineoblastoma is a rare tumor that is very likely to spread.

Meningeal tumors. A meningeal tumor, also called a meningioma, forms in the meninges (thin layers of tissue that cover the brain and spinal cord). It can form from different types of brain or spinal cord cells. Meningiomas are most common in adults. Types of meningeal tumors include the following:

- **Meningioma (grade I).** A grade I meningioma is the most common type of meningeal tumor. A grade I meningioma is a slow-growing tumor. It forms most often in the dura mater. A grade I meningioma can be cured if it is completely removed by surgery.

- **Meningioma (grade II and III).** This is a rare meningeal tumor. It grows quickly and is likely to spread within the brain and spinal cord. The prognosis is worse than a grade I meningioma because the tumor usually cannot be completely removed by surgery.

A hemangiopericytoma is not a meningeal tumor but is treated like a grade II or III meningioma. A hemangiopericytoma usually forms in the dura mater. The prognosis is worse than a grade I meningioma because the tumor usually cannot be completely removed by surgery.

Germ cell tumors. A germ cell tumor forms in germ cells, which are the cells that develop into sperm in men or ova (eggs) in women. There are different types of germ cell tumors. These include germinomas, teratomas, embryonal yolk sac carcinomas, and choriocarcinomas. Germ cell tumors can be either benign or malignant.

Craniopharyngioma (Grade I). A craniopharyngioma is a rare tumor that usually forms in the center of the brain just above the pituitary gland (a pea-sized organ at the bottom of the brain that controls other glands). Craniopharyngiomas can form from different types of brain or spinal cord cells.

Risk Factors for Adult Central Nervous System Tumor

Having certain genetic syndromes may increase the risk of a central nervous system tumor. Anything that increases your chance of getting a disease is called a risk factor. Having a risk factor does not mean that you will get cancer; not having risk factors doesn't mean that you will not get cancer.

Talk with your doctor if you think you may be at risk. There are few known risk factors for brain tumors. The following conditions may increase the risk of certain types of brain tumors:

- Being exposed to vinyl chloride may increase the risk of glioma.

- Infection with the Epstein-Barr virus, having AIDS (acquired immunodeficiency syndrome), or receiving an organ transplant may increase the risk of primary CNS lymphoma.

- Having certain genetic syndromes may increase the risk brain tumors:

  - Neurofibromatosis type 1 (NF1) or 2 (NF2)

  - von Hippel-Lindau disease

  - Tuberous sclerosis

  - Li-Fraumeni syndrome

  - Turcot syndrome type 1 or 2

  - Nevoid basal cell carcinoma syndrome

What Causes Adult Central Nervous System Tumor?

The cause of most adult brain and spinal cord tumors is not known.

What Are the Signs and Symptoms of Adult Central Nervous System Tumor?

The signs and symptoms of adult brain and spinal cord tumors are not the same in every person.

Signs and symptoms depend on the following:

- Where the tumor forms in the brain or spinal cord

- What the affected part of the brain controls

- The size of the tumor

Signs and symptoms may be caused by CNS tumors or by other conditions, including cancer that has spread to the brain. Check with your doctor if you have any of the following:

Brain Tumor Symptoms

- Morning headache or headache that goes away after vomiting

- Seizures

- Vision, hearing, and speech problems

- Loss of appetite

- Frequent nausea and vomiting

- Changes in personality, mood, ability to focus, or behavior

- Loss of balance and trouble walking

- Weakness

- Unusual sleepiness or change in activity level

Spinal Cord Tumor Symptoms

- Back pain or pain that spreads from the back towards the arms or legs

- A change in bowel habits or trouble urinating

- Weakness or numbness in the arms or legs

- Trouble walking

Diagnosis of Adult Central Nervous System Tumor

Diagnostic Tests

Tests that examine the brain and spinal cord are used to diagnose adult brain and spinal cord tumors.

The following tests and procedures may be used:

- **Physical exam and history.** An exam of the body to check general signs of health, including checking for signs of disease, such as lumps or anything else that seems unusual. A history of the patient's health habits and past illnesses and treatments will also be taken.

- **Neurological exam.** A series of questions and tests to check the brain, spinal cord, and nerve function. The exam checks a person's mental status, coordination, and ability to walk normally, and how well the muscles, senses, and reflexes work. This may also be called a neuro exam or a neurologic exam.

- **Visual field exam.** An exam to check a person's field of vision (the total area in which objects can be seen). This test measures both central vision (how much a person can see when looking straight ahead) and peripheral vision (how much a person can see in all other directions while staring straight ahead). Any loss of vision may be a sign of a tumor that has damaged or pressed on the parts of the brain that affect eyesight.

- **Tumor marker test.** A procedure in which a sample of blood, urine, or tissue is checked to measure the amounts of certain substances made by organs, tissues, or tumor cells in the body. Certain substances are linked to specific types of cancer when found in increased levels in the body. These are called tumor markers. This test may be done to diagnose a germ cell tumor.

- **Gene testing.** A laboratory test in which a sample of blood or tissue is tested for changes in a chromosome that has been linked with a certain type of brain tumor. This test may be done to diagnose an inherited syndrome.

- **Computed tomography (CT) scan (computerized axial tomography (CAT) scan).** A procedure that makes a series of detailed pictures of areas inside the body, taken from different angles. The pictures are made by a computer linked to an X-ray machine. A dye may be injected into a vein or swallowed to help the organs or tissues show up more clearly. This procedure is also called computed tomography, computerized tomography, or computerized axial tomography.

- **Magnetic resonance imaging (MRI) with gadolinium.** A procedure that uses a magnet, radio waves, and a computer to make a series of detailed pictures of the brain and spinal cord. A substance called gadolinium is injected into a vein. The gadolinium collects around the cancer cells so they show up brighter in the picture. This procedure is also called nuclear magnetic resonance imaging (NMRI). MRI is often used to diagnose tumors in the spinal cord. Sometimes a procedure called magnetic resonance spectroscopy (MRS) is done during the MRI scan. An MRS is used to diagnose tumors, based on their chemical makeup.

- **Single photon emission computed tomography (SPECT) scan.** A procedure that uses a special camera linked to a computer to make a 3-dimensional (3-D) picture of the brain. A very small amount of a radioactive substance is injected into a vein or inhaled through the nose. As the substance travels through the blood, the camera rotates around the head and takes pictures of the brain. Blood flow and metabolism are higher than normal in areas where cancer cells are growing. These areas will show up brighter in the picture. This procedure may be done just before or after a CT scan. SPECT is used to tell the difference between a primary tumor and a tumor that has spread to the brain from somewhere else in the body.

- **Positron emission tomography (PET) scan.** A procedure to find malignant tumor cells in the body. A small amount of radioactive glucose (sugar) is injected into a vein. The PET scanner rotates around the body and makes a picture of where glucose is being used in the brain. Malignant tumor cells show up brighter in the picture because they are more active and take up more glucose than normal cells do. PET is used to tell the difference between a primary tumor and a tumor that has spread to the brain from somewhere else in the body.

Biopsy

A biopsy is also used to diagnose a brain tumor. If imaging tests show there may be a brain tumor, a biopsy is usually done. One of the following types of biopsies may be used:

- **Stereotactic biopsy.** When imaging tests show there may be a tumor deep in the brain in a hard to reach place, a stereotactic brain biopsy may be done. This kind of biopsy uses a computer and a 3-dimensional (3D) scanning device to find the tumor and guide the needle used to remove the tissue. A small incision is made in the scalp and a small hole is drilled through the skull. A biopsy needle is inserted through the hole to remove cells or tissues so they can be viewed under a microscope by a pathologist to check for signs of cancer.

- **Open biopsy.** When imaging tests show that there may be a tumor that can be removed by surgery, an open biopsy may be done. A part of the skull is removed in an operation called a craniotomy. A sample of brain tissue is removed and viewed under a microscope by a pathologist. If cancer cells are found, some or all of the tumor may be removed during the same surgery. Tests are done before surgery to find the areas around the tumor that are important for normal brain function. There are also ways to test brain function during surgery. The doctor will use the results of these tests to remove as much of the tumor as possible with the least damage to normal tissue in the brain.

The pathologist checks the biopsy sample to find out the type and grade of brain tumor. The grade of the tumor is based on how the tumor cells look under a microscope and how quickly the tumor is likely to grow and spread.

The following tests may be done on the tumor tissue that is removed:

- **Immunohistochemistry.** A test that uses antibodies to check for certain antigens in a sample of tissue. The antibody is usually linked to a radioactive substance or a dye that causes the tissue to light up under a microscope. This type of test may be used to tell the difference between different types of cancer.

- **Light and electron microscopy.** A laboratory test in which cells in a sample of tissue are viewed under regular and high-powered microscopes to look for certain changes in the cells.

- **Cytogenetic analysis.** A laboratory test in which cells in a sample of tissue are viewed under a microscope to look for certain changes in the chromosomes.

Sometimes a biopsy or surgery cannot be done. For some tumors, a biopsy or surgery cannot be done safely because of where the tumor formed in the brain or spinal cord. These tumors are diagnosed and treated based on the results of imaging tests and other procedures.

Sometimes the results of imaging tests and other procedures show that the tumor is very likely to be benign and a biopsy is not done.

Treatment Options for Adult Brain and Spinal Cord Tumors

Five types of standard treatment are used:

1. **Active surveillance.** Active surveillance is closely watching a patient's condition but not giving any treatment unless there are changes in test results that show the condition is getting worse. Active surveillance may be used to avoid or delay the need for treatments such as radiation therapy or surgery, which can cause side effects or other problems. During active surveillance, certain exams and tests are done on a regular schedule. Active surveillance may be used for very slow-growing tumors that do not cause symptoms.

2. **Surgery.** Surgery may be used to diagnose and treat adult brain and spinal cord tumors. Removing tumor tissue helps decrease pressure of the tumor on nearby parts of the brain. Even if the doctor removes all the cancer that can be seen at the time of the surgery, some patients may be given chemotherapy or radiation therapy after surgery to kill any cancer cells that are left. Treatment given after the surgery, to lower the risk that the cancer will come back, is called adjuvant therapy.

3. **Radiation therapy.** Radiation therapy is a cancer treatment that uses high-energy X-rays or other types of radiation to kill cancer cells or keep them from growing. There are two types of radiation therapy:

    *   External radiation therapy
    *   Internal radiation therapy

    The way the radiation therapy is given depends on the type and grade of tumor and where it is in the brain or spinal cord. External radiation therapy is used to treat adult central nervous system tumors.

4. **Chemotherapy.** It is a cancer treatment that uses drugs to stop the growth of cancer cells, either by killing the cells or by stopping them from dividing.

5. **Targeted therapy.** It is a type of treatment that uses drugs or other substances to identify and attack specific cancer cells without harming normal cells. Monoclonal antibody therapy is a type of targeted therapy that uses antibodies made in the laboratory from a single type of immune system cell. These antibodies can identify substances on cancer cells or normal substances that may help cancer cells grow. Bevacizumab is a type of monoclonal antibody. Other types of targeted therapies are being studied for adult brain tumors, including tyrosine kinase inhibitors and new vascular endothelial growth factor (VEGF) inhibitors.

Prognosis for Primary Brain and Spinal Cord Tumors

The prognosis (chance of recovery) and treatment options for primary brain and spinal cord tumors depend on the following:

*   The type and grade of the tumor
*   Where the tumor is in the brain or spinal cord
*   Whether the tumor can be removed by surgery
*   Whether cancer cells remain after surgery
*   Whether there are certain changes in the chromosomes
*   Whether the cancer has just been diagnosed or has recurred (come back)
*   The patient's general health

The prognosis and treatment options for metastatic brain and spinal cord tumors depend on the following:

*   Whether there are more than two tumors in the brain or spinal cord
*   Where the tumor is in the brain or spinal cord
*   How well the tumor responds to treatment
*   Whether the primary tumor continues to grow or spread

Chapter 41

Pituitary Tumors

What Are Pituitary Tumors?

Pituitary tumors are abnormal growths of cells in the tissue of the pituitary gland. The pituitary gland is a bean shaped organ in the center of the brain, just behind and between the eyes. The pituitary gland causes the release of hormones in the body that control growth, metabolism, response to stress, and sexual and reproductive function.

Doctors and scientists classify pituitary tumors according to whether or not they spread beyond the pituitary gland:

- **Pituitary adenomas** are benign, meaning they are noncancerous and do not spread to other parts of the body. Most pituitary tumors fall into this category. Despite being benign, pituitary adenomas can make the pituitary gland produce too much or too little of certain hormones, causing health problems.

- **Pituitary carcinomas** are malignant. This means they can spread beyond the pituitary gland into the brain or spinal cord, or into other parts of the body. Very few pituitary tumors are carcinomas.

Because pituitary carcinomas are so rare, this health topic will cover only those pituitary tumors that are adenomas.

This chapter includes text excerpted from "Pituitary Tumors: Condition Information," *Eunice Kennedy Shriver* National Institute of Child Health and Human Development (NICHD), January 12, 2016.

- Their size:

  - **Microadenomas** are smaller than 1 centimeter. Most pituitary adenomas are microadenomas.

  - **Macroadenomas** are 1 centimeter or larger.

- Whether they secrete hormones:

  - **Functioning pituitary tumors (also called secretory tumors)** produce levels of hormones that are too high. Most pituitary tumors are functioning tumors. The symptoms they cause are due to the excessive levels of hormones they produce. These hormones play important roles in the healthy functioning of the body:

    - **Prolactin** causes a woman's breasts to make milk during and after pregnancy.

    - **Adrenocorticotropic hormone (ACTH)** is involved in the body's response to stress.

    - **Growth hormone** helps control body growth and metabolism.

    - **Thyroid stimulating hormone** is involved in growth, body temperature, and heart rate.

  - Nonfunctioning pituitary tumors (also called nonsecretory tumors) do not produce hormones. They can press on or damage the pituitary gland and prevent it from secreting adequate levels of hormones.

What Are the Symptoms of Pituitary Tumors?

Symptoms of Functioning Tumors

The symptoms of functioning tumors depend on the particular hormone the tumor is overproducing.

Prolactin

A pituitary tumor that produces too much prolactin may cause:

- Headache

- Some loss of vision

- Less frequent or no menstrual periods or menstrual periods with a very light flow

- Difficulty getting pregnant
- Impotence in men
- Lower sex drive
- The flow of breast milk in a woman who is not pregnant or breastfeeding

Adrenocorticotropic Hormone (ACTH)

A pituitary tumor that produces too much adrenocorticotropic hormone (ACTH) may cause:

- Headache
- Some loss of vision
- Weight gain reflected in the face, neck, and trunk of the body, but thin arms and legs
- A lump of fat on the back of the neck
- Thin skin that may include purple or pink stretch marks on the chest or abdomen
- Easy bruising
- Growth of fine hair on the face, upper back, or arms
- Bones that break easily
- Anxiety, irritability, depression
- Growth deceleration with weight gain in children
- Irregular menses

Growth Hormone

A pituitary tumor that produces too much growth hormone may cause:

- Headache
- Some loss of vision
- In adults, growth of the bones in the face, hands, and feet
- In children, excessive growth of the whole body
- Tingling or numbness in the hands and fingers

- Snoring or pauses in breathing during sleep
- Joint pain
- Sweating more than usual
- Extreme dislike of or concern about one or more parts of the body

Thyroid Stimulating Hormone (TSH)

A pituitary tumor that produces too much TSH (through high T4) may cause:

- Irregular heartbeat
- Shakiness
- Weight loss
- Trouble sleeping
- Frequent bowel movements
- Sweating

Symptoms of Nonfunctioning Tumors

Nonfunctioning tumors press on or damage the pituitary and prevent it from secreting enough hormones. If there is too little of a particular hormone, the gland or organ it normally controls will not function correctly. Symptoms of nonfunctioning pituitary tumors are:

- Headache
- Some loss of vision
- Loss of body hair
- In women, less frequent menstrual periods or no periods at all, or no milk from the breasts
- In men, loss of facial hair, growth of breast tissue, and impotence
- In women and men, lower sex drive
- In children, slowed growth and sexual development

Other General Symptoms of Pituitary Tumors

- Nausea and vomiting

- Confusion

- Dizziness

- Seizure

- Runny or drippy nose

How Many People Are Affected/At Risk for Pituitary Tumors?

It is estimated that up to 20 percent of people have pituitary tumors, but only about one third of these people experience symptoms that cause health problems. Most people with pituitary tumors never know they have them.

The highest incidence of pituitary tumors is in adults. These tumors are very rare in children and adolescents, with a prevalence of up to 1 per 1 million children. Studies suggest that only 3.5–8.5 percent of pituitary tumors are diagnosed before the age of 20.

What Causes Pituitary Tumors?

The exact cause of pituitary tumors is unknown.

In rare cases, inherited disorders may cause pituitary tumors. These diseases include multiple endocrine neoplasia type 1 (MEN 1) syndrome, Carney complex, and isolated familial acromegaly.

It is likely that pituitary tumors are caused by abnormalities in one or more genes, by hormonal abnormalities, or by a combination of these factors. Scientists, including the *Eunice Kennedy Shriver* National Institute of Child Health and Human Development (NICHD) researchers, are still working to figure out what causes pituitary tumors.

How Do Healthcare Providers Diagnose Pituitary Tumors?

A doctor will usually begin by giving you a physical exam and asking about your medical history. She or he will check your general health and examine your body for unusual things like lumps.

You might be given tests or procedures such as:

- Eye and visual field exam.

- Neurological exam. During this exam, the doctor gives you a series of tests and questions to check your coordination, mental status, reflexes, and muscle function.

- Magnetic resonance imaging (MRI) or computed tomography (CT) scan. MRI uses magnetic waves to produce detailed images of the inside of the body, while a CT scan uses X-rays to produce these pictures. These machines create images of the inside of the brain and spinal cord.

- Blood tests to check levels of hormones, blood sugar, and other substances.

- Urine tests to determine levels of certain hormones.

- Venous sampling. In this type of test, a sample of blood is taken from veins coming from the pituitary gland. Levels of certain hormones are measured in the blood sample.

- Biopsy. Cells or tissues are removed from the pituitary gland. They are then examined under a microscope to check for signs of cancer.

What Are the Treatments for Pituitary Tumors?

The most common treatments for pituitary tumors are:

- **Drug therapy.** Drugs can be given to treat the abnormal hormone levels caused by functioning pituitary tumors. The drug given depends on the hormone that is affected by the tumor.

- **Surgery.** The tumor is removed by performing an operation. The surgeon may reach the pituitary gland through a cut made under the upper lip or at the bottom of the nose between the nostrils. In other cases, the surgeon may cut through the skull to reach the pituitary tumor. Even if the tumor is completely removed, patients are commonly given radiation and chemotherapy after surgery to kill any tumor cells that might be present.

- **Radiation therapy.** Radiation therapy involves targeting a tumor with high energy X-rays that kill tumor cells or keep them from growing.

- **Chemotherapy.** Chemotherapy uses drugs that kill tumor cells or keep them from growing. Chemotherapy can be taken by mouth or injected.

The primary approach for treatment will depend on the type of pituitary tumor.

Is There a Cure for Pituitary Tumors?

Most pituitary tumors are curable. If a pituitary tumor is diagnosed early, the outlook for recovery is usually excellent. However, if tumors grow large enough, or grow rapidly, they are more likely to cause problems and will be more difficult to treat. Lifelong treatment or follow-up is often required, however, to make sure the tumor has not returned.

Chapter 42

Childhood Brain Tumors

Brain and Its Functions

The brain controls many important body functions. It has three major parts:

- The **cerebrum** is the largest part of the brain. It is at the top of the head. The cerebrum controls thinking, learning, problem solving, emotions, speech, reading, writing, and voluntary movement.

- The **cerebellum** is in the lower back of the brain (near the middle of the back of the head). It controls movement, balance, and posture.

- The **brainstem** connects the brain to the spinal cord. It is in the lowest part of the brain (just above the back of the neck). The brainstem controls breathing, heart rate, and the nerves and muscles used in seeing, hearing, walking, talking, and eating.

Spinal Cord and Its Function

The spinal cord connects the brain with nerves in most parts of the body. The spinal cord is a column of nerve tissue that runs from the brainstem down the center of the back. It is covered by three thin layers

This chapter includes text excerpted from "Childhood Brain and Spinal Cord Tumors Treatment Overview (PDQ®)—Patient Version," National Cancer Institute (NCI), February 5, 2018.

of tissue called membranes. These membranes are surrounded by the vertebrae (back bones). Spinal cord nerves carry messages between the brain and the rest of the body, such as a message from the brain to cause muscles to move or a message from the skin to the brain to feel touch.

What Is Childhood Brain or Spinal Cord Tumor?

A childhood brain or spinal cord tumor is a disease in which abnormal cells form in the tissues of the brain or spinal cord. There are many types of childhood brain and spinal cord tumors. The tumors may be benign (not cancer) or malignant (cancer). Benign brain tumors grow and press on nearby areas of the brain. They rarely spread into other tissues. Malignant brain tumors are likely to grow quickly and spread into other brain tissue. When a tumor grows into or presses on an area of the brain, it may stop that part of the brain from working the way it should. Both benign and malignant brain tumors can cause signs or symptoms and need treatment. Together, the brain and spinal cord make up the central nervous system (CNS).

Prevalence of Brain and Spinal Cord Cancer among Children

Although cancer is rare in children, brain and spinal cord tumors are the third most common type of childhood cancer, after leukemia and lymphoma. Brain tumors can occur in both children and adults. Treatment for children is usually different than treatment for adults.

Signs and Symptoms of Childhood Brain and Spinal Cord Tumors

The signs and symptoms of childhood brain and spinal cord tumors are not the same in every child.

Signs and symptoms depend on the following:

- Where the tumor forms in the brain or spinal cord.

- The size of the tumor.

- How fast the tumor grows.

- The child's age and development.

Signs and symptoms may be caused by childhood brain and spinal cord tumors or by other conditions, including cancer that has spread to the brain. Check with your child's doctor if your child has any of the following:

Brain tumor signs and symptoms:

- Morning headache or headache that goes away after vomiting.

- Frequent nausea and vomiting.

- Vision, hearing, and speech problems.

- Loss of balance and trouble walking.

- Unusual sleepiness or change in activity level.

- Unusual changes in personality or behavior.

- Seizures.

- Increase in the head size (in infants).

Spinal cord tumor signs and symptoms:

- Back pain or pain that spreads from the back towards the arms or legs.

- A change in bowel habits or trouble urinating.

- Weakness in the legs.

- Trouble walking.

In addition to these signs and symptoms of brain and spinal cord tumors, some children are unable to reach certain growth and development milestones such as sitting up, walking, and talking in sentences.

Causes

The cause of most childhood brain and spinal cord tumors is unknown.

Diagnosis

The following tests and procedures may be used:

- **Physical exam and history.** An exam of the body to check general signs of health, including checking for signs of disease, such as lumps or anything else that seems unusual. A history of the patient's health habits and past illnesses and treatments will also be taken.

- **Neurological exam.** A series of questions and tests to check the brain, spinal cord, and nerve function. The exam checks a person's mental status, coordination, and ability to walk normally, and how well the muscles, senses, and reflexes work. This may also be called a neuro exam or a neurologic exam.

- **Magnetic resonance imaging (MRI) with gadolinium.** A procedure that uses a magnet, radio waves, and a computer to make a series of detailed pictures of the brain and spinal cord. A substance called gadolinium is injected into a vein. The gadolinium collects around the cancer cells so they show up brighter in the picture. This procedure is also called nuclear magnetic resonance imaging (NMRI).

- **Serum tumor marker test.** A procedure in which a sample of blood is examined to measure the amounts of certain substances released into the blood by organs, tissues, or tumor cells in the body. Certain substances are linked to specific types of cancer when found in increased levels in the blood. These are called tumor markers.

Most childhood brain tumors are diagnosed and removed in surgery. If doctors think there might be a brain tumor, a biopsy may be done to remove a sample of tissue. For tumors in the brain, the biopsy is done by removing part of the skull and using a needle to remove a sample of tissue. A pathologist views the tissue under a microscope to look for cancer cells. If cancer cells are found, the doctor may remove as much tumor as safely possible during the same surgery. The pathologist checks the cancer cells to find out the type and grade of brain tumor. The grade of the tumor is based on how abnormal the cancer cells look under a microscope and how quickly the tumor is likely to grow and spread.

- **Immunohistochemistry.** A test that uses antibodies to check for certain antigens in a sample of tissue. The antibody is usually linked to a radioactive substance or a dye that causes the tissue to light up under a microscope. This type of test may be used to tell the difference between different types of cancer.

Imaging Tests

Sometimes a biopsy or surgery cannot be done safely because of where the tumor formed in the brain or spinal cord. These tumors are diagnosed based on the results of imaging tests and other procedures.

Treatment

Different types of treatment are available for children with brain and spinal cord tumors. Some treatments are standard and some are being tested in clinical trials.

Healthcare Team

Treatment will be overseen by a pediatric oncologist, a doctor who specializes in treating children with cancer. The pediatric oncologist works with other healthcare providers who are experts in treating children with brain tumors and who specialize in certain areas of medicine. These may include the following specialists:

- Pediatrician
- Neurosurgeon
- Neurologist
- Neuro-oncologist
- Neuropathologist
- Neuroradiologist
- Radiation oncologist
- Endocrinologist
- Psychologist
- Ophthalmologist
- Rehabilitation specialist
- Social worker
- Nurse specialist

Standard Treatment

Three types of standard treatment are used:

Surgery

Surgery may be used to diagnose and treat childhood brain and spinal cord tumors.

Radiation Therapy

Radiation therapy is a cancer treatment that uses high energy X-rays or other types of radiation to kill cancer cells or keep them from growing. There are two types of radiation therapy:

- **External radiation** therapy uses a machine outside the body to send radiation toward the cancer.

- **Internal radiation** therapy uses a radioactive substance sealed in needles, seeds, wires, or catheters that are placed directly into or near the cancer.

The way the radiation therapy is given depends on the type of cancer being treated. External radiation therapy is used to treat childhood brain and spinal cord tumors.

Chemotherapy

Chemotherapy is a cancer treatment that uses drugs to stop the growth of cancer cells, either by killing the cells or by stopping them from dividing. When chemotherapy is taken by mouth or injected into a vein or muscle, the drugs enter the bloodstream and can reach cancer cells throughout the body (systemic chemotherapy). When chemotherapy is placed directly in the cerebrospinal fluid, an organ, or a body cavity such as the abdomen, the drugs mainly affect cancer cells in those areas (regional chemotherapy). The way the chemotherapy is given depends on the type and stage of the cancer being treated.

Anticancer drugs given by mouth or vein to treat brain and spinal cord tumors cannot cross the blood-brain barrier and enter the fluid that surrounds the brain and spinal cord. Instead, an anticancer drug is injected into the fluid filled space to kill cancer cells there. This is called intrathecal chemotherapy (IC).

Side Effects

Some cancer treatments cause side effects months or years after treatment has ended. These are called late effects. Late effects of cancer treatment may include the following:

- Physical problems.

- Changes in mood, feelings, thinking, learning, or memory.

- Second cancers (new types of cancer).

Some late effects may be treated or controlled. It is important to talk with your child's doctors about the effects cancer treatment can have on your child.

Prognosis

Certain factors affect prognosis (chance of recovery). It depends on the following:

- Whether there are any cancer cells left after surgery.
- The type of tumor.
- Where the tumor is in the body.
- The child's age.
- Whether the tumor has just been diagnosed or has recurred (come back).

Chapter 43

Living with a Brain Tumor

Nutrition

It's important for you to take care of yourself by eating well. You need the right amount of calories to maintain a good weight. You also need enough protein to keep up your strength. Eating well may help you feel better and have more energy.

Sometimes, especially during or soon after treatment, you may not feel like eating. You may be uncomfortable or tired. You may find that foods don't taste as good as they used to. In addition, the side effects of treatment (such as poor appetite, nausea, vomiting, or mouth blisters) can make it hard to eat well. Your doctor, a registered dietitian, or another healthcare provider can suggest ways to deal with these problems. Also, the National Cancer Institute (NCI) booklet *Eating Hints* (www.cancer.gov/publications/patient-education/eatinghints.pdf) has many useful ideas and recipes.

Supportive Care

A brain tumor and its treatment can lead to other health problems. You may receive supportive care to prevent or control these problems.

You can have supportive care before, during, and after cancer treatment. It can improve your comfort and quality of life during treatment.

This chapter includes text excerpted from "What You Need to Know about Brain Tumors," National Cancer Institute (NCI), May 2009. Reviewed February 2018.

Your healthcare team can help you with the following problems:

- **Swelling of the brain:** Many people with brain tumors need steroids to help relieve swelling of the brain.

- **Seizures:** Brain tumors can cause seizures (convulsions). Certain drugs can help prevent or control seizures.

- **Fluid buildup in the skull:** If fluid builds up in the skull, the surgeon may place a shunt to drain the fluid.

- **Sadness and other feelings:** It's normal to feel sad, anxious, or confused after a diagnosis of a serious illness. Some people find it helpful to talk about their feelings.

Many people with brain tumors receive supportive care along with treatments intended to slow the progress of the disease. Some decide not to have antitumor treatment and receive only supportive care to manage their symptoms.

Follow-Up Care

You'll need regular checkups after treatment for a brain tumor. For example, for certain types of brain tumors, checkups may be every 3 months. Checkups help ensure that any changes in your health are noted and treated if needed. If you have any health problems between checkups, you should contact your doctor.

Your doctor will check for return of the tumor. Also, checkups help detect health problems that can result from cancer treatment.

Checkups may include careful physical and neurologic exams, as well as magnetic resonance imaging (MRI) or computed tomography (CT) scans. If you have a shunt, your doctor checks to see that it's working well.

Sources of Support

Learning you have a brain tumor can change your life and the lives of those close to you. These changes can be hard to handle. It's normal for you, your family, and your friends to need help coping with the feelings that such a diagnosis can bring.

Concerns about treatments and managing side effects, hospital stays, and medical bills are common. You may also worry about caring for your family, keeping your job, or continuing daily activities.

Here's where you can go for support:

- Doctors, nurses, and other members of your healthcare team can answer questions about treatment, working, or other activities.

- Social workers, counselors, or members of the clergy can be helpful if you want to talk about your feelings or concerns. Often, social workers can suggest resources for financial aid, transportation, home care, or emotional support.

- Support groups also can help. In these groups, people with brain tumors or their family members meet with other patients or their families to share what they have learned about coping with the disease and the effects of treatment. Groups may offer support in person, over the telephone, or on the Internet. You may want to talk with a member of your healthcare team about finding a support group.

- Information specialists at 800-4-CANCER (800-422-6237) and at LiveHelp (livehelp.cancer.gov/app/chat/chat_launch) can help you locate programs, services, and publications. They can send you a list of organizations that offer services to people with cancer.

Part Seven

Degenerative Brain Disorders

Chapter 44

Dementias

Chapter Contents

Section 44.1

Dementia Types, Causes, and Treatments

This section includes text excerpted from "Dementia:
Hope through Research," National Institute of Neurological
Disorders and Stroke (NINDS), December 2017.

Dementia is the loss of cognitive functioning—the ability to think, remember, or reason—to such an extent that it interferes with a person's daily life and activities. These functions include memory, language skills, visual perception, problem solving, self-management, and the ability to focus and pay attention. Some people with dementia cannot control their emotions, and their personalities may change. Dementia ranges in severity from the mildest stage, when it is just beginning to affect a person's functioning, to the most severe stage, when the person must depend completely on others for basic activities of daily living.

Age is the primary risk factor for developing dementia. For that reason, the number of people living with dementia could double in the next 40 years as the number of Americans age 65 and older increases from 48 million today to more than 88 million in 2050. Regardless of the form of dementia, the personal, economic, and societal demands can be devastating.

Dementia is not the same as age-related cognitive decline—when certain areas of thinking, memory, and information processing slow with age, but intelligence remains unchanged. Unlike dementia, age-related memory loss isn't disabling. Occasional lapses of forgetfulness are normal in elderly adults. While dementia is more common with advanced age (as many as half of all people age 85 or older may have some form of dementia), it is not an inevitable part of aging. Many people live into their 90s and beyond without any signs of dementia.

Dementia is also not the same as delirium, which is usually a short-term complication of a medical condition and most often can be treated successfully. Signs and symptoms of dementia result when once-healthy neurons (nerve cells) in the brain stop working, lose connections with other brain cells, and die. While everyone loses some neurons as they age, people with dementia experience far greater loss.

Causes of Dementia Disorders

Alzheimer disease (AD) is the most common cause of dementia in older adults. As many as 5 million Americans age 65 and older may have the disease. In most neurodegenerative diseases, certain proteins abnormally clump together and are thought to damage healthy neurons, causing them to stop functioning and die. In Alzheimer, fragments of a protein called amyloid form abnormal clusters called plaques between brain cells, and a protein called tau forms tangles inside nerve cells.

It seems likely that damage to the brain starts a decade or more before memory and other cognitive problems appear. The damage often initially appears in the hippocampus, the part of the brain essential in forming memories. Ultimately, the abnormal plaques and tangles spread throughout the brain, and brain tissue significantly shrinks.

As AD progresses, people experience greater memory loss and other cognitive difficulties. Problems can include wandering and getting lost, trouble handling money and paying bills, repeating questions, taking longer to complete normal daily tasks, and personality and behavior changes.

People are often diagnosed in this stage. Memory loss and confusion worsen, and people begin to have problems recognizing family and friends. They may be unable to learn new things, carry out multi-step tasks such as getting dressed, or cope with new situations. In addition, people at this stage may have hallucinations, delusions, and paranoia, and may behave impulsively.

People with severe Alzheimer cannot communicate and are completely dependent on others for their care. Near the end, the person may be in bed most or all of the time as body functions shut down. Certain drugs can temporarily slow some symptoms of Alzheimer from getting worse, but currently there are no treatments that stop the progression of the disease.

Researchers have not found a single gene solely responsible for AD; rather, multiple genes are likely involved. One genetic risk factor—having one form of the apolipoprotein E (*APOE*) gene on chromosome 19—does increase a person's risk for developing Alzheimer. People who inherit one copy of this *APOE ε4* allele have an increased chance of developing the disease; those who inherit two copies of the allele are at even greater risk. (An allele is a variant form of a pair of genes that are located on a particular chromosome and control the same trait.) The *APOE ε4* allele may also be associated with an earlier onset of memory loss and other symptoms. Researchers have found that this allele is associated with an increased number of amyloid plaques in the brain tissue of affected people.

Frontotemporal disorders (FTD) are forms of dementia caused by a family of neurodegenerative brain diseases collectively called frontotemporal lobar degeneration. They primarily affect the frontal and temporal lobes of the brain, rather than the widespread shrinking and wasting away (atrophy) of brain tissue seen in AD. In these disorders, changes to nerve cells in the brain's frontal lobes affect the ability to reason and make decisions, prioritize and multitask, act appropriately, and control movement. Changes to the temporal lobes affect memory and how people understand words, recognize objects, and recognize and respond to emotions. Some people decline rapidly over 2–3 years, while others show only minimal changes for many years. People can live with FTD for 2–10 years, sometimes longer, but it is difficult to predict the time course for an affected individual. The signs and symptoms may vary greatly among individuals as different parts of the brain are affected. No treatment that can cure or reverse FTD is currently available.

Clinically, FTD is classified into two main types of syndromes:

- **Behavioral variant frontotemporal dementia (bvFTD)** involves changes in behavior, judgment, and personality. People with this disorder may have problems with cognition, but their memory may stay relatively intact. They may do impulsive things that are out of character or may engage in repetitive, unusual behaviors. People with bvFTD also may say or do inappropriate things or become uncaring. Over time, language and/or movement problems may occur.

- **Primary progressive aphasia (PPA)** involves changes in the ability to speak, understand, and express thoughts and/or words and to write and read. Many people with PPA, though not all, develop symptoms of dementia. Problems with memory, reasoning, and judgment are not apparent at first but can develop and progress over time. Sometimes a person with PPA cannot recognize the faces of familiar people and common objects (called semantic PPA). Other individuals have increasing trouble producing speech and may eventually be unable to speak at all (called agrammatic PPA). PPA is a language disorder that is not the same as the problems with speech and ability to read and write (called aphasia) that can result from a stroke.

Other types of FTDs include:

- **Corticobasal degeneration (CBD)** involves progressive nerve-cell loss and atrophy of specific areas of the brain, which can affect memory, behavior, thinking, language, and movement. The disease is named after parts of the brain that are affected—the cerebral cortex (the outer part of the brain) and the basal ganglia (structures deep in the brain involved with movement). Not everyone who has CBD has problems with memory, cognition, language, or behavior. The disease tends to progress gradually, with early symptoms beginning around age 60. Some of the movement symptoms of CBD are similar to those seen in Parkinson disease (PD).

- **Frontotemporal dementia with motor neuron disease (FTD/MND, also called FTD-ALS)** is a combination of behavioral variant frontotemporal dementia and the progressive neuromuscular weakness typically seen in amyotrophic lateral sclerosis (ALS). ALS is a neurodegenerative disease that attacks nerve cells responsible for controlling voluntary muscles (muscle action that can be controlled, such as that in the arms, legs, and face). Symptoms of either disease may appear first, with other symptoms developing over time.

- **Pick disease** is characterized by Pick bodies—masses comprised of the protein tau that accumulate inside nerve cells, causing them to appear enlarged or balloon-like. It is usually seen with bvFTD but sometimes with PPA. Some symptoms are similar to those of AD, including loss of speech, changes in behavior, and trouble with thinking. However, while inappropriate behavior characterizes the early stages of Pick disease, memory loss is often the first symptom of Alzheimer. Antidepressants and antipsychotics can control some of the behavioral symptoms of Pick disease, but no treatment is available to stop the disease from progressing.

- **Progressive supranuclear palsy (PSP)** is a brain disease that can cause problems with thinking, memory, behavior, problem solving, and judgment. It also affects the control of eye movements, mood, speech, swallowing, vision, concentration, and language. Because certain parts of the brain that control movement are damaged, this disease shares some of the problems with movement seen in people with corticobasal degeneration and PD.

Lewy body dementia (LBD) is one of the most common causes of dementia after AD and vascular disease. It typically begins after age 50, but can occur earlier. It involves abnormal protein deposits called Lewy bodies, which are balloon-like structures that form inside nerve cells. The abnormal buildup of the protein alpha-synuclein and other proteins causes neurons to work less effectively and die. Initial symptoms may vary, but over time, people with these disorders develop similar cognitive, behavioral, physical, and sleep-related symptoms.

LBD includes two related conditions—dementia with Lewy bodies (DLB) and Parkinson disease dementia (PDD). In DLB, the cognitive symptoms are seen within a year of movement symptoms called parkinsonism (including tremor, difficulty with walking and posture, and rigid muscles). In PDD, the cognitive symptoms develop more than a year after movement problems begin.

- **DLB** is one of the more common forms of progressive dementia. Neurons in the outer layer of the brain (cortex) and in the substantia nigra (a region involved with the production of dopamine) degenerate. Many neurons that remain contain Lewy bodies. Symptoms such as difficulty sleeping, loss of smell, and visual hallucinations often precede movement and other problems by as many as 10 years. Later in the course of DLB, some signs and symptoms are similar to AD and may include memory loss, poor judgment, and confusion. Other signs and symptoms of DLB are similar to those of PD, including difficulty with movement and posture, a shuffling walk, and changes in alertness and attention. There is no cure for DLB, but there are drugs that control some symptoms.

- **PDD** can occur in people with PD, but not all people with PD will develop dementia. PDD may affect memory, social judgment, language, or reasoning. Autopsy studies show that people with PDD often have Lewy bodies in the cortex and other brain areas, and many have amyloid plaques and tau tangles like those found in people with AD, though it is not understood what these similarities mean. The time from the onset of movement symptoms to the onset of dementia symptoms varies greatly from person to person. Risk factors for developing PDD include the onset of Parkinson-related movement symptoms followed by mild cognitive impairment and rapid eye movement (REM) sleep behavior disorder, which involves having frequent nightmares and hallucinations.

Vascular contributions to cognitive impairment and dementia (VCID) cause significant changes to memory, thinking, and behavior. Cognition and brain function can be significantly affected by the size, location, and number of brain injuries. Vascular dementia and vascular cognitive impairment arise as a result of risk factors that similarly increase the risk for cerebrovascular disease (stroke), including atrial fibrillation, hypertension, diabetes, and high cholesterol. Symptoms of VCID can begin suddenly and progress or subside during one's lifetime. VCID can occur along with AD. Persons with VCID almost always have abnormalities in the brain on magnetic resonance imaging scans (MRI). These include evidence of prior strokes, often small and asymptomatic, as well as diffuse changes in the brain's "white matter"—the connecting "wires" of the brain that are critical for relaying messages between brain regions. Microscopic brain examination shows thickening of blood vessel walls called arteriosclerosis and thinning or loss of components of the white matter.

Forms of VCID include:

- **Vascular dementia** refers to progressive loss of memory and other cognitive functions caused by vascular injury or disease within the brain. Symptoms of vascular dementia may sometimes be difficult to distinguish from AD. Problems with organization, attention, slowed thinking, and problem solving are all more prominent in VCID, while memory loss is more prominent in Alzheimer.

- **Vascular cognitive impairment** involves changes with language, attention, and the ability to think, reason, and remember that are noticeable but are not significant enough to greatly impact daily life. These changes, caused by vascular injury or disease within the brain, progress slowly over time.

- **Poststroke dementia** can develop months after a major stroke. Not everyone who has had a major stroke will develop vascular dementia, but the risk for dementia is significantly higher in someone who has had a stroke.

- **Multi-infarct dementia (MID)** is the result of many small strokes (infarcts) and mini-strokes. Language or other functions may be impaired, depending on the region of the brain that is affected. The risk for dementia is significantly higher in someone who has had a stroke. Dementia is more likely when strokes affect both sides of the brain. Even strokes that don't show any noticeable symptoms can increase the risk of dementia.

- **Cerebral autosomal dominant arteriopathy with subcortical infarcts and leukoencephalopathy (CADASIL)** is an extremely rare inherited disorder caused by a thickening of the walls of small- and medium-sized blood vessels, which reduces the flow of blood to the brain. CADASIL is associated with multi-infarct dementia, stroke, and other disorders. The first symptoms can appear in people between ages 20 and 40. CADASIL may have symptoms that can be confused with multiple sclerosis (MS). Many people with CADASIL are undiagnosed.

- **Subcortical vascular dementia,** previously called Binswanger disease (BD), involves extensive microscopic damage to the small blood vessels and nerve fibers that make up white matter. Some consider it an aggressive form of multi-infarct dementia. Cognitive changes include problems with short-term memory, organization, attention, decision making, and behavior. Symptoms tend to begin after age 60, and they progress in a stepwise manner. People with subcortical vascular disease often have high blood pressure, a history of stroke, or evidence of disease of the large blood vessels in the neck or heart valves.

- **Cerebral amyloid angiopathy (CAA)** is a buildup of amyloid plaques in the walls of blood vessels in the brain. It is generally diagnosed when multiple tiny bleeds in the brain are discovered using magnetic resonance imaging (MRI).

Risk Factors for Dementia

The following risk factors may increase a person's chance of developing one or more kinds of dementia. Some of these factors can be modified, while others cannot.

- **Age.** Advancing age is the best known risk factor for developing dementia.

- **Hypertension.** High blood pressure has been linked to cognitive decline, stroke, and types of dementia that damage the white matter regions of the brain. High blood pressure causes "wear-and-tear" to brain blood vessel walls called arteriosclerosis.

- **Stroke.** A single major stroke or a series of smaller strokes increases a person's risk of developing vascular dementia. A person who has had a stroke is at an increased risk of having additional strokes, which further increases the risk of developing dementia.

- **Alcohol use.** Most studies suggest that regularly drinking large amounts of alcohol increases the risk of dementia. Specific dementias are associated with alcohol abuse, such as Wernicke-Korsakoff syndrome.

- **Atherosclerosis.** The accumulation of fats and cholesterol in the lining of arteries, coupled with an inflammatory process that leads to a thickening of the vessel walls (known as atherosclerosis), can lead to stroke, which raises the risk for vascular dementia.

- **Diabetes.** People with diabetes appear to have a higher risk for dementia. Poorly controlled diabetes is a risk factor for stroke and cardiovascular disease, which in turn increase the risk for vascular dementia.

- **Down syndrome.** Many people with Down syndrome develop symptoms of AD by the time they reach middle age.

- **Genetics.** The chance of developing a genetically linked form of dementia increases when more than one family member has the disorder. In many dementias, there can be a family history of a similar disease. In some cases, such as with the FTDs, having just one parent who carries a mutation increases the risk of inheriting the condition. A very small proportion of dementia is inherited.

- **Head injury.** An impact to the head can cause a traumatic brain injury (TBI). Certain types of TBI, or repeated TBIs, can cause dementia and other severe cognitive problems.

- **PD.** The degeneration and death of nerve cells in the brain in people with PD can cause dementia and significant memory loss.

- **Smoking.** Smoking increases the risk of developing cardiovascular diseases that slow or stop blood from getting to the brain.

Diagnosis

To diagnose dementia, doctors first assess whether an individual has an underlying treatable condition such as abnormal thyroid function, vitamin deficiency, or normal pressure hydrocephalus that may relate to cognitive difficulties. Early detection of symptoms is important, as some causes can be treated. In many cases, the specific type of dementia may not be confirmed until after the person has died and the brain is examined.

447

An assessment generally includes:

- **Medical history and physical exam.** Assessing a person's medical and family history, current symptoms and medication, and vital signs can help the doctor detect conditions that might cause or occur with dementia. Some conditions may be treatable.

- **Neurological evaluations.** Assessing balance, sensory response, reflexes, and other functions helps the doctor identify signs of conditions that may affect the diagnosis or are treatable with drugs. Doctors also might use an electroencephalogram, a test that records patterns of electrical activity in the brain, to check for abnormal electrical brain activity.

- **Brain scans.** Computed tomography (CT) and MRI scans can detect structural abnormalities and rule out other causes of dementia. Positron emission tomography (PET) can look for patterns of altered brain activity that are common in dementia. It can detect amyloid plaques and tau tangles in AD.

- **Cognitive and neuropsychological tests.** These tests are used to assess memory, language skills, math skills, problem-solving, and other abilities related to mental functioning.

- **Laboratory tests.** Testing a person's blood and other fluids, as well as checking levels of various chemicals, hormones, and vitamin levels, can identify or rule out conditions that may contribute to dementia.

- **Presymptomatic tests.** Genetic testing can help some people who have a strong family history of dementia identify risk for a dementia with a known gene defect.

- **Psychiatric evaluation.** This evaluation will help determine if depression or another mental health condition is causing or contributing to a person's symptoms.

The *Guidelines* prepared by the National Institute on Aging (NIA) and the Alzheimer Association (AA) focus on three stages of AD:

1. Dementia due to Alzheimer,

2. Mild cognitive impairment (MCI) due to Alzheimer, and

3. Preclinical (presymptomatic) Alzheimer. (Presymptomatic identification is exclusively used as a research diagnosis at this point and has no relevance to routine clinical practice.)

The *Guidelines* also include biomarker tests used in studies to measure biological changes in the brain associated with AD and criteria for documenting and reporting Alzheimer-related changes observed during an autopsy.

Treatment and Management

There are currently no treatments to stop or slow dementia in neurodegenerative diseases. Some diseases that occur at the same time as dementia (such as diabetes and depression) can be treated. Other symptoms that may occur in dementia-like conditions can also be treated, although some symptoms may only respond to treatment for a period of time. A team of specialists—doctors, nurses, and speech, physical, and other therapists—familiar with these disorders can help guide patient care.

Medications are available to treat certain behavioral symptoms, as well as delusions, depression, muscle stiffness, and risk factors for vascular cognitive impairment such as high blood pressure. Always consult with a doctor, as some medications may make symptoms worse.

AD. Most drugs for dementia are used to treat symptoms in AD. One class of drugs, called cholinesterase inhibitors, can temporarily improve or stabilize memory and thinking skills in some people by increasing the activity of the cholinergic brain network—a subsystem in the brain that is highly involved with memory and learning. These drugs include donepezil, rivastigmine, and galantamine. The drug memantine is in another class of medications called N-methyl-D-aspartate (NMDA) receptor antagonists, which prevent declines in learning and memory. Memantine may be combined with a cholinesterase inhibitor for added benefits. These drugs are sometimes used to treat other dementias in which AD is believed to co-occur.

FTD. There are no medications approved to treat or prevent FTD and most other types of progressive dementia. Sedatives, antidepressants, and other drugs used to treat Parkinson and Alzheimer symptoms may help manage certain symptoms and behavioral problems associated with the disorders.

DLB. Medicines available for managing DLB are aimed at relieving symptoms such as gait and balance disturbances, stiffness, hallucinations, and delusions. Studies suggest that the cholinesterase inhibitor drugs for AD may offer some benefit to people with DLB.

PDD. Some studies suggest that the cholinesterase inhibitors used to treat people with AD might improve cognitive, behavioral, and psychotic symptoms in people with PDD. Unfortunately, many of the medications used to treat the motor symptoms of PD worsen the cognitive problems. The U.S. Food and Drug Administration (FDA) has approved rivastigmine (an Alzheimer drug) to treat cognitive symptoms in PDD.

Vascular contributions to cognitive impairment and dementia. This type of dementia is often managed with drugs to prevent strokes or reduce the risk of additional brain damage. Some studies suggest that drugs that improve memory in AD might benefit people with early vascular dementia. Treating the modifiable risk factors can help prevent additional stroke.

A team of therapists can help with maintaining physical movement, address speech and swallowing issues, and help people learn new ways to handle loss of skills with everyday tasks such as feeding oneself. It is important to educate family, friends, and caregivers about a loved one's medical issues. Also, in-person and online support groups available through many disease awareness and caregiver advocacy organizations can give families and other caregivers additional resources, as well as opportunities to share experiences and express concerns.

Section 44.2

Alzheimer Disease

This section includes text excerpted from "Alzheimer's Disease Fact Sheet," National Institute on Aging (NIA), National Institutes of Health (NIH), August 17, 2016.

Alzheimer disease (AD) is an irreversible, progressive brain disorder that slowly destroys memory and thinking skills, and eventually the ability to carry out the simplest tasks. In most people with Alzheimer, symptoms first appear in their mid-60s. Estimates vary, but experts suggest that more than 5 million Americans may have Alzheimer.

Changes in the Brain

Scientists continue to unravel the complex brain changes involved in the onset and progression of AD. It seems likely that damage to the brain starts a decade or more before memory and other cognitive problems appear. During this preclinical stage of AD, people seem to be symptom-free, but toxic changes are taking place in the brain. Abnormal deposits of proteins form amyloid plaques and tau tangles throughout the brain, and once-healthy neurons stop functioning, lose connections with other neurons, and die.

The damage initially appears to take place in the hippocampus, the part of the brain essential in forming memories. As more neurons die, additional parts of the brain are affected, and they begin to shrink. By the final stage of Alzheimer, damage is widespread, and brain tissue has shrunk significantly.

Signs and Symptoms

Memory problems are typically one of the first signs of cognitive impairment related to AD. Some people with memory problems have a condition called mild cognitive impairment (MCI). In MCI, people have more memory problems than normal for their age, but their symptoms do not interfere with their everyday lives. Movement difficulties and problems with the sense of smell have also been linked to MCI. Older people with MCI are at greater risk for developing Alzheimer, but not all of them do. Some may even go back to normal cognition.

The first symptoms of Alzheimer vary from person to person. For many, decline in nonmemory aspects of cognition, such as word-finding, vision/spatial issues, and impaired reasoning or judgment, may signal the very early stages of AD. Researchers are studying biomarkers (biological signs of disease found in brain images, cerebrospinal fluid, and blood) to see if they can detect early changes in the brains of people with MCI and in cognitively normal people who may be at greater risk for Alzheimer. Studies indicate that such early detection may be possible, but more research is needed before these techniques can be relied upon to diagnose AD in everyday medical practice.

Mild AD

As AD progresses, people experience greater memory loss and other cognitive difficulties. Problems can include wandering and getting lost, trouble handling money and paying bills, repeating questions, taking longer to complete normal daily tasks, and personality and behavior changes. People are often diagnosed in this stage.

Moderate AD

In this stage, damage occurs in areas of the brain that control language, reasoning, sensory processing, and conscious thought. Memory loss and confusion grow worse, and people begin to have problems recognizing family and friends. They may be unable to learn new things, carry out multistep tasks such as getting dressed, or cope with new situations. In addition, people at this stage may have hallucinations, delusions, paranoia, and may behave impulsively.

Severe AD

Ultimately, plaques and tangles spread throughout the brain, and brain tissue shrinks significantly. People with severe Alzheimer cannot communicate and are completely dependent on others for their care. Near the end, the person may be in bed most or all of the time as the body shuts down.

What Causes Alzheimer

Scientists don't yet fully understand what causes AD in most people. There is a genetic component to some cases of early-onset AD. Late-onset Alzheimer arises from a complex series of brain changes that occur over decades. The causes probably include a combination of genetic, environmental, and lifestyle factors. The importance of any one of these factors in increasing or decreasing the risk of developing Alzheimer may differ from person to person.

What the Research Says

Scientists are conducting studies to learn more about plaques, tangles, and other biological features of AD. Advances in brain imaging techniques allow researchers to see the development and spread of abnormal amyloid and tau proteins in the living brain, as well as changes in brain structure and function. Scientists are also exploring the very earliest steps in the disease process by studying changes in the brain and body fluids that can be detected years before Alzheimer symptoms appear. Findings from these studies will help in understanding the causes of Alzheimer and make diagnosis easier.

One of the great mysteries of AD is why it largely strikes older adults. Research on normal brain aging is shedding light on this question. For example, scientists are learning how age-related changes in the brain may harm neurons and contribute to Alzheimer damage. These age-related changes include atrophy (shrinking) of certain parts of the brain, inflammation, production of unstable molecules called free radicals, and mitochondrial dysfunction (a breakdown of energy production within a cell).

Genetics

Most people with Alzheimer have the late-onset form of the disease, in which symptoms become apparent in their mid-60s. The apolipoprotein E (*APOE*) gene is involved in late-onset Alzheimer. This gene has several forms. One of them, *APOE ε4*, increases a person's risk of developing the disease and is also associated with an earlier age of disease onset. However, carrying the *APOE ε4* form of the gene does not mean that a person will definitely develop AD, and some people with no *APOE ε4* may also develop the disease.

Also, scientists have identified a number of regions of interest in the genome (an organism's complete set of deoxyribonucleic acid (DNA)) that may increase a person's risk for late-onset Alzheimer to varying degrees.

Early-onset AD occurs between a person's 30s–mid-60s and represents less than 10 percent of all people with Alzheimer. Some cases are caused by an inherited change in one of three genes, resulting in a type known as early-onset familial AD, or FAD. For other cases of early-onset Alzheimer, research suggests there may be a genetic component related to factors other than these three genes.

Most people with Down syndrome develop Alzheimer. This may be because people with Down syndrome have an extra copy of chromosome 21, which contains the gene that generates harmful amyloid.

Health, Environmental, and Lifestyle Factors

Research suggests that a host of factors beyond genetics may play a role in the development and course of AD. There is a great deal of interest, for example, in the relationship between cognitive decline and vascular conditions such as heart disease, stroke, and high blood pressure, as well as metabolic conditions such as diabetes and obesity. Ongoing research will help us understand whether and how reducing risk factors for these conditions may also reduce the risk of Alzheimer.

A nutritious diet, physical activity, social engagement, and mentally stimulating pursuits have all been associated with helping people stay healthy as they age. These factors might also help reduce the risk of cognitive decline and AD. Clinical trials are testing some of these possibilities.

Diagnosis of Alzheimer Disease

Doctors use several methods and tools to help determine whether a person who is having memory problems has "possible Alzheimer dementia" (dementia may be due to another cause) or "probable Alzheimer dementia" (no other cause for dementia can be found).

To diagnose Alzheimer, doctors may:

- Ask the person and a family member or friend questions about overall health, past medical problems, ability to carry out daily activities, and changes in behavior and personality

- Conduct tests of memory, problem solving, attention, counting, and language

- Carry out standard medical tests, such as blood and urine tests, to identify other possible causes of the problem

- Perform brain scans, such as computed tomography (CT), magnetic resonance imaging (MRI), or positron emission tomography (PET), to rule out other possible causes for symptoms

These tests may be repeated to give doctors information about how the person's memory and other cognitive functions are changing over time.

AD can be definitely diagnosed only after death, by linking clinical measures with an examination of brain tissue in an autopsy.

People with memory and thinking concerns should talk to their doctor to find out whether their symptoms are due to Alzheimer or another cause, such as stroke, tumor, Parkinson disease (PD), sleep disturbances, side effects of medication, an infection, or a non-Alzheimer dementia. Some of these conditions may be treatable and possibly reversible.

If the diagnosis is Alzheimer, beginning treatment early in the disease process may help preserve daily functioning for some time, even though the underlying disease process cannot be stopped or reversed. An early diagnosis also helps families plan for the future. They can take care of financial and legal matters, address potential safety issues, learn about living arrangements, and develop support networks.

In addition, an early diagnosis gives people greater opportunities to participate in clinical trials that are testing possible new treatments for AD or other research studies.

Treatment of AD

AD is complex, and it is unlikely that any one drug or other intervention can successfully treat it. Current approaches focus on helping people maintain mental function, manage behavioral symptoms, and slow down certain problems, such as memory loss. Researchers hope to develop therapies targeting specific genetic, molecular, and cellular mechanisms so that the actual underlying cause of the disease can be stopped or prevented.

Maintaining Mental Function

Several medications are approved by the U.S. Food and Drug Administration (FDA) to treat symptoms of Alzheimer. Donepezil (Aricept®), rivastigmine (Exelon®), and galantamine (Razadyne®) are used to treat mild to moderate Alzheimer (donepezil can be used for severe Alzheimer as well). Memantine (Namenda®) is used to treat moderate to severe Alzheimer. These drugs work by regulating neurotransmitters, the chemicals that transmit messages between neurons. They may help reduce symptoms and help with certain behavioral problems. However, these drugs don't change the underlying disease process. They are effective for some but not all people, and may help only for a limited time. The FDA has also approved Aricept® and Namzaric®, a combination of Namenda® and Aricept®, for the treatment of moderate to severe AD.

Managing Behavior

Common behavioral symptoms of Alzheimer include sleeplessness, wandering, agitation, anxiety, and aggression. Scientists are learning why these symptoms occur and are studying new treatments—drug and nondrug—to manage them. Research has shown that treating behavioral symptoms can make people with Alzheimer more comfortable and makes things easier for caregivers.

Section 44.3

Vascular Dementia

This section includes text excerpted from "What Is
Vascular Dementia?" National Institute on Aging (NIA),
National Institutes of Health (NIH), May 17, 2017.

Vascular dementia, considered the second most common form of
dementia after Alzheimer disease (AD), and vascular cognitive impairment (VCI) result from injuries to the vessels supplying blood to the
brain, often after a stroke or series of strokes. Vascular dementia and
VCI arise as a result of risk factors that similarly increase the risk for
cerebrovascular disease (such as stroke), including atrial fibrillation,
hypertension (high blood pressure), diabetes, and high cholesterol.

Symptoms

The symptoms of vascular dementia can be similar to those of Alzheimer, and both conditions can occur at the same time. Symptoms of
vascular dementia can begin suddenly and worsen or improve during
one's lifetime. This type of dementia is often managed with drugs
to prevent strokes. The aim is to reduce the risk of additional brain
damage. Some studies suggest that drugs that improve memory in
AD might benefit people with early vascular dementia. Interventions
that address risk factors may be incorporated into the management
of vascular dementia.

Types of Vascular Dementia

Some types of vascular dementia include:

Multi-infarct dementia. This type of dementia occurs when a person has had many small strokes that damage brain cells. One side of
the body may be disproportionately affected, and multi-infarct dementia may impair language or other functions, depending on the region
of the brain that is affected. When the strokes occur on both sides of
the brain, dementia is more likely than when stroke occurs on one
side of the brain. In some cases, a single stroke can damage the brain

enough to cause dementia. This so-called single-infarct dementia is more common when stroke affects the left side of the brain—where speech centers are located—and/or when it involves the hippocampus, the part of the brain that is vital for memory.

Cerebral autosomal dominant arteriopathy with subcortical infarcts and leukoencephalopathy (CADASIL). This inherited form of cardiovascular disease results in a thickening of the walls of small- and medium-sized blood vessels, eventually stemming the flow of blood to the brain. It is associated with mutations of a gene called *Notch3*. CADASIL is associated with multi-infarct dementia, stroke, migraine with aura (migraine preceded by visual symptoms), and mood disorders. The first symptoms can appear in people between ages 20 and 40. Many people with CADASIL are undiagnosed. People with first-degree relatives who have CADASIL can be tested for genetic mutations to the *Notch3* gene to determine their own risk of developing CADASIL.

Subcortical vascular dementia, also called Binswanger disease. This rare form of dementia involves extensive damage to the small blood vessels and nerve fibers that make up white matter, the "network" part of the brain believed to be critical for relaying messages between regions. The symptoms of Binswanger are related to the disruption of subcortical neural circuits involving short-term memory, organization, mood, attention, decision making, and appropriate behavior. A characteristic feature of this disease is psychomotor slowness, such as an increase in the time it takes for a person to think of a letter and then write it on a piece of paper.

Managing Vascular Dementia

This type of dementia is often managed with drugs to prevent strokes. The aim is to reduce the risk of additional brain damage. Some studies suggest that drugs that improve memory in AD might benefit people with early vascular dementia. Interventions that address risk factors may be incorporated into the management of vascular dementia.

Section 44.4

Lewy Body Dementia

This section includes text excerpted from "Lewy Body Dementia:
Hope through Research," National Institute of Neurological
Disorders and Stroke (NINDS), September 2015.

Lewy body dementia (LBD) is a complex and challenging brain disorder. It is complex because it affects many parts of the brain in ways that scientists are trying to understand more fully. It is challenging because its many possible symptoms make it hard to do everyday tasks that once came easily.

Although less known than its "cousins" Alzheimer disease (AD) and Parkinson disease (PD), LBD is not a rare disorder. More than 1 million Americans, most of them older adults, are affected by its disabling changes in the ability to think and move.

As researchers seek better ways to treat LBD—and ultimately to find a cure—people with LBD and their families struggle day to day to get an accurate diagnosis, find the best treatment, and manage at home.

This section is meant to help people with LBD, their families, and professionals learn more about the disease and resources for coping. It explains what is known about the different types of LBD and how they are diagnosed. Most importantly, it describes how to treat and manage this difficult disease, with practical advice for both people with LBD and their caregivers.

The Basics of Lewy Body Dementia

LBD is a disease associated with abnormal deposits of a protein called alpha-synuclein in the brain. These deposits, called Lewy bodies, affect chemicals in the brain whose changes, in turn, can lead to problems with thinking, movement, behavior, and mood. LBD is one of the most common causes of dementia, after Alzheimer disease and vascular disease.

Dementia is a severe loss of thinking abilities that interferes with a person's capacity to perform daily activities such as household tasks, personal care, and handling finances. Dementia has many possible causes, including stroke, brain tumor, depression, and vitamin deficiency, as well as disorders such as LBD, Parkinson, and Alzheimer.

Diagnosing LBD can be challenging for a number of reasons. Early LBD symptoms are often confused with similar symptoms found in other brain diseases like Alzheimer. Also, LBD can occur alone or along with Alzheimer or Parkinson disease (PD).

There are two types of LBD—dementia with Lewy bodies and Parkinson disease dementia. The earliest signs of these two diseases differ but reflect the same biological changes in the brain. Over time, people with dementia with Lewy bodies or Parkinson disease dementia may develop similar symptoms

Who Is Affected by LBD?

LBD affects more than 1 million individuals in the United States. LBD typically begins at age 50 or older, although sometimes younger people have it. LBD appears to affect slightly more men than women.

LBD is a progressive disease, meaning symptoms start slowly and worsen over time. The disease lasts an average of 5–7 years from the time of diagnosis to death, but the time span can range from 2–20 years. How quickly symptoms develop and change varies greatly from person to person, depending on overall health, age, and severity of symptoms.

In the early stages of LBD, usually before a diagnosis is made, symptoms can be mild, and people can function fairly normally. As the disease advances, people with LBD require more and more help due to a decline in thinking and movement abilities. In the later stages of the disease, they may depend entirely on others for assistance and care.

Some LBD symptoms may respond to treatment for a period of time. Currently, there is no cure for the disease. Research is improving our understanding of this challenging condition, and advances in science may one day lead to better diagnosis, improved care, and new treatments.

What Are Lewy Bodies?

Lewy bodies are named for Dr. Friederich Lewy, a German neurologist. In 1912, he discovered abnormal protein deposits that disrupt the brain's normal functioning in people with PD. These abnormal deposits are now called "Lewy bodies."

Lewy bodies are made of a protein called alpha-synuclein. In the healthy brain, alpha-synuclein plays a number of important roles in neurons (nerve cells) in the brain, especially at synapses, where brain cells communicate with each other. In LBD, alpha-synuclein forms into clumps inside neurons, starting in particular regions of the brain. This process causes neurons to work less effectively and, eventually, to die. The activities of brain chemicals important to brain function are also affected. The result is widespread damage to certain parts of the brain and a decline in abilities affected by those brain regions.

Lewy bodies affect several different brain regions in LBD:

- the cerebral cortex, which controls many functions, including information processing, perception, thought, and language

- the limbic cortex, which plays a major role in emotions and behavior

- the hippocampus, which is essential to forming new memories

- the midbrain, including the substantia nigra, which is involved in movement

- the brainstem, which is important in regulating sleep and maintaining alertness

- brain regions important in recognizing smells (olfactory pathways)

Types of LBD

LBD includes two related conditions—dementia with Lewy bodies and Parkinson disease dementia (PDD). The difference between them lies largely in the timing of cognitive (thinking) and movement symptoms. In dementia with Lewy bodies, cognitive symptoms are noted within a year of parkinsonism, any condition that involves the types of movement changes, such as tremor or muscle stiffness, seen in PD. In PDD, movement symptoms are pronounced in the early stages, with cognitive symptoms developing years later.

Dementia with Lewy Bodies

People with dementia with Lewy bodies have a decline in thinking ability that may look somewhat like AD. But over time they also develop movement and other distinctive symptoms that suggest dementia with Lewy bodies. Symptoms that distinguish this form of dementia from others may include:

- visual hallucinations early in the course of dementia

- fluctuations in cognitive ability, attention, and alertness

- slowness of movement, difficulty walking, or rigidity (parkinsonism)

- sensitivity to medications used to treat hallucinations

- rapid eye movement (REM) sleep behavior disorder, in which people physically act out their dreams by yelling, flailing, punching bed partners, and falling out of bed

- more trouble with complex mental activities, such as multi-tasking, problem solving, and analytical thinking, than with memory

PDD

This type of LBD starts as a movement disorder, with symptoms such as slowed movement, muscle stiffness, tremor, and a shuffling walk. These symptoms are consistent with a diagnosis of PD. Later on, cognitive symptoms of dementia and changes in mood and behavior may arise. Not all people with Parkinson develop dementia, and it is difficult to predict who will. Being diagnosed with Parkinson late in life is a risk factor for PDD.

Causes and Risk Factors

The precise cause of LBD is unknown, but scientists are learning more about its biology and genetics. For example, they know that an accumulation of Lewy bodies is associated with a loss of certain neurons in the brain that produce two important neurotransmitters, chemicals that act as messengers between brain cells. One of these messengers, acetylcholine, is important for memory and learning. The other, dopamine, plays an important role in behavior, cognition, movement, motivation, sleep, and mood.

Scientists are also learning about risk factors for LBD. Age is considered the greatest risk factor. Most people who develop the disorder are over age 50.

Other known risk factors for LBD include the following:

- **Diseases and health conditions.** Certain diseases and health conditions, particularly Parkinson disease and REM sleep behavior disorder, are linked to a higher risk of LBD.

- **Genetics.** While having a family member with LBD may increase a person's risk, LBD is not normally considered a genetic disease. A small percentage of families with dementia with Lewy bodies has a genetic association, such as a variant of the GBA gene, but in most cases, the cause is unknown. At this time, no genetic test can accurately predict whether someone will develop LBD. Future genetic research may reveal more information about causes and risk.

- **Lifestyle.** No specific lifestyle factor has been proven to increase one's risk for LBD. However, some studies suggest that a healthy lifestyle—including regular exercise, mental stimulation, and a healthy diet—might reduce the chance of developing age-associated dementias.

Common Symptoms

People with LBD may not have every LBD symptom, and the severity of symptoms can vary greatly from person to person. Throughout the course of the disease, any sudden or major change in functional ability or behavior should be reported to a doctor.

The most common symptoms include changes in cognition, movement, sleep, and behavior.

Cognitive Symptoms

LBD causes changes in thinking abilities. These changes may include:

- **Dementia.** Severe loss of thinking abilities that interferes with a person's capacity to perform daily activities. Dementia is a primary symptom in LBD and usually includes trouble with visual and spatial abilities (judging distance and depth or misidentifying objects), planning, multitasking, problem solving, and reasoning. Memory problems may not be evident at first but often arise as LBD progresses. Dementia can also include changes in mood and behavior, poor judgment, loss of initiative, confusion about time and place, and difficulty with language and numbers.

- **Cognitive fluctuations.** Unpredictable changes in concentration, attention, alertness, and wakefulness from day to day and sometimes throughout the day. A person with LBD may stare into space for periods of time, seem drowsy and lethargic, or sleep for several hours during the day despite getting enough sleep the night before. His or her flow of ideas may be disorganized, unclear, or illogical at times. The person may seem better one day, then worse the next day. These cognitive fluctuations are common in LBD but are not always easy for a doctor to identify.

- **Hallucinations.** Seeing or hearing things that are not present. Visual hallucinations occur in up to 80 percent of people with LBD, often early on. They are typically realistic and detailed, such as images of children or animals. Auditory hallucinations are less common than visual ones but may also occur. Hallucinations that are not disruptive may not require treatment. However, if they are frightening or dangerous (for example, if the person attempts to fight a perceived intruder), then a doctor may prescribe medication.

Movement Symptoms

Some people with LBD may not experience significant movement problems for several years. Others may have them early on. At first, signs of movement problems, such as a change in handwriting, may be very mild and thus overlooked. Parkinsonism is seen early on in PDD but can also develop later on in dementia with Lewy bodies. Specific signs of parkinsonism may include:

- muscle rigidity or stiffness
- shuffling gait, slow movement, or frozen stance
- tremor or shaking, most commonly at rest
- balance problems and falls
- stooped posture
- loss of coordination
- smaller handwriting than was usual for the person
- reduced facial expression
- difficulty swallowing
- a weak voice

Sleep Disorders

Sleep disorders are common in people with LBD but are often undiagnosed. A sleep specialist can play an important role on a treatment team, helping to diagnose and treat sleep disorders. Sleep-related disorders seen in people with LBD may include:

- **REM sleep behavior disorder.** A condition in which a person seems to act out dreams. It may include vivid dreaming, talking in one's sleep, violent movements, or falling out of bed. Sometimes only the bed partner of the person with LBD is aware of these symptoms. REM sleep behavior disorder appears in some people years before other LBD symptoms.

- **Excessive daytime sleepiness.** Sleeping 2 or more hours during the day.

- **Insomnia.** Difficulty falling or staying asleep, or waking up too early.

- **Restless leg syndrome (RLS).** A condition in which a person, while resting, feels the urge to move his or her legs to stop unpleasant or unusual sensations. Walking or moving usually relieves the discomfort.

Behavioral and Mood Symptoms

Changes in behavior and mood are possible in LBD. These changes may include:

- **Depression.** A persistent feeling of sadness, inability to enjoy activities, or trouble with sleeping, eating, and other normal activities.

- **Apathy.** A lack of interest in normal daily activities or events; less social interaction.

- **Anxiety.** Intense apprehension, uncertainty, or fear about a future event or situation. A person may ask the same questions over and over or be angry or fearful when a loved one is not present.

- **Agitation.** Restlessness, as seen by pacing, hand wringing, an inability to get settled, constant repeating of words or phrases, or irritability.

- **Delusions.** Strongly held false beliefs or opinions not based on evidence. For example, a person may think his or her spouse is having an affair or that relatives long dead are still living. Another delusion that may be seen in people with LBD is Capgras syndrome, in which the person believes a relative or friend has been replaced by an imposter.

- **Paranoia.** An extreme, irrational distrust of others, such as suspicion that people are taking or hiding things.

Other LBD Symptoms

People with LBD can also experience significant changes in the part of the nervous system that regulates automatic functions such as those of the heart, glands, and muscles. The person may have:

- changes in body temperature
- problems with blood pressure
- dizziness
- fainting
- frequent falls
- sensitivity to heat and cold
- sexual dysfunction
- urinary incontinence
- constipation
- a poor sense of smell

Diagnosis

It's important to know which type of LBD a person has, both to tailor treatment to particular symptoms and to understand how the disease will likely progress. Clinicians and researchers use the "1-year rule" to diagnose which form of LBD a person has. If cognitive symptoms appear within a year of movement problems, the diagnosis is dementia with Lewy bodies. If cognitive problems develop more than a year after the onset of movement problems, the diagnosis is PDD.

Regardless of the initial symptoms, over time people with LBD often develop similar symptoms due to the presence of Lewy bodies in the brain. But there are some differences. For example, dementia with Lewy bodies may progress more quickly than PDD.

Dementia with Lewy bodies is often hard to diagnose because its early symptoms may resemble those of Alzheimer, PD, or a psychiatric illness. As a result, it is often misdiagnosed or missed altogether. As additional symptoms appear, it is often easier to make an accurate diagnosis.

The good news is that doctors are increasingly able to diagnose LBD earlier and more accurately as researchers identify which symptoms help distinguish it from similar disorders.

No single test, such as a blood test, can be used to diagnose a frontotemporal disorder. A definitive diagnosis can be confirmed only by a genetic test in familial cases or a brain autopsy after a person dies. To diagnose a probable frontotemporal disorder in a living person, a doctor—usually a neurologist, psychiatrist, or psychologist—will:

Difficult as it is, getting an accurate diagnosis of LBD early on is important so that a person:

- gets the right medical care and avoids potentially harmful treatment

- has time to plan medical care and arrange legal and financial affairs

- can build a support team to stay independent and maximize quality of life

While a diagnosis of LBD can be distressing, some people are relieved to know the reason for their troubling symptoms. It is important to allow time to adjust to the news. Talking about a diagnosis can help shift the focus toward developing a care plan.

Who Can Diagnose LBD?

Many physicians and other medical professionals are not familiar with LBD, so patients may consult several doctors before receiving a diagnosis. Visiting a family doctor is often the first step for people who are experiencing changes in thinking, movement, or behavior. However, neurologists—doctors who specialize in disorders of the brain and nervous system—generally have the expertise needed to diagnose LBD. Geriatric psychiatrists, neuropsychologists, and geriatricians may also be skilled in diagnosing the condition.

If a specialist cannot be found in your community, ask the neurology department of the nearest medical school for a referral. A hospital affiliated with a medical school may also have a dementia or movement disorders clinic that provides expert evaluation.

Tests Used to Diagnose LBD

Doctors perform physical and neurological examinations and various tests to distinguish LBD from other illnesses. An evaluation may include:

- **Medical history and examination.** A review of previous and current illnesses, medications, and current symptoms and tests of movement and memory give the doctor valuable information.

- **Medical tests.** Laboratory studies can help rule out other diseases and hormonal or vitamin deficiencies that can be associated with cognitive changes.

- **Brain imaging.** Computed tomography (CT) or magnetic resonance imaging (MRI) can detect brain shrinkage or structural abnormalities and help rule out other possible causes of dementia or movement symptoms.

- **Neuropsychological tests.** These tests are used to assess memory and other cognitive functions and can help identify affected brain regions.

There are no brain scans or medical tests that can definitively diagnose LBD. Currently, LBD can be diagnosed with certainty only by a brain autopsy after death.

However, researchers are studying ways to diagnose LBD more accurately in the living brain. Certain types of neuroimaging—positron emission tomography (PET) and single-photon emission computed tomography—have shown promise in detecting differences between dementia with Lewy bodies and AD. These methods may help diagnose certain features of the disorder, such as dopamine deficiencies. Researchers are also investigating the use of lumbar puncture (spinal tap) to measure proteins in cerebrospinal fluid that might distinguish dementia with Lewy bodies from AD and other brain disorders.

Other Helpful Information

It is important for the patient and a close family member or friend to tell the doctor about any symptoms involving thinking, movement, sleep, behavior, or mood. Also, discuss other health problems and provide a list of all current medications, including prescriptions, over-the-counter drugs, vitamins, and supplements. Certain medications can worsen LBD symptoms.

Caregivers may be reluctant to talk about a person's symptoms when that person is present. Ask to speak with the doctor privately if necessary. The more information a doctor has, the more accurate a diagnosis can be.

467

Treatment and Management

While LBD currently cannot be prevented or cured, some symptoms may respond to treatment for a period of time. A comprehensive treatment plan may involve medications, physical and other types of therapy, and counseling. Changes to make the home safer, equipment to make everyday tasks easier, and social support are also very important.

A skilled care team often can provide suggestions to help improve quality of life for both people with LBD and their caregivers.

Building a Care Team

After receiving a diagnosis, a person with LBD may benefit from seeing a neurologist who specializes in dementia and/or movement disorders. A good place to find an LBD specialist is at a dementia or movement disorders clinic in an academic medical center in your community. If such a specialist cannot be found, a general neurologist should be part of the care team. Ask a primary care physician for a referral.

A doctor can work with other types of healthcare providers. Depending on an individual's particular symptoms, other professionals may be helpful:

- **Physical therapists** can help with movement problems through cardiovascular, strengthening, and flexibility exercises, as well as gait training and general physical fitness programs.

- **Speech therapists** may help with low voice volume, voice projection, and swallowing difficulties.

- **Occupational therapists** help identify ways to more easily carry out everyday activities, such as eating and bathing, to promote independence.

- **Music or expressive arts therapists** may provide meaningful activities that can reduce anxiety and improve well-being.

- **Mental health counselors** can help people with LBD and their families learn how to manage difficult emotions and behaviors and plan for the future.

Support groups are another valuable resource for both people with LBD and caregivers. Sharing experiences and tips with others in the same situation can help people identify practical solutions to day-to-day challenges and get emotional and social support.

Medications

Several drugs and other treatments are available to treat LBD symptoms. It is important to work with a knowledgeable health professional because certain medications can make some symptoms worse. Some symptoms can improve with nondrug treatments.

Cognitive Symptoms

Some medications used to treat AD also may be used to treat the cognitive symptoms of LBD. These drugs, called cholinesterase inhibitors, act on a chemical in the brain that is important for memory and thinking. They may also improve behavioral symptoms. The U.S. Food and Drug Administration (FDA) approves specific drugs for certain uses after rigorous testing and review. The FDA has approved one Alzheimer drug, rivastigmine (Exelon®), to treat cognitive symptoms in Parkinson disease dementia. This and other Alzheimer drugs can have side effects such as nausea and diarrhea.

Movement Symptoms

LBD-related movement symptoms may be treated with a Parkinson medication called carbidopa-levodopa (Sinemet®, Parcopa®, Stalevo®). This drug can help improve functioning by making it easier to walk, get out of bed, and move around. However, it cannot stop or reverse the progress of the disease.

Side effects of this medication can include hallucinations and other psychiatric or behavioral problems. Because of this risk, physicians may recommend not treating mild movement symptoms with medication. If prescribed, carbidopa-levodopa usually begins at a low dose and is increased gradually. Other Parkinson medications are less commonly used in people with LBD due to a higher frequency of side effects.

A surgical procedure called deep brain stimulation, which can be very effective in treating the movement symptoms of PD, is not recommended for people with LBD because it can result in greater cognitive impairment.

People with LBD may benefit from physical therapy and exercise. Talk with your doctor about what physical activities are best.

Sleep Disorders

Sleep problems may increase confusion and behavioral problems in people with LBD and add to a caregiver's burden. A physician can order a sleep study to identify any underlying sleep disorders such as sleep apnea, RLS, and REM sleep behavior disorder.

REM sleep behavior disorder, a common LBD symptom, involves acting out one's dreams, leading to lost sleep and even injuries to sleep partners. Clonazepam (Klonopin®), a drug used to control seizures and relieve panic attacks, is often effective for the disorder at very low dosages. However, it can have side effects such as dizziness, unsteadiness, and problems with thinking. Melatonin, a naturally occurring hormone used to treat insomnia, may also offer some benefit when taken alone or with clonazepam.

Excessive daytime sleepiness is also common in LBD. If it is severe, a sleep specialist may prescribe a stimulant to help the person stay awake during the day.

Some people with LBD may have difficulty falling asleep. If trouble sleeping at night (insomnia) persists, a physician may recommend a prescription medication to promote sleep. It is important to note that treating insomnia and other sleep problems in people with LBD has not been extensively studied, and that treatments may worsen daytime sleepiness and should be used with caution.

Certain sleep problems can be addressed without medications. Increasing daytime exercise or activities and avoiding lengthy or frequent naps can promote better sleep. Avoiding alcohol, caffeine, or chocolate late in the day can help, too. Some over-the-counter medications can also affect sleep, so review all medications and supplements with a physician.

Behavioral and Mood Problems

Behavioral and mood problems in people with LBD can arise from hallucinations or delusions. They may also be a result of pain, illness, stress or anxiety, and the inability to express frustration, fear, or feeling overwhelmed. The person may resist care or lash out verbally or physically. Caregivers must try to be patient and use a variety of strategies to handle such challenging behaviors. Some behavioral problems can be managed by making changes in the person's environment and/or treating medical conditions. Other problems may require medication.

The first step is to visit a doctor to see if a medical condition unrelated to LBD is causing the problem. Injuries, fever, urinary tract or pulmonary infections, pressure ulcers (bed sores), and constipation can worsen behavioral problems. Increased confusion can also occur.

Certain medications used to treat LBD symptoms or other diseases may also cause behavioral problems. For example, some sleep aids, pain medications, bladder control medications, and drugs used to treat

LBD-related movement symptoms can cause confusion, agitation, hallucinations, and delusions. Similarly, some anti-anxiety medicines can actually increase anxiety in people with LBD. Review your medications with your doctor to determine if any changes are needed.

Not all behavioral problems are caused by illness or medication. A person's surroundings—including levels of stimulation or stress, lighting, daily routines, and relationships—can lead to behavior issues. Caregivers can alter the home environment to try to minimize anxiety and stress for the person with LBD. In general, people with LBD benefit from having simple tasks, consistent schedules, regular exercise, and adequate sleep. Large crowds or overly stimulating environments can increase confusion and anxiety.

Hallucinations and delusions are among the biggest challenges for LBD caregivers. The person with LBD may not understand or accept that the hallucinations are not real and become agitated or anxious. Caregivers can help by responding to the fears expressed instead of arguing or responding factually to comments that may not be true. By tuning in to the person's emotions, caregivers can offer empathy and concern, maintain the person's dignity, and limit further tension.

Cholinesterase inhibitors may reduce hallucinations and other psychiatric symptoms of LBD. These medications may have side effects, such as nausea, and are not always effective. However, they can be a good first choice to treat behavioral symptoms. Cholinesterase inhibitors do not affect behavior immediately, so they should be considered part of a long-term strategy.

Antidepressants can be used to treat depression and anxiety, which are common in LBD. Two types of antidepressants, called selective serotonin reuptake inhibitors and serotonin and norepinephrine reuptake inhibitors, are often well tolerated by people with LBD.

In some cases, antipsychotic medications are necessary to treat LBD-related behavioral symptoms to improve both the quality of life and safety of the person with LBD and his or her caregiver. These types of medications must be used with caution because they can cause severe side effects and can worsen movement symptoms.

If antipsychotics are prescribed, it is very important to use the newer kind, called atypical antipsychotics. These medications should be used at the lowest dose possible and for the shortest time possible to control symptoms. Many LBD experts prefer quetiapine (Seroquel®) or clozapine (Clozaril®, FazaClo®) to control difficult behavioral symptoms. Typical (or traditional) antipsychotics, such as haloperidol (Haldol®), generally should not be prescribed for people with LBD. They can cause dangerous side effects.

Other Treatment Considerations

LBD affects the part of the nervous system that regulates automatic actions like blood pressure and digestion. One common symptom is orthostatic hypotension, low blood pressure that can cause dizziness and fainting. Simple measures such as leg elevation, elastic stockings, and, when recommended by a doctor, increasing salt and fluid intake can help.

If these measures are not enough, a doctor may prescribe medication. Urinary incontinence (loss of bladder control) should be treated cautiously because certain medications used to treat this condition may worsen cognition or increase confusion. Consider seeing a urologist. Constipation can often be treated by exercise and changes in diet, though laxatives and stool softeners may be necessary.

People with LBD are often sensitive to prescription and over-the-counter medications for other medical conditions. Talk with your doctor about any side effects seen in a person with LBD.

If surgery is planned and the person with LBD is told to stop taking all medications beforehand, ask the doctor to consult the person's neurologist in developing a plan for careful withdrawal. In addition, be sure to talk with the anesthesiologist in advance to discuss medication sensitivities and risks unique to LBD. People with LBD who receive certain anesthetics may become confused or delirious and have a sudden, significant decline in functional abilities, which may become permanent.

Depending on the procedure, possible alternatives to general anesthesia may include a spinal or regional block. These methods are less likely to result in confusion after surgery. Caregivers should also discuss the use of strong pain relievers after surgery, since people with LBD can become delirious if these drugs are used too freely.

Advice for People Living with LBD

Coping with a diagnosis of LBD and all that follows can be challenging. Getting support from family, friends, and professionals is critical to ensuring the best possible quality of life. Creating a safe environment and preparing for the future are important, too. Take time to focus on your strengths, enjoy each day, and make the most of your time with family and friends. Here are some ways to live with LBD day to day.

Getting Help

Your family and close friends are likely aware of changes in your thinking, movement, or behavior. You may want to tell others about your diagnosis so they can better understand the reason for these changes and learn more about LBD. For example, you could say that you have been diagnosed with a brain disorder called LBD, which can affect thinking, movement, and behavior. You can say that you will need more help over time. By sharing your diagnosis with those closest to you, you can build a support team to help you manage LBD.

As LBD progresses, you will likely have more trouble managing everyday tasks such as taking medication, paying bills, and driving. You will gradually need more assistance from family members, friends, and perhaps professional caregivers. Although you may be reluctant to get help, try to let others partner with you so you can manage responsibilities together. Remember, LBD affects your loved ones, too. You can help reduce their stress when you accept their assistance.

Finding someone you can talk with about your diagnosis—a trusted friend or family member, a mental health professional, or a spiritual advisor—may be helpful.

Consider Safety

The changes in thinking and movement that occur with LBD require attention to safety issues. Consider these steps:

- Fill out and carry the LBD Medical Alert Wallet Card and present it any time you are hospitalized, require emergency medical care, or meet with your doctors. It contains important information about medication sensitivities.

- Consider subscribing to a medical alert service, in which you push a button on a bracelet or necklace to access 911 if you need emergency help.

- Address safety issues in your home, including areas of fall risk, poor lighting, stairs, or cluttered walkways. Think about home modifications that may be needed, such as installing grab bars in the bathroom or modifying stairs with ramps. Ask your doctor to refer you to a home health agency for a home safety evaluation.

- Talk with your doctor about LBD and driving, and have your driving skills evaluated, if needed.

Plan for Your Future

There are many ways to plan ahead. Here are some things to consider:

- If you are working, consult with a legal and financial expert about planning for disability leave or retirement. Symptoms of LBD will interfere with work performance over time, and it is essential to plan now to obtain benefits you are entitled to.

- Consult with an attorney who specializes in elder law or estate planning to help you write or update important documents, such as a living will, healthcare power of attorney, and will.

- Identify local resources for home care, meals, and other services before you need them so you know whom to call when the time comes.

- Explore moving to a retirement or continuing care community where activities and varying levels of care can be provided over time, as needed. Ask about staff members' experience caring for people with LBD.

Find Enjoyment Everyday

It is important to focus on living with LBD. Your attitude can help you find enjoyment in daily life. Despite the many challenges and adjustments, you can have moments of humor, tenderness, and gratitude with the people closest to you.

Make a list of events and activities you can still enjoy—then find a way to do them! For example, listening to music, exercising, or going out for a meal allows you to enjoy time with family and friends. If you can't find pleasure in daily life, consult your doctor or another healthcare professional to discuss effective ways to cope and move forward. Let your family know if you are struggling emotionally so they can offer support.

Caring for a Person with LBD

As someone who is caring for a person with LBD, you will take on many different responsibilities over time. You do not have to face these responsibilities alone. Many sources of help are available, from adult day centers and respite care to online and in-person support groups.

Below are some important actions you can take to adjust to your new roles, be realistic about your situation, and care for yourself.

Educate Others about LBD

Most people, including many healthcare professionals, are not familiar with LBD. In particular, emergency room physicians and other hospital workers may not know that people with LBD are extremely sensitive to antipsychotic medications. Caregivers can educate healthcare professionals and others by:

- Informing hospital staff of the LBD diagnosis and medication sensitivities, and requesting that the person's neurologist be consulted
- before giving any drugs to control behavior problems.
- Sharing educational pamphlets and other materials with doctors, nurses, and other healthcare professionals who care for the person with LBD.
- Teaching family and friends about LBD so they can better understand your situation.

Adjust Expectations

You will likely experience a wide range of emotions as you care for the person with LBD. Sometimes, caregiving will feel loving and rewarding. Other times, it will lead to anger, impatience, resentment, or fatigue. You must recognize your strengths and limitations, especially in light of your past relationship with the person. Roles may change between a husband and wife or between a parent and adult children. Adjusting expectations can allow you to approach your new roles realistically and to seek help as needed.

People approach challenges at varied paces. Some people want to learn everything possible and be prepared for every scenario, while others manage best by taking one day at a time. Caring for someone with LBD requires a balance. On one hand, you should plan for the future. On the other hand, you may want to make each day count in personal ways and focus on creating enjoyable and meaningful moments.

Care for Yourself

As a caregiver, you play an essential role in the life of the person with LBD, so it is critical for you to maintain your own health and well-being. You may be at increased risk for poor sleep, depression, or illness as a result of your responsibilities. Watch for signs of physical or emotional fatigue such as irritability, withdrawal from friends and family, and changes in appetite or weight.

All caregivers need time away from caregiving responsibilities to maintain their well-being. Learn to accept help when it's offered and learn to ask family and friends for help. One option is professional respite care, which can be obtained through home care agencies and adult day programs. Similarly, friends or family can come to the home or take the person with LBD on an outing to give you a break.

Address Family Concerns

Not all family members may understand or accept LBD at the same time, and this can create conflict. Some adult children may deny that parents have a problem, while others may be supportive. It can take a while to learn new roles and responsibilities.

Family members who visit occasionally may not see the symptoms that primary caregivers see daily and may underestimate or minimize your responsibilities or stress. Professional counselors can help with family meetings or provide guidance on how families can work together to manage LBD.

Helping Children and Teens Cope with LBD

When someone has LBD, it affects the whole family, including children and grandchildren. Children notice when something "doesn't seem right." Telling them in age-appropriate language that someone they know or love has been diagnosed with a brain disorder can help them make sense of the changes they see. Give them enough information to answer questions or provide explanations without overwhelming them.

Children and teens may feel a loss of connection with the person with LBD who has problems with attention or alertness. They may also resent the loss of a parent caregiver's attention and may need special time with him or her. Look for signs of stress in children, such as poor grades at school, withdrawal from friendships, or unhealthy behaviors at home. Parents may want to notify teachers or counselors of the LBD diagnosis in the family so they can watch for changes in the young person that warrant attention.

Here are some other ways parents can help children and teens adjust to a family member with LBD:

- Help them keep up with normal activities such as sports, clubs, and other hobbies outside the home. Suggest ways for kids to engage with the relative with LBD through structured activities or play. For example, the child or teen can make a cup of tea for the person with LBD.

• Find online resources for older children and teens so they can learn about dementia and LBD.

It is important for families to make time for fun. Many challenges can be faced when they are balanced with enjoyable times. While LBD creates significant changes in family routines, children and teens will cope more effectively if the disorder becomes part of, but not all of, their lives.

Section 44.5

Frontotemporal Disorders

This section includes text excerpted from "What Are Frontotemporal Disorders?" National Institute on Aging (NIA), National Institutes of Health (NIH), May 17, 2017.

Damage to the brain's frontal and temporal lobes causes forms of dementia called frontotemporal disorders (FTD).

FDs are the result of damage to neurons (nerve cells) in parts of the brain called the frontal and temporal lobes. As neurons die in the frontal and temporal regions, these lobes atrophy, or shrink. Gradually, this damage causes difficulties in thinking and behaviors normally controlled by these parts of the brain. Many possible symptoms can result, including unusual behaviors, emotional problems, trouble communicating, difficulty with work, or difficulty with walking.

FDs are forms of dementia caused by a family of brain diseases known as frontotemporal lobar degeneration (FTLD). Dementia is a severe loss of thinking abilities that interferes with a person's ability to perform daily activities such as working, driving, and preparing meals. Other brain diseases that can cause dementia include Alzheimer disease (AD) and multiple strokes. Scientists estimate that FTLD may cause up to 10 percent of all cases of dementia and is the second most common cause of dementia, after Alzheimer, in people younger than age 65. Roughly 60 percent of people with FTLD are 45–64 years old.

People can live with FTDs for up to 10 years, sometimes longer, but it is difficult to predict the time course for an individual patient. The disorders are progressive, meaning symptoms get worse over time. In the early stages, people may have just one type of symptom. As the disease progresses, other types of symptoms appear as more parts of the brain are affected. No cure or treatments that slow or stop the progression of FTDs are available today. However, research is improving awareness and understanding of these challenging conditions. This progress is opening doors to better diagnosis, improved care, and, eventually, new treatments.

Changes in the Brain

FTDs affect the frontal and temporal lobes of the brain. They can begin in the frontal lobe, the temporal lobe, or both. Initially, FTDs leave other brain regions untouched, including those that control short-term memory.

The frontal lobes, situated above the eyes and behind the forehead both on the right and left sides of the brain, direct executive functioning. This includes planning and sequencing (thinking through which steps come first, second, third, and so on), prioritizing (doing more important activities first and less important activities last), multitasking (shifting from one activity to another as needed), and monitoring and correcting errors.

When functioning well, the frontal lobes also help manage emotional responses. They enable people to avoid inappropriate social behaviors, such as shouting loudly in a library or at a funeral. They help people make decisions that make sense for a given situation. When the frontal lobes are damaged, people may focus on insignificant details and ignore important aspects of a situation or engage in purposeless activities. The frontal lobes are also involved in language, particularly linking words to form sentences, and in motor functions, such as moving the arms, legs, and mouth.

The temporal lobes, located below and to the side of each frontal lobe on the right and left sides of the brain, contain essential areas for memory but also play a major role in language and emotions. They help people understand words, speak, read, write, and connect words with their meanings. They allow people to recognize objects and to relate appropriate emotions to objects and events. When the temporal lobes are dysfunctional, people may have difficulty recognizing emotions and responding appropriately to them.

Which lobe—and part of the lobe—is affected first determines which symptoms appear first. For example, if the disease starts in the part of the frontal lobe responsible for decision-making, then the first symptom might be trouble managing finances. If it begins in the part of the temporal lobe that connects emotions to objects, then the first symptom might be an inability to recognize potentially dangerous objects—a person might reach for a snake or plunge a hand into boiling water, for example.

Section 44.6

Mixed Dementia

This section includes text excerpted from "What Is Mixed Dementia?" National Institute on Aging (NIA), National Institutes of Health (NIH), May 17, 2017.

It is common for people to have mixed dementia—a combination of two or more disorders, at least one of which is dementia. A number of combinations are possible. For example, some people have both Alzheimer disease (AD) and vascular dementia.

Some studies indicate that mixed dementia is the most common cause of dementia in the elderly. For example, autopsy studies looking at the brains of people who had dementia indicate that most people age 80 and older had mixed dementia—a combination of brain changes related to AD (amyloid and tau), cerebrovascular disease (such as stroke), and, in some instances, Lewy body dementia (LBD) (Lewy bodies). These studies suggest that mixed dementia is caused by both Alzheimer-related neurodegenerative processes and vascular disease-related processes.

In a person with mixed dementia, it may not be clear exactly how many of a person's symptoms are due to Alzheimer or another type of dementia. In one study, approximately 40 percent of people who were thought to have Alzheimer were found after autopsy to also have some form of cerebrovascular disease. In addition, several studies have found that many of the major risk factors for vascular disease also may be risk factors for AD.

Researchers are still working to understand how underlying disease processes in mixed dementia influence each other. It is not clear, for example, if symptoms are likely to be worse when a person has brain changes reflecting multiple types of dementia. Nor do we know if a person with multiple dementias can benefit from treating one type, for example, when a person with Alzheimer controls high blood pressure and other vascular disease risk factors.

Chapter 45

Amyotrophic Lateral Sclerosis (ALS)

What Is Amyotrophic Lateral Sclerosis (ALS)?

- Amyotrophic lateral sclerosis (ALS) is a rare group of neurological diseases that mainly involve the nerve cells (neurons)
  responsible for controlling voluntary muscle movement. Voluntary muscles produce movements like chewing, walking,
  breathing, and talking. The disease is progressive, meaning the
  symptoms get worse over time. There is no cure for ALS and
  no effective treatment to halt, or reverse, the progression of the
  disease.

- ALS belongs to a wider group of disorders known as motor
  neuron diseases, which are caused by gradual deterioration
  (degeneration) and death of motor neurons. Motor neurons are
  nerve cells that extend from the brain to the spinal cord and to
  muscles throughout the body. These motor neurons initiate and
  provide vital communication links between the brain and the
  voluntary muscles.

This chapter includes text excerpted from "Amyotrophic Lateral Sclerosis (ALS)
Fact Sheet," National Institute of Neurological Disorders and Stroke (NINDS),
June 2013. Reviewed February 2018.

- Messages from motor neurons in the brain (called upper motor neurons) are transmitted to motor neurons in the spinal cord and to motor nuclei of brain (called lower motor neurons) and from the spinal cord and motor nuclei of brain to a particular muscle or muscles.

- In ALS, both the upper motor neurons and the lower motor neurons degenerate or die, and stop sending messages to the muscles. Unable to function, the muscles gradually weaken, start to twitch (called fasciculations), and waste away (atrophy). Eventually, the brain loses its ability to initiate and control voluntary movements.

- Early symptoms of ALS usually include muscle weakness or stiffness. Gradually all muscles under voluntary control are affected, and individuals lose their strength and the ability to speak, eat, move, and even breathe. Most people with ALS die from respiratory failure, usually within 3–5 years from when the symptoms first appear. However, about 10 percent of people with ALS survive for 10 or more years.

Who Gets ALS?

- Centers for Disease Control and Prevention (CDC) estimated that between 14,000–15,000 Americans have ALS. ALS is a common neuromuscular disease worldwide. It affects people of all races and ethnic backgrounds.

- There are several potential risk factors for ALS including:

- **Age.** Although the disease can strike at any age, symptoms most commonly develop between the ages of 55 and 75.

- **Gender.** Men are slightly more likely than women to develop ALS. However, as age the difference between men and women disappears.

- **Race and ethnicity.** Most likely to develop the disease are Caucasians and non-Hispanics.

- Some studies suggest that military veterans are about 1.5–2 times more likely to develop ALS. Although the reason for this is unclear, possible risk factors for veterans include exposure to lead, pesticides, and other environmental toxins. ALS is recognized as a service-connected disease by the U.S. Department of Veterans Affairs (VA).

Sporadic ALS

- The majority of ALS cases (90 percent or more) are considered sporadic. This means the disease seems to occur at random with no clearly associated risk factors and no family history of the disease. Although family members of people with sporadic ALS are at an increased risk for the disease, the overall risk is very low and most will not develop ALS.

Familial (Genetic) ALS

- About 5–10 percent of all ALS cases are familial, which means that an individual inherits the disease from his or her parents. The familial form of ALS usually only requires one parent to carry the gene responsible for the disease. Mutations in more than a dozen genes have been found to cause familial ALS. About 25–40 percent of all familial cases (and a small percentage of sporadic cases) are caused by a defect in a gene known as "chromosome 9 open reading frame 72," or *C9ORF72*. Interestingly, the same mutation can be associated with atrophy of frontal-temporal lobes of the brain causing frontal-temporal lobe dementia. Some individuals carrying this mutation may show signs of both motor neuron and dementia symptoms (ALS-FTD). Another 12–20 percent of familial cases result from mutations in the gene that provides instructions for the production of the enzyme copper-zinc superoxide dismutase 1 (SOD1).

What Are the Symptoms?

- The onset of ALS can be so subtle that the symptoms are overlooked but gradually these symptoms develop into more obvious weakness or atrophy that may cause a physician to suspect ALS. Some of the early symptoms include:

- fasciculations (muscle twitches) in the arm, leg, shoulder, or tongue

- muscle cramps

- tight and stiff muscles (spasticity)

- muscle weakness affecting an arm, a leg, neck, or diaphragm.

- slurred and nasal speech

- difficulty chewing or swallowing

For many individuals the first sign of ALS may appear in the hand or arm as they experience difficulty with simple tasks such as buttoning a shirt, writing, or turning a key in a lock. In other cases, symptoms initially affect one of the legs, and people experience awkwardness when walking or running or they notice that they are tripping or stumbling more often. When symptoms begin in the arms or legs, it is referred to as "limb onset" ALS. Other individuals first notice speech or swallowing problems, termed "bulbar onset" ALS.

Regardless of where the symptoms first appear, muscle weakness and atrophy spread to other parts of the body as the disease progresses. Individuals may develop problems with moving, swallowing (dysphagia), speaking or forming words (dysarthria), and breathing (dyspnea).

Although the sequence of emerging symptoms and the rate of disease progression vary from person to person, eventually individuals will not be able to stand or walk, get in or out of bed on their own, or use their hands and arms.

Individuals with ALS usually have difficulty swallowing and chewing food, which makes it hard to eat normally and increases the risk of choking. They also burn calories at a faster rate than most people without ALS. Due to these factors, people with ALS tend to lose weight rapidly and can become malnourished.

Because people with ALS usually retain their ability to perform higher mental processes such as reasoning, remembering, understanding, and problem solving, they are aware of their progressive loss of function and may become anxious and depressed.

A small percentage of individuals may experience problems with language or decision-making, and there is growing evidence that some may even develop a form of dementia over time. Individuals with ALS will have difficulty breathing as the muscles of the respiratory system weaken. They eventually lose the ability to breathe on their own and must depend on a ventilator. Affected individuals also face an increased risk of pneumonia during later stages of the disease. Besides muscle cramps that may cause discomfort, some individuals with ALS may develop painful neuropathy (nerve disease or damage).

How Is ALS Diagnosed?

- No one test can provide a definitive diagnosis of ALS. ALS is primarily diagnosed based on detailed history of the symptoms and signs observed by a physician during physical examination along with a series of tests to rule out other mimicking diseases.

However, the presence of upper and lower motor neuron symptoms strongly suggests the presence of the disease.

- Physicians will review an individual's full medical history and conduct a neurologic examination at regular intervals to assess whether symptoms such as muscle weakness, atrophy of muscles, and spasticity are getting progressively worse. ALS symptoms in the early stages of the disease can be similar to those of a wide variety of other, more treatable diseases or disorders. Appropriate tests can exclude the possibility of other conditions.

Muscle and Imaging Tests

- Electromyography (EMG), a special recording technique that detects electrical activity of muscle fibers, can help diagnose ALS. Another common test is a nerve conduction study (NCS), which measures electrical activity of the nerves and muscles by assessing the nerve's ability to send a signal along the nerve or to the muscle. Specific abnormalities in the NCS and EMG may suggest, for example, that the individual has a form of peripheral neuropathy (damage to peripheral nerves outside of the brain and spinal cord) or myopathy (muscle disease) rather than ALS.

- A physician may also order a magnetic resonance imaging (MRI) test, a noninvasive procedure that uses a magnetic field and radio waves to produce detailed images of the brain and spinal cord. Standard MRI scans are generally normal in people with ALS. However, they can reveal other problems that may be causing the symptoms, such as a spinal cord tumor, a herniated disk in the neck that compresses the spinal cord, syringomyelia (a cyst in the spinal cord), or cervical spondylosis (abnormal wear affecting the spine in the neck).

Laboratory Tests

- Based on the person's symptoms, test results, and findings from the examination, a physician may order tests on blood and urine samples to eliminate the possibility of other diseases.

Tests for Other Diseases and Disorders

- Infectious diseases such as human immunodeficiency virus (HIV), human T-cell leukemia virus (HTLV), polio, and West Nile virus can, in some cases, cause ALS-like symptoms.

Neurological disorders such as multiple sclerosis, postpolio syndrome, multifocal motor neuropathy, and spinal and bulbar muscular atrophy (Kennedy disease) also can mimic certain features of the disease and should be considered by physicians attempting to make a diagnosis. Fasciculations and muscle cramps also occur in benign conditions. Because of the prognosis carried by this diagnosis and the variety of diseases or disorders that can resemble ALS in the early stages of the disease, individuals may wish to obtain a second neurological opinion.

What Causes ALS?

- The cause of ALS is not known, and scientists do not yet know why ALS strikes some people and not others. However, evidence from scientific studies suggests that both genetics and environment play a role in the development of ALS.

Genetics

- An important step toward determining ALS risk factors was made in 1993 when scientists supported by the National Institute of Neurological Disorders and Stroke (NINDS) discovered that mutations in the *SOD1* gene were associated with some cases of familial ALS. Although it is still not clear how mutations in the *SOD1* gene lead to motor neuron degeneration, there is increasing evidence that the gene playing a role in producing mutant *SOD1* protein can become toxic.

- Since then, more than a dozen additional genetic mutations have been identified and each of these gene discoveries is providing new insights into possible mechanisms of ALS. The discovery of certain genetic mutations involved in ALS suggests that changes in the processing of ribonucleic acid (RNA) molecules may lead to ALS-related motor neuron degeneration. RNA molecules are one of the major macromolecules in the cell involved in directing the synthesis of specific proteins as well as gene regulation and activity.

- Other gene mutations indicate defects in the natural process in which malfunctioning proteins are broken down and used to build new ones, known as protein recycling. Still others point to possible defects in the structure and shape of motor neurons, as well as increased susceptibility to environmental toxins. Overall, it is becoming increasingly clear that a number of cellular defects can lead to motor neuron degeneration in ALS.

- Another important discovery was made when scientists found that a defect in the *C9ORF72* gene is not only present in a significant subset of individuals with ALS but also in some people with a type of frontotemporal dementia (FTD). This observation provides evidence for genetic ties between these two neurodegenerative disorders. Most researchers now believe ALS and some forms of FTD are related disorders.

Environmental Factors

- In searching for the cause of ALS, researchers are also studying the impact of environmental factors. Researchers are investigating a number of possible causes such as exposure to toxic or infectious agents, viruses, physical trauma, diet, and behavioral and occupational factors. For example, researchers have suggested that exposure to toxins during warfare, or strenuous physical activity, are possible reasons for why some veterans and athletes may be at increased risk of developing ALS.

- Although there has been no consistent association between any environmental factor and the risk of developing ALS, future research may show that some factors are involved in the development or progression of the disease.

How Is ALS Treated?

- No cure has yet been found for ALS. However, there are treatments available that can help control symptoms, prevent unnecessary complications, and make living with the disease easier. Supportive care is best provided by multidisciplinary teams of healthcare professionals such as physicians; pharmacists; physical, occupational, and speech therapists; nutritionists; social workers; respiratory therapists and clinical psychologists; and home care and hospice nurses. These teams can design an individualized treatment plan and provide special equipment aimed at keeping people as mobile, comfortable, and independent as possible.

Medication

- The U.S. Food and Drug Administration (FDA) has approved the drugs riluzole (Rilutek) and edaravone (Radicava) to treat ALS. Riluzole is believed to reduce damage to motor neurons by decreasing levels of glutamate, which transports messages between nerve cells and motor neurons. Clinical trials in people with ALS showed that riluzole prolongs survival by a few months, particularly in the bulbar form of the disease, but does not reverse the damage already done to motor neurons. Edaravone has been shown to slow the decline in clinical assessment of daily functioning in persons with ALS.

- Physicians can also prescribe medications to help manage symptoms of ALS, including muscle cramps, stiffness, excess saliva, and phlegm, and the pseudobulbar affect (involuntary or uncontrollable episodes of crying and/or laughing, or other emotional displays). Drugs also are available to help individuals with pain, depression, sleep disturbances, and constipation. Pharmacists can give advice on the proper use of medications and monitor a person's prescriptions to avoid risks of drug interactions.

Physical Therapy

- Physical therapy and special equipment can enhance an individual's independence and safety throughout the course of ALS. Gentle, low-impact aerobic exercise such as walking, swimming, and stationary bicycling can strengthen unaffected muscles, improve cardiovascular health, and help people fight fatigue and depression. Range of motion and stretching exercises can help prevent painful spasticity and shortening (contracture) of muscles.

- Physical therapists can recommend exercises that provide these benefits without overworking muscles. Occupational therapists can suggest devices such as ramps, braces, walkers, and wheelchairs that help individuals conserve energy and remain mobile.

Speech Therapy

- People with ALS who have difficulty speaking may benefit from working with a speech therapist, who can teach adaptive strategies to speak louder and more clearly. As ALS progresses, speech therapists can help people maintain the ability to communicate. They can recommend aids such as computer-based speech synthesizers that use eye-tracking technology and can help people develop ways for responding to yes-or-no questions with their eyes or by other nonverbal means.

- Some people with ALS may choose to use voice banking while they are still able to speak as a process of storing their own voice for future use in computer-based speech synthesizers. These methods and devices help people communicate when they can no longer speak or produce vocal sounds.

Nutritional Support

- Nutritional support is an important part of the care of people with ALS. It has been shown that individuals with ALS will get weaker if they lose weight. Nutritionists can teach individuals and caregivers how to plan and prepare small meals throughout the day that provide enough calories, fiber, and fluid and how to avoid foods that are difficult to swallow. People may begin using suction devices to remove excess fluids or saliva and prevent choking. When individuals can no longer get enough nourishment from eating, doctors may advise inserting a feeding tube into the stomach. The use of a feeding tube also reduces the risk of choking and pneumonia that can result from inhaling liquids into the lungs.

Breathing Support

- As the muscles responsible for breathing start to weaken, people may experience shortness of breath during physical activity and difficulty breathing at night or when lying down. Doctors may test an individual's breathing to determine when to recommend a treatment called noninvasive ventilation (NIV). NIV refers to breathing support that is usually delivered through a mask over the nose and/or mouth. Initially, NIV may only be necessary at night. When muscles are no longer able to maintain normal oxygen and carbon dioxide levels, NIV may be used full-time. NIV improves the quality of life and prolongs survival for many people with ALS. Because the muscles that control breathing become weak, individuals with ALS may also have trouble generating a strong cough. There are several techniques to help people increase forceful coughing, including mechanical cough assist devices and breath stacking. In breath stacking, a person takes a series of small breaths without exhaling until the lungs are full, briefly holds the breath, and then expels the air with a cough.

- As the disease progresses and muscles weaken further, individuals may consider forms of mechanical ventilation (respirators) in which a machine inflates and deflates the lungs. Doctors may place a breathing tube through the mouth or may surgically create a hole at the front of the neck and insert a tube leading to the windpipe (tracheostomy). The tube is connected to a respirator.

• Individuals with ALS and their families often consider several factors when deciding whether and when to use ventilation support. These devices differ in their effect on a person's quality of life and in cost. Although ventilation support can ease problems with breathing and prolong survival, it does not affect the progression of ALS. People may choose to be fully informed about these considerations and the long-term effects of life without movement before they make decisions about ventilation support.

What Research Is Being Done?

Cellular Defects

• Scientists are seeking to understand the mechanisms that selectively trigger motor neurons to degenerate in ALS, and to find effective approaches to halt the processes leading to cell death. Using both animal models and cell culture systems, scientists are trying to determine how and why ALS-causing gene mutations lead to the destruction of neurons. These animal models include fruit flies, zebrafish, and rodents.

• Initially, genetically modified animal models focused on mutations in the *SOD1* gene but more recently, models have been developed for defects in the *C9ORF72, TARDP, FUS, PFN1, TUBA4A,* and *UBQLN2* genes. Research in these models suggests that, depending on the gene mutation, motor neuron death is caused by a variety of cellular defects, including in the processing of RNA molecules and recycling of proteins, and structural impairments of motor neurons. Increasing evidence also suggests that various types of glial support cells and inflammation cells of the nervous system may play an important role in the disease.

Stem Cells

• In addition to animal models, scientists are also using innovative stem cells models to study ALS. Scientists have developed ways to take skin or blood cells from individuals with ALS and turn them into stem cells, which are capable of becoming any cell type in the body, including motor neurons and other cell types that may be involved in the disease. NINDS is supporting research on the development of stem cell lines for a number of neurodegenerative diseases, including ALS.

Familial versus Sporadic ALS

- Overall, the work in familial ALS is already leading to a greater understanding of the more common sporadic form of the disease. Because familial ALS and sporadic ALS show many of the same signs and symptoms, some researchers believe that some familial ALS, genes may also be involved in sporadic ALS.

- Clinical research studies supported by NINDS are looking into how ALS symptoms change over time in people with *C9ORF72* mutations. Other NINDS-supported research studies are working to identify additional genes that may cause or put a person at risk for either familial or sporadic ALS.

- Additionally, researchers are looking at the potential role of epigenetics in the development of ALS. Epigenetic changes can switch genes on and off, and thus can profoundly affect the human condition in both health and disease. These changes can occur in response to multiple factors, including external or environmental conditions and events. Although this research is still at a very exploratory stage, scientists hope that understanding epigenetics can offer new information about how ALS develops.

Biomarkers

- Biomarkers are biological measures that help to identify the presence or rate of progression of a disease or the effectiveness of a therapeutic intervention. Since ALS is difficult to diagnose, biomarkers could potentially help clinicians diagnose ALS earlier and faster.

- Additionally, biomarkers are needed to help predict and accurately measure disease progression and enhance clinical studies aimed at developing more effective treatments. Biomarkers can be molecules derived from a bodily fluid (such as those in the blood and cerebrospinal fluid), an image of the brain or spinal cord, or a measure of the ability of a nerve or muscle to process electrical signals. The NINDS is supporting research on the development biomarkers for ALS.

New Treatment Options

- Potential therapies for ALS are being investigated in a range of disease models. This work involves tests of drug-like compounds, gene therapy approaches, antibodies, and cell-based therapies. For example, NINDS-supported scientists are investigating whether lowering levels of the *SOD1* enzyme in the brain and spinal cord of individuals with *SOD1* gene mutations would slow the rate of disease progression.

- Other NINDS scientists are studying the use of glial-restricted progenitor cells (which have the ability to develop into other support cells) to slow disease progression and improve respiratory function. Additionally, a number of exploratory treatments are being tested in people with ALS. Investigators are optimistic that these and other basic, translational, and clinical research studies will eventually lead to new and more effective treatments for ALS.

Chapter 46

Creutzfeldt-Jakob Disease

What Is Creutzfeldt-Jakob Disease (CJD)?

Creutzfeldt-Jakob disease (CJD) is a rare disorder of the brain, degenerative and invariably fatal. It affects approximately one in a million people around the world and about 200 people in the United States. CJD usually appears in more advanced stages of life and maintains a rapid trajectory. Typically, symptoms begin around the age of 60 and 90 percent of patients die within a year. In the initial stages of the disease, patients suffer from memory failure, behavioral changes, lack of coordination and visual disturbances. As the disease progresses, mental deterioration becomes pronounced and involuntary movements, blindness, weakness of the extremities and coma may occur.

There are three main categories of CJD:

- In **sporadic CJD,** the disease appears even when the person does not have known risk factors for the disease. This is the most common type of CJD, occurring in at least 85 percent of cases.

- In **hereditary CJD,** the person has a family history of the disease or positive genetic mutation tests associated with CJD. About 5–10 percent of CJD cases in the United States are hereditary.

This chapter includes text excerpted from "Creutzfeldt-Jakob Disease Fact Sheet," National Institute of Neurological Disorders and Stroke (NINDS), May 10, 2017.

- In **acquired CJD,** the disease is transmitted by exposure to brain tissue or the nervous system, commonly by certain medical procedures. There is no evidence that CJD is contagious through casual contact with a CJD patient. Since CJD was first described in the year 1920, less than 1 percent of cases have been CJD acquired.

CJD belongs to a family of diseases of humans and animals known as transmissible spongiform encephalopathies (TSE). Spongiform refers to the characteristic appearance of infected brains, which fill with holes or holes until they resemble sponges under a microscope. CJD is the most common of the known human transmissible spongiform encephalopathies (TSEs). Other human TSEs include kuru, fatal familial insomnia (IFF) and Gerstmann-Straussler-Scheinker disease (GSS). The kuru was identified in people of an isolated tribe of Papua New Guinea and has almost disappeared. IFF and GSS are extremely rare hereditary diseases, found only in a few families around the world. We can find other TSE cases in specific types of animals. These include bovine spongiform encephalopathy (BSE), which is found in cows and is often called scrapie "mad cow" disease, which affects sheep, and mink encephalopathy. Similar diseases have occurred in moose, deer, and exotic zoo animals.

What Are the Symptoms of the Disease?

CJD is characterized by rapidly progressive dementia. Initially, individuals experience problems with muscular coordination; personality changes, including impaired memory, judgment, and thinking; and impaired vision. People with the disease also may experience insomnia, depression, or unusual sensations. CJD does not cause a fever or other flu-like symptoms. As the illness progresses, mental impairment becomes severe. Individuals often develop involuntary muscle jerks called myoclonus, and they may go blind. They eventually lose the ability to move and speak and enter a coma. Pneumonia and other infections often occur in these individuals and can lead to death.

There are several known variants of CJD. These variants differ somewhat in the symptoms and course of the disease. For example, a variant form of the disease-called new variant or variant (nv-CJD, v-CJD), described in Great Britain and France-begins primarily with psychiatric symptoms, affects younger individuals than other types of CJD, and has a longer than usual duration from onset of symptoms to death. Another variant, called the panencephalopathic form, occurs primarily in Japan and has a relatively long course, with symptoms often progressing for several years. Scientists are trying to learn what causes these variations in the symptoms and course of the disease.

Some symptoms of CJD can be similar to symptoms of other progressive neurological disorders, such as Alzheimer or Huntington disease. However, CJD causes unique changes in brain tissue which can be seen at autopsy. It also tends to cause more rapid deterioration of a person's abilities than Alzheimer disease or most other types of dementia.

How Is CJD Diagnosed?

There is currently no single diagnostic test for CJD. When a doctor suspects CJD, the first concern is to rule out treatable forms of dementia such as encephalitis (inflammation of the brain) or chronic meningitis. A neurological examination will be performed and the doctor may seek consultation with other physicians. Standard diagnostic tests will include a spinal tap to rule out more common causes of dementia and an electroencephalogram (EEG) to record the brain's electrical pattern, which can be particularly valuable because it shows a specific type of abnormality in CJD. Computerized tomography of the brain can help rule out the possibility that the symptoms result from other problems such as stroke or a brain tumor. Magnetic resonance imaging (MRI) brain scans also can reveal characteristic patterns of brain degeneration that can help diagnose CJD.

The only way to confirm a diagnosis of CJD is by brain biopsy or autopsy. In a brain biopsy, a neurosurgeon removes a small piece of tissue from the patient's brain so that it can be examined by a neuropathologist. This procedure may be dangerous for the individual, and the operation does not always obtain tissue from the affected part of the brain. Because a correct diagnosis of CJD does not help the person, a brain biopsy is discouraged unless it is needed to rule out a treatable disorder. In an autopsy, the whole brain is examined after death. Both brain biopsy and autopsy pose a small, but definite, risk that the surgeon or others who handle the brain tissue may become accidentally infected by self-inoculation. Special surgical and disinfection procedures can minimize this risk. A fact sheet with guidance on these procedures is available from the National Institute of Neurological Disorders and Stroke (NINDS) and the World Health Organization (WHO).

Scientists are working to develop laboratory tests for CJD. One such test, developed at NINDS, is performed on a person's cerebrospinal fluid and detects a protein marker that indicates neuronal degeneration. This can help diagnose CJD in people who already show the clinical symptoms of the disease. This test is much easier and safer than a brain biopsy. The false positive rate is about 5–10 percent. Scientists are working to develop this test for use in commercial laboratories. They are also working to develop other tests for this disorder.

How Is CJD Disease Treated?

There is no treatment that can cure or control CJD. Researchers have tested many drugs, including amantadine, steroids, interferon, acyclovir, antiviral agents, and antibiotics. Studies of a variety of other drugs are now in progress. However, so far none of these treatments has shown any consistent benefit in humans. Current treatment for CJD is aimed at alleviating symptoms and making the individual as comfortable as possible. Opiate drugs can help relieve pain if it occurs, and the drugs clonazepam and sodium valproate may help relieve myoclonus. During later stages of the disease, changing the person's position frequently can keep him or her comfortable and helps prevent bedsores. A catheter can be used to drain urine if the individual cannot control bladder function, and intravenous fluids and artificial feeding also may be used.

What Causes CJD?

Some researchers believe an unusual "slow virus" or another organism causes CJD. However, they have never been able to isolate a virus or other organism in people with the disease. Furthermore, the agent that causes CJD has several characteristics that are unusual for known organisms such as viruses and bacteria. It is difficult to kill, it does not appear to contain any genetic information in the form of nucleic acids (Deoxyribonucleic acid (DNA) or Ribonucleic acid (RNA)), and it usually has a long incubation period before symptoms appear. In some cases, the incubation period may be as long as 50 years. The leading scientific theory at this time maintains that CJD and the other TSEs are caused by a type of protein called a prion.

Prion proteins occur in both a normal form, which is a harmless protein found in the body's cells, and in an infectious form, which causes disease. The harmless and infectious forms of the prion protein have the same sequence of amino acids (the "building blocks" of proteins) but the infectious form of the protein takes a different folded shape than the normal protein. Sporadic CJD may develop because some of a person's normal prions spontaneously change into the infectious form of the protein and then alter the prions in other cells in a chain reaction.

Once they appear, abnormal prion proteins aggregate, or clump together. Investigators think these protein aggregates may lead to the neuron loss and other brain damage seen in CJD. However, they do not know exactly how this damage occurs.

About 5–10 percent of all CJD cases are inherited. These cases arise from a mutation, or change, in the gene that controls formation of the normal prion protein. While prions themselves do not contain genetic information and do not require genes to reproduce themselves, infectious prions can arise if a mutation occurs in the gene for the body's normal prion protein. If the prion protein gene is altered in a person's sperm or egg cells, the mutation can be transmitted to the person's offspring. All mutations in the prion protein gene are inherited as dominant traits. Therefore, family history is helpful in considering the diagnosis. Several different mutations in the prion gene have been identified. The particular mutation found in each family affects how frequently the disease appears and what symptoms are most noticeable. However, not all people with mutations in the prion protein gene develop CJD.

How Is CJD Transmitted?

CJD cannot be transmitted through the air or through touching or most other forms of casual contact. Spouses and other household members of sporadic CJD patients have no higher risk of contracting the disease than the general population. However, exposure to brain tissue and spinal cord fluid from infected individuals should be avoided to prevent transmission of the disease through these materials.

In some cases, CJD has spread to other people from grafts of dura mater (a tissue that covers the brain), transplanted corneas, implantation of inadequately sterilized electrodes in the brain, and injections of contaminated pituitary growth hormone derived from human pituitary glands taken from cadavers. Doctors call these cases that are linked to medical procedures *iatrogenic* cases. Since 1985, all human growth hormone used in the United States has been synthesized by recombinant DNA procedures, which eliminates the risk of transmitting CJD by this route.

The appearance of the new variant of CJD (nv-CJD or v-CJD) in several younger than average people in Great Britain and France has led to concern that BSE may be transmitted to humans through consumption of contaminated beef. Although laboratory tests have shown a strong similarity between the prions causing BSE and v-CJD, there is no direct proof to support this theory.

Many people are concerned that it may be possible to transmit CJD through blood and related blood products such as plasma. Some animal studies suggest that contaminated blood and related products may transmit the disease, although this has never been shown in humans. If there are infectious agents in these fluids, they are probably in very low concentrations. Scientists do not know how many abnormal prions a person must receive before he or she develops CJD, so they do not know whether these fluids are potentially infectious or not. They do know that, even though millions of people receive blood transfusions each year, there are no reported cases of someone contracting CJD from a transfusion. Even among people with hemophilia, who sometimes receive blood plasma concentrated from thousands of donors, there are no reported cases of CJD.

While there is no evidence that blood from people with sporadic CJD is infectious, studies have found that infectious prions from BSE and vCJD may accumulate in the lymph nodes (which produce white blood cells), the spleen, and the tonsils. These findings suggest that blood transfusions from people with vCJD might transmit the disease. The possibility that blood from people with vCJD may be infectious has led to a policy preventing people in the United States from donating blood if they have resided for more than 3 months in a country or countries where BSE is common.

How Can People Avoid Spreading the Disease?

To reduce the already very low risk of CJD transmission from one person to another, people should never donate blood, tissues, or organs if they have suspected or confirmed CJD, or if they are at increased risk because of a family history of the disease, a dura mater graft, or other factor.

Normal sterilization procedures such as cooking, washing, and boiling do not destroy prions. Caregivers, healthcare workers, and undertakers should take the following precautions when they are working with a person with CJD:

- Cover cuts and abrasions with waterproof dressings.
- Wear surgical gloves when handling a patient's tissues and fluids or dressing the patient's wounds.

- Avoid cutting or sticking themselves with instruments contaminated by the patient's blood or other tissues.

- Use disposable bedclothes and other cloth for contact with the patient. If disposable materials are not available, regular cloth should be soaked in undiluted chlorine bleach for an hour or more, and then washed in a normal fashion after each use.

- Use face protection if there is a risk of splashing contaminated material such as blood or cerebrospinal fluid.

- Soak instruments that have come in contact with the patient in undiluted chlorine bleach for an hour or more, then use an autoclave (pressure cooker) to sterilize them in distilled water for at least one hour at 132–134 degrees Centigrade.

Chapter 47

Friedreich Ataxia

What Is Friedreich Ataxia?

Friedreich ataxia is an inherited condition that affects the nervous system and causes movement problems. People with this condition develop impaired muscle coordination (ataxia) that worsens over time. Other features include the gradual loss of strength and sensation in the arms and legs, muscle stiffness (spasticity), and impaired speech. Many individuals have a form of heart disease called hypertrophic cardiomyopathy. Some develop diabetes, impaired vision, hearing loss, or an abnormal curvature of the spine (scoliosis). Most people with Friedreich ataxia begin to experience the signs and symptoms around puberty. This condition is caused by mutations in the *FXN* gene and is inherited in an autosomal recessive pattern.

What Are the Signs and Symptoms of Friedreich Ataxia?

- Symptoms usually begin between the ages of 5 and 15 but can, on occasion, appear in adulthood or even as late as age 75. The first symptom is usually difficulty walking (gait ataxia). The ataxia gradually worsens and slowly spreads to the arms and

This chapter includes text excerpted from "Friedreich Ataxia," Genetic and Rare Diseases Information Center (GARD), National Center for Advancing Translational Sciences (NCATS), May 22, 2015.

then the trunk. Over time, muscles begin to weaken and waste away, especially in the feet, lower legs, and hands. Other symptoms include loss of tendon reflexes, especially in the knees and ankles. There is often a gradual loss of sensation in the extremities, which may spread to other parts of the body. Slurred speech (dysarthria), fatigue, and involuntary eye movements (nystagmus) are also common. Most people with Friedreich ataxia develop scoliosis (a curving of the spine to one side), which, if severe, may impair breathing.

- Other symptoms that may occur include chest pain, shortness of breath, and heart palpitations. These symptoms are the result of various forms of heart disease that often accompany Friedreich ataxia, such as cardiomyopathy (enlargement of the heart), myocardial fibrosis (formation of fiber-like material in the muscles of the heart), and cardiac failure. Heart rhythm abnormalities such as tachycardia (fast heart rate) and heart block (impaired conduction of cardiac impulses within the heart) are also common. About 20 percent of people with Friedreich ataxia develop carbohydrate intolerance and 10 percent develop diabetes mellitus. Some people lose hearing or eyesight.

- The rate of progression varies from person to person. Generally, within 10–20 years after the first symptoms appear, people with Friedreich ataxia need to consistently use a wheelchair. Life expectancy may be affected, and many people with Friedreich ataxia die in adulthood from the associated heart disease. However, some people with less severe symptoms of Friedreich ataxia live much longer, sometimes into their sixties or seventies.

What Causes Friedreich Ataxia?

- Friedreich ataxia is caused by mutations in the *FXN* gene. This gene provides instructions for making a protein called frataxin. One region of the *FXN* gene contains a segment of deoxyribonucleic acid (DNA) known as a GAA trinucleotide repeat. This segment is made up of a series of three DNA building blocks (one guanine and two adenines) that appear multiple times in a row. Normally, this segment is repeated 5–33 times within the *FXN* gene. In people with Friedreich ataxia, the GAA segment is repeated 66 to more than 1,000 times. The length of the GAA trinucleotide repeat appears to be related to the age at which the symptoms of Friedreich ataxia appear.

- The abnormally long GAA trinucleotide repeat disrupts the production of frataxin, which severely reduces the amount of this protein in cells. Certain nerve and muscle cells cannot function properly with a shortage of frataxin, leading to the characteristic signs and symptoms of Friedreich ataxia.

Is Friedreich Ataxia Inherited?

Friedreich ataxia is inherited in an autosomal recessive manner. This means that to be affected, a person must have a mutation in both copies of the responsible gene in each cell. The parents of an affected person usually each carry one mutated copy of the gene and are referred to as carriers. Carriers typically do not show signs or symptoms of the condition. When two carriers of an autosomal recessive condition have children, each child has a 25 percent (1 in 4) risk to have the condition, a 50 percent (1 in 2) risk to be a carrier like each of the parents, and a 25 percent chance to not have the condition and not be a carrier.

What Is the Diagnosis for Friedreich Ataxia?

Making a diagnosis for a genetic or rare disease can often be challenging. Healthcare professionals typically look at a person's medical history, symptoms, physical exam, and laboratory test results in order to make a diagnosis. The following resources provide information relating to diagnosis and testing for this condition. If you have questions about getting a diagnosis, you should contact a healthcare professional.

Chapter 48

Huntington Disease

In 1872, the American physician George Huntington wrote about an illness that he called "an heirloom from generations away back in the dim past." He was not the first to describe the disorder, which has been traced back to the Middle Ages at least. One of its earliest names was chorea, which, as in "choreography," is the Greek word for dance. The term chorea describes how people affected with the disorder writhe, twist, and turn in a constant, uncontrollable dance-like motion. Later, other descriptive names evolved. "Hereditary chorea" emphasizes how the disease is passed from parent to child. "Chronic progressive chorea" stresses how symptoms of the disease worsen over time. Today, physicians commonly use the simple term Huntington disease (HD) to describe this highly complex disorder that causes untold suffering for thousands of families. More than 15,000 Americans have HD. At least 150,000 others have a 50 percent risk of developing the disease and thousands more of their relatives live with the possibility that they, too, might develop HD.

What Is Huntington Disease?

Huntington disease (HD) is a progressive brain disorder that causes uncontrolled movements, emotional problems, and loss of thinking ability (cognition).

This chapter contains text excerpted from the following sources: Text in this chapter begins with excerpts from "Huntington's Disease: Hope through Research," National Institute of Neurological Disorders and Stroke (NINDS), June 6, 2017; Text beginning with the heading "What Is Huntington Disease?" is excerpted from "Huntington Disease," Genetics Home Reference (GHR), National Institutes of Health (NIH), June 2013. Reviewed February 2018.

Adult-onset HD, the most common form of this disorder, usually appears in a person's thirties or forties. Early signs and symptoms can include irritability, depression, small involuntary movements, poor coordination, and trouble learning new information or making decisions. Many people with Huntington disease develop involuntary jerking or twitching movements known as chorea. As the disease progresses, these movements become more pronounced. Affected individuals may have trouble walking, speaking, and swallowing. People with this disorder also experience changes in personality and a decline in thinking and reasoning abilities. Individuals with the adult-onset form of Huntington disease usually live about 15–20 years after signs and symptoms begin.

A less common form of Huntington disease known as the juvenile form begins in childhood or adolescence. It also involves movement problems and mental and emotional changes. Additional signs of the juvenile form include slow movements, clumsiness, frequent falling, rigidity, slurred speech, and drooling. School performance declines as thinking and reasoning abilities become impaired. Seizures occur in 30–50 percent of children with this condition. Juvenile HD tends to progress more quickly than the adult-onset form; affected individuals usually live 10–15 years after signs and symptoms appear.

How Common Is HD?

HD affects an estimated 3–7 per 100,000 people of European ancestry. The disorder appears to be less common in some other populations, including people of Japanese, Chinese, and African descent.

What Are the Genetic Changes Related to HD?

Mutations in the *HTT* gene cause HD. The *HTT* gene provides instructions for making a protein called huntingtin. Although the function of this protein is unknown, it appears to play an important role in nerve cells (neurons) in the brain. The *HTT* mutation that causes HD involves a deoxyribonucleic acid (DNA) segment known as a cytosine-adenine-guanine (CAG) trinucleotide repeat. This segment is made up of a series of three DNA building blocks (cytosine, adenine, and guanine) that appear multiple times in a row. Normally, the CAG segment is repeated 10–35 times within the gene. In people with HD, the CAG segment is repeated 36 to more than 120 times. People with 36–39 CAG repeats may or may not develop the signs and symptoms of HD, while people with 40 or more repeats almost always develop the disorder. An increase in the size of the CAG segment leads to the production of an abnormally long version of the huntingtin protein. The elongated protein is cut into smaller, toxic fragments that bind together and accumulate in neurons, disrupting the normal functions of these cells. The dysfunction and eventual death of neurons in certain areas of the brain underlie the signs and symptoms of HD.

Can HD Be Inherited?

This condition is inherited in an autosomal dominant pattern, which means one copy of the altered gene in each cell is sufficient to cause the disorder. An affected person usually inherits the altered gene from one affected parent. In rare cases, an individual with HD does not have a parent with the disorder. As the altered *HTT* gene is passed from one generation to the next, the size of the CAG trinucleotide repeat often increases in size. A larger number of repeats is usually associated with an earlier onset of signs and symptoms. This phenomenon is called anticipation. People with the adult-onset form of HD typically have 40–50 CAG repeats in the *HTT* gene, while people with the juvenile form of the disorder tend to have more than 60 CAG repeats. Individuals who have 27–35 CAG repeats in the *HTT* gene do not develop HD, but they are at risk of having children who will develop the disorder. As the gene is passed from parent to child, the size of the CAG trinucleotide repeat may lengthen into the range associated with HD (36 repeats or more).

Chapter 49

Multiple Sclerosis (MS)

What Is Multiple Sclerosis (MS)?

Multiple sclerosis (MS) is a neuroinflammatory disease that affects myelin, a substance that makes up the membrane (called the myelin sheath) that wraps around nerve fibers (axons). Myelinated axons are commonly called white matter. Researchers have learned that MS also damages the nerve cell bodies, which are found in the brain's gray matter, as well as the axons themselves in the brain, spinal cord, and optic nerve (the nerve that transmits visual information from the eye to the brain). As the disease progresses, the brain's cortex shrinks (cortical atrophy).

The term multiple sclerosis refers to the distinctive areas of scar tissue (sclerosis or plaques) that are visible in the white matter of people who have MS. Plaques can be as small as a pinhead or as large as the size of a golf ball. Doctors can see these areas by examining the brain and spinal cord using a type of brain scan called magnetic resonance imaging (MRI). While MS sometimes causes severe disability, it is only rarely fatal and most people with MS have a normal life expectancy.

This chapter includes text excerpted from "Multiple Sclerosis: Hope through Research," National Institute of Neurological Disorders and Stroke (NINDS), June 2012. Reviewed February 2018.

What Are Plaques Made of and Why Do They Develop?

Plaques, or lesions, are the result of an inflammatory process in the brain that causes immune system cells to attack myelin. The myelin sheath helps to speed nerve impulses traveling within the nervous system. Axons are also damaged in MS, although not as extensively, or as early in the disease, as myelin.

Under normal circumstances, cells of the immune system travel in and out of the brain patrolling for infectious agents (viruses, for example) or unhealthy cells. This is called the "surveillance" function of the immune system.

Surveillance cells usually won't spring into action unless they recognize an infectious agent or unhealthy cells. When they do, they produce substances to stop the infectious agent. If they encounter unhealthy cells, they either kill them directly or clean out the dying area and produce substances that promote healing and repair among the cells that are left.

Researchers have observed that immune cells behave differently in the brains of people with MS. They become active and attack what appears to be healthy myelin. It is unclear what triggers this attack. MS is one of many autoimmune disorders, such as rheumatoid arthritis, and lupus, in which the immune system mistakenly attacks a person's healthy tissue as opposed to performing its normal role of attacking foreign invaders like viruses and bacteria. Whatever the reason, during these periods of immune system activity, most of the myelin within the affected area is damaged or destroyed. The axons also may be damaged. The symptoms of MS depend on the severity of the immune reaction as well as the location and extent of the plaques, which primarily appear in the brainstem, cerebellum, spinal cord, optic nerves, and the white matter of the brain around the brain ventricles (fluid filled spaces inside of the brain).

What Are the Signs and Symptoms of MS?

The symptoms of MS usually begin over one to several days, but in some forms, they may develop more slowly. They may be mild or severe and may go away quickly or last for months. Sometimes the initial symptoms of MS are overlooked because they disappear in a day or so and normal function returns. Because symptoms come and go in the majority of people with MS, the presence of symptoms is called an attack, or in medical terms, an exacerbation. Recovery from symptoms is referred to as remission, while a return of symptoms is called a relapse. This form of MS is therefore called relapsing-remitting MS, in contrast to a more slowly developing form called primary progressive MS. Progressive MS can also be a second stage of the illness that follows years of relapsing-remitting symptoms.

A diagnosis of MS is often delayed because MS shares symptoms with other neurological conditions and diseases.

The first symptoms of MS often include:

- vision problems such as blurred or double vision or optic neuritis, which causes pain in the eye and a rapid loss of vision
- weak, stiff muscles, often with painful muscle spasms
- tingling or numbness in the arms, legs, trunk of the body, or face
- clumsiness, particularly difficulty staying balanced when walking
- bladder control problems, either inability to control the bladder or urgency
- dizziness that doesn't go away
- MS may also cause later symptoms such as:
- mental or physical fatigue which accompanies the above symptoms during an attack
- mood changes such as depression or euphoria
- changes in the ability to concentrate or to multitask effectively
- difficulty making decisions, planning, or prioritizing at work or in private life

Some people with MS develop *transverse myelitis*, a condition caused by inflammation in the spinal cord. Transverse myelitis causes loss of spinal cord function over a period of time lasting from several hours to several weeks. It usually begins as a sudden onset of lower back pain, muscle weakness, or abnormal sensations in the toes, and feet, and can rapidly progress to more severe symptoms, including paralysis. In most cases of transverse myelitis, people recover at least some function within the first 12 weeks after an attack begins. Transverse myelitis can also result from viral infections, arteriovenous malformations, or neuroinflammatory problems unrelated to MS. In such instances, there are no plaques in the brain that suggest previous MS attacks.

Neuromyelitis optica is a disorder associated with transverse myelitis as well as optic nerve inflammation. Patients with this disorder usually have antibodies against a particular protein in their spinal cord, called the aquaporin channel. These patients respond differently to treatment than most people with MS.

Most individuals with MS have muscle weakness, often in their hands and legs. Muscle stiffness and spasms can also be a problem. These symptoms may be severe enough to affect walking or standing. In some cases, MS leads to partial or complete paralysis. Many people with MS find that weakness and fatigue are worse when they have a fever or when they are exposed to heat. MS exacerbations may occur following common infections.

Tingling and burning sensations are common, as well as the opposite, numbness and loss of sensation. Moving the neck from side to side or flexing it back and forth may cause "Lhermitte sign," a characteristic sensation of MS that feels like a sharp spike of electricity coursing down the spine.

While it is rare for pain to be the first sign of MS, pain often occurs with optic neuritis and trigeminal neuralgia, a neurological disorder that affects one of the nerves that runs across the jaw, cheek, and face. Painful spasms of the limbs and sharp pain shooting down the legs or around the abdomen can also be symptoms of MS.

Most individuals with MS experience difficulties with coordination and balance at some time during the course of the disease. Some may have a continuous trembling of the head, limbs, and body, especially during movement, although such trembling is more common with other disorders such as Parkinson disease.

Fatigue is common, especially during exacerbations of MS. A person with MS may be tired all the time or may be easily fatigued from mental or physical exertion.

Urinary symptoms, including loss of bladder control and sudden attacks of urgency, are common as MS progresses. People with MS sometimes also develop constipation or sexual problems.

Depression is a common feature of MS. A small number of individuals with MS may develop more severe psychiatric disorders such as bipolar disorder, and paranoia, or experience inappropriate episodes of high spirits, known as euphoria. People with MS, especially those who have had the disease for a long time, can experience difficulty with thinking, learning, memory, and judgment. The first signs of what doctors call cognitive dysfunction (CD) may be subtle. The person may have problems finding the right word to say, or trouble remembering how to do routine tasks on the job or at home. Day to day decisions that once came easily may now be made more slowly and show poor judgment. Changes may be so small or happen so slowly that it takes a family member or friend to point them out.

How Many People Have MS?

No one knows exactly how many people have MS. Experts think there are currently 250,000–350,000 people in the United States diagnosed with MS. This estimate suggests that approximately 200 new cases are diagnosed every week. Studies of the prevalence (the proportion of individuals in a population having a particular disease) of MS indicate that the rate of the disease increased steadily during the 20th century.

As with most autoimmune disorders, twice as many women are affected by MS as men. MS is more common in colder climates. People of Northern European descent appear to be at the highest risk for the disease, regardless of where they live. Native Americans of North and South America, as well as Asian American populations, have relatively low rates of MS.

What Causes MS?

The ultimate cause of MS is damage to myelin, nerve fibers, and neurons in the brain and spinal cord, which together make up the central nervous system (CNS). But how that happens, and why, are questions that challenge researchers. Evidence appears to show that MS is a disease caused by genetic vulnerabilities combined with environmental factors.

Although there is little doubt that the immune system contributes to the brain and spinal cord tissue destruction of MS, the exact target of the immune system attacks and which immune system cells cause the destruction isn't fully understood.

Researchers have several possible explanations for what might be going on. The immune system could be:

- fighting some kind of infectious agent (for example, a virus) that has components which mimic components of the brain (molecular mimicry)
- destroying brain cells because they are unhealthy
- mistakenly identifying normal brain cells as foreign

The last possibility has been the favored explanation for many years. Research now suggests that the first two activities might also play a role in the development of MS. There is a special barrier, called the blood-brain barrier, which separates the brain and spinal cord from the immune system. If there is a break in the barrier, it exposes the brain to the immune system for the first time. When this happens, the immune system may misinterpret the brain as "foreign."

Genetic Susceptibility

Susceptibility to MS may be inherited. Studies of families indicate that relatives of an individual with MS have an increased risk for developing the disease. Experts estimate that about 15 percent of individuals with MS have one or more family members or relatives who also have MS. But even identical twins, whose deoxyribonucleic acid (DNA) is exactly the same, have only a 1 in 3 chance of both having the disease. This suggests that MS is not entirely controlled by genes. Other factors must come into play.

Current research suggests that dozens of genes and possibly hundreds of variations in the genetic code (called gene variants) combine to create vulnerability to MS. Some of these genes have been identified. Most of the genes identified so far are associated with functions of the immune system. Additionally, many of the known genes are similar to those that have been identified in people with other autoimmune diseases as type 1 diabetes, rheumatoid arthritis, or lupus. Researchers continue to look for additional genes and to study how they interact with each other to make an individual vulnerable to developing MS.

Sunlight and Vitamin D

A number of studies have suggested that people who spend more time in the sun and those with relatively high levels of vitamin D are less likely to develop MS. Bright sunlight helps human skin produce vitamin D. Researchers believe that vitamin D may help regulate the immune system in ways that reduce the risk of MS. People from regions near the equator, where there is a great deal of bright sunlight, generally have a much lower risk of MS than people from temperate areas such as the United States and Canada. Other studies suggest that people with higher levels of vitamin D generally have less severe MS and fewer relapses.

Smoking

A number of studies have found that people who smoke are more likely to develop MS. People who smoke also tend to have more brain lesions and brain shrinkage than nonsmokers. The reasons for this are currently unclear.

Infectious Factors and Viruses

A number of viruses have been found in people with MS, but the virus most consistently linked to the development of MS is Epstein Barr virus (EBV), the virus that causes mononucleosis.

Only about 5 percent of the population has not been infected by EBV. These individuals are at a lower risk for developing MS than those who have been infected. People who were infected with EBV in adolescence or adulthood and who therefore develop an exaggerated immune response to EBV are at a significantly higher risk for developing MS than those who were infected in early childhood. This suggests that it may be the type of immune response to EBV that predisposes to MS, rather than EBV infection itself. However, there is still no proof that EBV causes MS.

Autoimmune and Inflammatory Processes

Tissue inflammation and antibodies in the blood that fight normal components of the body and tissue in people with MS are similar to those found in other autoimmune diseases. Along with overlapping evidence from genetic studies, these findings suggest that MS results from some kind of disturbed regulation of the immune system.

How Is MS Diagnosed?

There is no single test used to diagnose MS. Doctors use a number of tests to rule out or confirm the diagnosis. There are many other disorders that can mimic MS. Some of these other disorders can be cured, while others require different treatments than those used for MS. Therefore it is very important to perform a thorough investigation before making a diagnosis.

In addition to a complete medical history, physical examination, and a detailed neurological examination, a doctor will order an MRI scan of the head and spine to look for the characteristic lesions of MS. MRI is used to generate images of the brain and/or spinal cord. Then a special dye or contrast agent is injected into a vein and the MRI is repeated. In regions with active inflammation in MS, there is disruption of the blood-brain barrier and the dye will leak into the active MS lesion.

Doctors may also order evoked potential tests, which use electrodes on the skin and painless electric signals to measure how quickly and accurately the nervous system responds to stimulation. In addition, they may request a lumbar puncture (sometimes called a "spinal tap") to obtain a sample of cerebrospinal fluid. This allows them to look for proteins and inflammatory cells associated with the disease and to rule out other diseases that may look similar to MS, including some infections and other illnesses. MS is confirmed when positive signs of the disease are found in different parts of the nervous system at more than one time interval and there is no alternative diagnosis.

What Is the Course of MS?

The course of MS is different for each individual, which makes it difficult to predict. For most people, it starts with a first attack, usually (but not always) followed by a full to almost full recovery. Weeks, months, or even years may pass before another attack occurs, followed again by a period of relief from symptoms. This characteristic pattern is called relapsing-remitting MS.

Primary-progressive MS is characterized by a gradual physical decline with no noticeable remissions, although there may be temporary or minor relief from symptoms. This type of MS has a later onset, usually after age 40, and is just as common in men as in women.

Secondary progressive MS begins with a relapsing-remitting course, followed by a later primary progressive course. The majority of individuals with severe relapsing-remitting MS will develop secondary progressive MS if they are untreated.

Finally, there are some rare and unusual variants of MS. One of these is Marburg variant MS (also called malignant MS), which causes a swift and relentless decline resulting in significant disability or even death shortly after disease onset. Balo Concentric Sclerosis (BCS), which causes concentric rings of demyelination that can be seen on an MRI, is another variant type of MS that can progress rapidly. Determining the particular type of MS is important because the current disease modifying drugs have been proven beneficial only for the relapsing-remitting types of MS.

What Is an Exacerbation or Attack of MS?

An exacerbation—which is also called a relapse, flare up, or attack—is a sudden worsening of MS symptoms, or the appearance of new symptoms that lasts for at least 24 hours. MS relapses are thought to be associated with the development of new areas of damage in the brain. Exacerbations are characteristic of relapsing-remitting MS, in which attacks are followed by periods of complete or partial recovery with no apparent worsening of symptoms.

An attack may be mild or its symptoms may be severe enough to significantly interfere with life's daily activities. Most exacerbations last from several days to several weeks, although some have been known to last for months.

When the symptoms of the attack subside, an individual with MS is said to be in remission. However, MRI data have shown that this is somewhat misleading because MS lesions continue to appear during these remission periods. Patients do not experience symptoms during remission because the inflammation may not be severe or it may occur in areas of the brain that do not produce obvious symptoms. Research suggests that only about 1 out of every 10 MS lesions is perceived by a person with MS. Therefore, MRI examination plays a very important role in establishing an MS diagnosis, deciding when the disease should be treated, and determining whether treatments work effectively or not. It also has been a valuable tool to test whether an experimental new therapy is effective at reducing exacerbations.

Are There Treatments Available for MS?

There is still no cure for MS, but there are treatments for initial attacks, medications and therapies to improve symptoms, and recently developed drugs to slow the worsening of the disease. These new drugs have been shown to reduce the number and severity of relapses and to delay the long-term progression of MS.

Table 49.1. Disease Modifying Drugs

Trade Name	Generic Name
Avonex	interferon beta-1a
Betaseron	interferon beta-1b
Rebif	interferon beta-1a
Copaxone	glatiramer acetate
Tysabri	natalizumab
Novantrone	mitoxantrone
Gilenya	fingolimod

How Do Doctors Treat the Symptoms of MS?

MS causes a variety of symptoms that can interfere with daily activities but which can usually be treated or managed to reduce their impact. Many of these issues are best treated by neurologists who have advanced training in the treatment of MS and who can prescribe specific medications to treat the problems.

Vision Problems

Eye and vision problems are common in people with MS but rarely result in permanent blindness. Inflammation of the optic nerve or damage to the myelin that covers the optic nerve and other nerve fibers can cause a number of symptoms, including blurring, or graying of vision, blindness in one eye, loss of normal color vision, depth perception, or a dark spot in the center of the visual field (scotoma).

Uncontrolled horizontal or vertical eye movements (nystagmus) and "jumping vision" (opsoclonus) are common to MS, and can be either mild or severe enough to impair vision.

Double vision (diplopia) occurs when the two eyes are not perfectly aligned. This occurs commonly in MS when a pair of muscles that control a specific eye movement aren't coordinated due to weakness in one or both muscles. Double vision may increase with fatigue or as the result of spending too much time reading or on the computer. Periodically resting the eyes may be helpful.

Weak Muscles, Stiff Muscles, Painful Muscle Spasms, and Weak Reflexes

Muscle weakness is common in MS, along with muscle spasticity. Spasticity refers to muscles that are stiff or that go into spasms without any warning. Spasticity in MS can be as mild as a feeling of tightness in the muscles or so severe that it causes painful, uncontrolled spasms. It can also cause pain or tightness in and around the joints. It also frequently affects walking, reducing the normal flexibility, or "bounce" involved in taking steps.

Tremor

People with MS sometimes develop tremor, or uncontrollable shaking, often triggered by movement. Tremor can be very disabling. Assistive devices and weights attached to limbs are sometimes helpful for people with tremor. Deep brain stimulation and drugs such as clonazepam also may be useful.

Problems with Walking and Balance

Many people with MS experience difficulty walking. In fact, studies indicate that half of those with relapsing-remitting MS will need some kind of help walking within 15 years of their diagnosis if they remain untreated. The most common walking problem in people with MS experience is ataxia—unsteady, uncoordinated movements—due to damage with the areas of the brain that coordinate movement of muscles. People with severe ataxia generally benefit from the use of a cane, walker, or other assistive device. Physical therapy can also reduce walking problems in many cases.

In 2010, the U.S. Food and Drug Administration (FDA) approved the drug dalfampridine to improve walking in patients with MS. It is the first drug approved for this use. Clinical trials showed that patients treated with dalfampridine had faster walking speeds than those treated with a placebo pill.

Fatigue

Fatigue is a common symptom of MS and may be both physical (for example, tiredness in the legs) and psychological (due to depression). Probably the most important measures people with MS can take to counter physical fatigue are to avoid excessive activity and to stay out of the heat, which often aggravates MS symptoms. On the other hand, daily physical activity programs of mild to moderate intensity can significantly reduce fatigue. An antidepressant such as fluoxetine may be prescribed if the fatigue is caused by depression. Other drugs that may reduce fatigue in some individuals include amantadine and modafinil.

Fatigue may be reduced if the person receives occupational therapy to simplify tasks and/or physical therapy to learn how to walk in a way that saves physical energy or that takes advantage of an assistive device. Some people benefit from stress management programs, relaxation training, membership in an MS support group, or individual psychotherapy. Treating sleep problems and MS symptoms that interfere with sleep (such as spastic muscles) may also help.

Pain

People with MS may experience several types of pain during the course of the disease.

Trigeminal neuralgia is a sharp, stabbing, facial pain caused by MS affecting the trigeminal nerve as it exits the brainstem on its way to

the jaw and cheek. It can be treated with anticonvulsant or antispas-
modic drugs, alcohol injections, or surgery.

People with MS occasionally develop central pain, a syndrome
caused by damage to the brain and/or spinal cord. Drugs such as gabapentin and nortriptyline sometimes help to reduce central pain.

Burning, tingling, and prickling (commonly called "pins and needles") are sensations that happen in the absence of any stimulation.
The medical term for them is "dysesthesias" They are often chronic
and hard to treat.

Chronic back or other musculoskeletal pain may be caused by walking problems or by using assistive aids incorrectly. Treatments may
include heat, massage, ultrasound treatments, and physical therapy
to correct faulty posture and strengthen and stretch muscles.

Problems with Bladder Control and Constipation

The most common bladder control problems encountered by people
with MS are urinary frequency, urgency, or the loss of bladder control. The same spasticity that causes spasms in legs can also affect
the bladder. A small number of individuals will have the opposite
problem—retaining large amounts of urine. Urologists can help with
treatment of bladder related problems. A number of medical treatments are available. Constipation is also common and can be treated
with a high fiber diet, laxatives, and other measures.

Sexual Issues

People with MS sometimes experience sexual problems. Sexual
arousal begins in the central nervous system, as the brain sends messages to the sex organs along nerves running through the spinal cord.
If MS damages these nerve pathways, sexual response—including
arousal and orgasm—can be directly affected. Sexual problems may
also stem from MS symptoms such as fatigue, cramped or spastic
muscles, and psychological factors related to lowered self-esteem or
depression. Some of these problems can be corrected with medications.
Psychological counseling also may be helpful.

Depression

Studies indicate that clinical depression is more frequent among
people with MS than it is in the general population or in persons with
many other chronic, disabling conditions. MS may cause depression
as part of the disease process, since it damages myelin and nerve

fibers inside the brain. If the plaques are in parts of the brain that are involved in emotional expression and control, a variety of behavioral changes can result, including depression. Depression can intensify symptoms of fatigue, pain, and sexual dysfunction. It is most often treated with selective serotonin reuptake inhibitor (SSRI) antidepressant medications, which are less likely than other antidepressant medications to cause fatigue.

Inappropriate Laughing or Crying

MS is sometimes associated with a condition called pseudobulbar affect that causes inappropriate and involuntary expressions of laughter, crying, or anger. These expressions are often unrelated to mood; for example, the person may cry when they are actually very happy, or laugh when they are not especially happy. In 2010 the FDA approved the first treatment specifically for pseudobulbar affect, a combination of the drugs dextromethorphan and quinidine. The condition can also be treated with other drugs such as amitriptyline or citalopram.

Cognitive Changes

Half to three quarters of people with MS experience cognitive impairment, which is a phrase doctors use to describe a decline in the ability to think quickly and clearly and to remember easily. These cognitive changes may appear at the same time as the physical symptoms or they may develop gradually over time. Some individuals with MS may feel as if they are thinking more slowly, are easily distracted, have trouble remembering, or are losing their way with words. The right word may often seem to be on the tip of their tongue.

Some experts believe that it is more likely to be cognitive decline, rather than physical impairment, that causes people with MS to eventually withdraw from the workforce. A number of neuropsychological tests have been developed to evaluate the cognitive status of individuals with MS. Based on the outcomes of these tests, a neuropsychologist can determine the extent of strengths and weaknesses in different cognitive areas. Drugs such as donepezil, which is usually used for Alzheimer disease, may be helpful in some cases.

Complementary and Alternative Therapies

Many people with MS use some form of complementary or alternative medicine. These therapies come from many disciplines, cultures, and traditions and encompass techniques as different as acupuncture, aromatherapy, ayurvedic medicine, touch and energy therapies, physical movement disciplines such as yoga, and tai chi, herbal supplements, and biofeedback. Because of the risk of interactions between alternative and more conventional therapies, people with MS should discuss all the therapies they are using with their doctor, especially herbal supplements. Although herbal supplements are considered "natural," they have biologically active ingredients that could have harmful effects on their own or interact harmfully with other medications.

Chapter 50

Parkinson Disease

Parkinson disease is a brain disorder that leads to shaking, stiffness, and difficulty with walking, balance, and coordination. Parkinson symptoms usually begin gradually and get worse over time. As the disease progresses, people may have difficulty walking and talking. They may also have mental and behavioral changes, sleep problems, depression, memory difficulties, and fatigue. Both men and women can have Parkinson disease. However, the disease affects about 50 percent more men than women.

One clear risk factor for Parkinson is age. Although most people with Parkinson first develop the disease at about age 60, about 5–10 percent of people with Parkinson have "early-onset" disease, which begins before the age of 50. Early-onset forms of Parkinson are often, but not always, inherited, and some forms have been linked to specific gene mutations.

What Causes Parkinson Disease?

Parkinson disease occurs when nerve cells, or neurons, in an area of the brain that controls movement become impaired and/or die. Normally, these neurons produce an important brain chemical known as dopamine. When the neurons die or become impaired, they produce less dopamine, which causes the movement problems of Parkinson. Scientists still do not know what causes cells that produce dopamine to die.

This chapter includes text excerpted from "Parkinson's Disease," National Institute on Aging (NIA), National Institutes of Health (NIH), May 16, 2017.

People with Parkinson also lose the nerve endings that produce nor-epinephrine, the main chemical messenger of the sympathetic nervous system, which controls many automatic functions of the body, such as heart rate and blood pressure. The loss of norepinephrine might help explain some of the nonmovement features of Parkinson, such as fatigue, irregular blood pressure, decreased movement of food through the digestive tract, and sudden drop in blood pressure when a person stands up from a sitting or lying-down position.

Many brain cells of people with Parkinson contain Lewy bodies, unusual clumps of the protein alpha-synuclein. Scientists are trying to better understand the normal and abnormal functions of alpha-synuclein and its relationship to genetic mutations that impact Parkinson disease and Lewy body dementia.

Although some cases of Parkinson appear to be hereditary, and a few can be traced to specific genetic mutations, in most cases the disease occurs randomly and does not seem to run in families. Many researchers now believe that Parkinson disease results from a combination of genetic factors and environmental factors such as exposure to toxins.

Symptoms of Parkinson Disease

Parkinson disease has four main symptoms:

- Tremor (trembling) in hands, arms, legs, jaw, or head

- Stiffness of the limbs and trunk

- Slowness of movement

- Impaired balance and coordination, sometimes leading to falls

Other symptoms may include depression and other emotional changes; difficulty swallowing, chewing, and speaking; urinary problems or constipation; skin problems; and sleep disruptions.

Symptoms of Parkinson and the rate of progression differ among individuals. Sometimes people dismiss early symptoms of Parkinson as the effects of normal aging. In most cases, there are no medical tests to definitively detect the disease, so it can be difficult to diagnose accurately.

Early symptoms of Parkinson disease are subtle and occur gradually. For example, affected people may feel mild tremors or have difficulty getting out of a chair. They may notice that they speak too softly, or that their handwriting is slow and looks cramped or small.

Friends or family members may be the first to notice changes in someone with early Parkinson. They may see that the person's face lacks expression and animation, or that the person does not move an arm or leg normally.

People with Parkinson often develop a parkinsonian gait that includes a tendency to lean forward, small quick steps as if hurrying forward, and reduced swinging of the arms. They also may have trouble initiating or continuing movement.

Symptoms often begin on one side of the body or even in one limb on one side of the body. As the disease progresses, it eventually affects both sides. However, the symptoms may still be more severe on one side than on the other. Many people with Parkinson note that prior to experiencing stiffness and tremor, they had sleep problems, constipation, decreased ability to smell, and restless legs.

Diagnosis of Parkinson Disease

A number of disorders can cause symptoms similar to those of Parkinson disease. People with Parkinson-like symptoms that result from other causes are sometimes said to have parkinsonism. While these disorders initially may be misdiagnosed as Parkinson, certain medical tests, as well as response to drug treatment, may help to distinguish them from Parkinson. Since many other diseases have similar features but require different treatments, it is important to make an exact diagnosis as soon as possible. There are currently no blood or laboratory tests to diagnose nongenetic cases of Parkinson disease. Diagnosis is based on a person's medical history and a neurological examination. Improvement after initiating medication is another important hallmark of Parkinson disease.

Treatment of Parkinson Disease

Although there is no cure for Parkinson disease, medicines, surgical treatment, and other therapies can often relieve some symptoms.

Medicines for Parkinson Disease

- Medicines prescribed for Parkinson include:
- Drugs that increase the level of dopamine in the brain
- Drugs that affect other brain chemicals in the body
- Drugs that help control nonmotor symptoms

The main therapy for Parkinson is levodopa, also called L-dopa. Nerve cells use levodopa to make dopamine to replenish the brain's dwindling supply. Usually, people take levodopa along with another medication called carbidopa. Carbidopa prevents or reduces some of the side effects of levodopa therapy—such as nausea, vomiting, low blood pressure, and restlessness—and reduces the amount of levodopa needed to improve symptoms.

People with Parkinson should never stop taking levodopa without telling their doctor. Suddenly stopping the drug may have serious side effects, such as being unable to move or having difficulty breathing.

Other medicines used to treat Parkinson symptoms include:

- Dopamine agonists to mimic the role of dopamine in the brain

- MAO-B inhibitors to slow down an enzyme that breaks down dopamine in the brain

- Catechol-O-methyltransferase (COMT) inhibitors to help break down dopamine

- Amantadine, an old antiviral drug, to reduce involuntary movements

- Anticholinergic drugs to reduce tremors and muscle rigidity

Deep Brain Stimulation (DBS)

For people with Parkinson who do not respond well to medications, deep brain stimulation, or DBS, may be appropriate. DBS is a surgical procedure that surgically implants electrodes into part of the brain and connects them to a small electrical device implanted in the chest. The device and electrodes painlessly stimulate the brain in a way that helps stop many of the movement-related symptoms of Parkinson, such as tremor, slowness of movement, and rigidity.

Other Therapies

Other therapies may be used to help with Parkinson disease symptoms. They include physical, occupational, and speech therapies, which help with gait and voice disorders, tremors and rigidity, and decline in mental functions. Other supportive therapies include a healthy diet and exercises to strengthen muscles and improve balance.

Chapter 51

Progressive Supranuclear Palsy (PSP)

What Is Progressive Supranuclear Palsy (PSP)?

Progressive supranuclear palsy (PSP) is an uncommon brain disorder that affects movement, control of walking (gait) and balance, speech, swallowing, vision, mood and behavior, and thinking. The disease results from damage to nerve cells in the brain. Its long name indicates that the disease worsens (progressive) and causes weakness (palsy) by damaging certain parts of the brain above nerve cell clusters called nuclei (supranuclear). These nuclei particularly control eye movements. One of the classic signs of the disease is an inability to aim and move the eyes properly, which individuals may experience as blurring of vision.

Estimates vary, but only about 3–6 in every 100,000 people worldwide, or approximately 20,000 Americans, have PSP—making it much less common than Parkinson disease (PD) (another movement disorder in which an estimated 50,000 Americans are diagnosed each year). Symptoms of PSP begin on average after age 60, but may occur earlier. Men are affected more often than women.

PSP was first described as a distinct disorder in 1964, when three scientists published a paper that distinguished the condition from PD.

This chapter includes text excerpted from "Progressive Supranuclear Palsy Fact Sheet," National Institute of Neurological Disorders and Stroke (NINDS), September 2015.

It was sometimes referred to as Steele-Richardson-Olszewski syndrome, reflecting the combined names of the scientists who defined the disorder. Currently there is no effective treatment for PSP, but some symptoms can be managed with medication or other interventions.

What Are the Symptoms?

The pattern of signs and symptoms can be quite different from person to person. The most frequent first symptom of PSP is a loss of balance while walking. Individuals may have unexplained falls or a stiffness and awkwardness in gait. As the disease progresses, most people will begin to develop a blurring of vision and problems controlling eye movement. In fact, eye problems, in particular slowness of eye movements, usually offer the first definitive clue that PSP is the proper diagnosis. Individuals affected by PSP especially have trouble voluntarily shifting their gaze vertically (i.e., downward and/or upward) and also can have trouble controlling their eyelids. This can lead to a need to move the head to look in different directions, involuntary closing of the eyes, prolonged or infrequent blinking, or difficulty in opening the eyes. Another common visual problem is an inability to maintain eye contact during a conversation. This can give the mistaken impression that the person is hostile or uninterested.

People with PSP often show alterations of mood and behavior, including depression and apathy. Some show changes in judgment, insight, and problem solving, and may have difficulty finding words. They may lose interest in ordinary pleasurable activities or show increased irritability and forgetfulness. Individuals may suddenly laugh or cry for no apparent reason, they may be apathetic, or they may have occasional angry outbursts, also for no apparent reason. Speech usually becomes slower and slurred and swallowing solid foods or liquids can be difficult. Other symptoms include slowed movement, monotone speech, and a mask-like facial expression. Since many symptoms of PSP are also seen in individuals with PD, particularly early in the disorder, PSP is often misdiagnosed as PD.

How Is PSP Different from PD?

Both PSP and PD cause stiffness, movement difficulties, and clumsiness, but PSP is more rapidly progressive as compared to PD. People with PSP usually stand exceptionally straight or occasionally even tilt their heads backward (and tend to fall backward). This is termed "axial rigidity." Those with PD usually bend forward. Problems with speech and swallowing are much more common and severe in PSP than in PD, and tend to show up earlier in the course of the disease. Eye movements are abnormal in PSP but close to normal in PD. Both diseases share other features: onset in late middle age, bradykinesia (slow movement), and rigidity of muscles. Tremor, very common in individuals with PD, is rare in PSP. Although individuals with PD markedly benefit from the drug levodopa, people with PSP respond minimally and only briefly to this drug. Also, people with PSP show accumulation of the protein tau in affected brain cells, while people with PD show accumulation of a different protein, called alpha-synuclein.

What Causes PSP?

The exact cause of PSP is unknown. The symptoms of PSP are caused by a gradual deterioration of brain cells in a few specific areas in the brain, mainly in the region called the brainstem. One of these areas, the substantia nigra, is also affected in PD, and damage to this region of the brain accounts in part for the motor symptoms that PSP and PD have in common.

The hallmark of the disease is the accumulation of abnormal deposits of the protein tau in nerve cells in the brain, so that the cells do not work properly and die. The protein tau is associated with microtubules—structures that support a nerve cell's long processes, or axons, that transmit information to other nerve cells. The accumulation of tau puts PSP in the group of disorders called the tauopathies, which also includes other disorders such as Alzheimer disease (AD), corticobasal degeneration, and some forms of frontotemporal degeneration. Scientists are looking at ways to prevent the harmful clumping of tau in treating each of these disorders.

PSP is usually sporadic, meaning that occurs infrequently and without known cause; in very few cases the disease results from mutations in the *MAPT* gene, which then provides faulty instructions for making tau to the nerve cell. Genetic factors have not been implicated in most individuals.

There are several theories about PSP's cause. A central hypothesis in many neurodegenerative diseases is that once the abnormal aggregates of proteins like tau form in a cell, they can affect a connected cell to also form the protein clumps. In this way the toxic protein aggregates spreads through the nervous system. How this process is triggered remains unknown. One possibility is that an unconventional infectious agent takes years or decades to start producing visible effects (as is seen in disorders like Creutzfeldt-Jakob Disease (CJD)).

Another possibility is that random genetic mutations, of the kind that occur in all of us all the time, happen to occur in particular cells or certain genes, in just the right combination to injure these cells. A third possibility is that there is exposure to some unknown chemical in the food, air, or water which slowly damages certain vulnerable areas of the brain. This theory stems from a clue found on the Pacific island of Guam, where a common neurological disease occurring only there and on a few neighboring islands shares some of the characteristics of PSP, AD, PD, and amyotrophic lateral sclerosis (ALS). Its cause is thought to be a dietary factor or toxic substance found only in that area.

Another possible cause of PSP is cellular damage caused by free radicals, which are reactive molecules produced continuously by all cells during normal metabolism. Although the body has built-in mechanisms for clearing free radicals from the system, scientists suspect that, under certain circumstances, free radicals can react with and damage other molecules. A great deal of research is directed at understanding the role of free radical damage in human diseases.

How Is PSP Diagnosed?

No specific laboratory tests or imaging approaches currently exist to definitively diagnose PSP. The disease is often difficult to diagnose because its symptoms can be very much like those of other movement disorders, and because some of the most characteristic symptoms may develop late or not at all. Initial complaints in PSP are typically vague and fall into these categories:

- Symptoms of disequilibrium, such as unsteady walking or abrupt and unexplained falls without loss of consciousness;
- Visual complaints, including blurred vision, difficulties in looking up or down, double vision, light sensitivity, burning eyes, or other eye trouble;
- Slurred speech; and
- Various mental complaints such as slowness of thought, impaired memory, personality changes, and changes in mood.

An initial diagnosis is based on the person's medical history and a physical and neurological exam. Diagnostic scans such as magnetic resonance imaging (MRI) may show shrinkage at the top of the brainstem. Other imaging tests can look at brain activity in known areas of degeneration.

PSP is often misdiagnosed because it is relatively rare and some of its symptoms are very much like those of PD. Memory problems and personality changes may also lead a physician to mistake PSP for depression, or even attribute symptoms to some form of dementia. The key to diagnosing PSP is identifying early gait instability and difficulty moving the eyes, speech and swallow abnormalities, as well as ruling out other similar disorders, some of which are treatable.

Is There Any Treatment?

There is currently no effective treatment for PSP, although scientists are searching for better ways to manage the disease. PSP symptoms usually do not respond to medications. Drugs prescribed to treat PD, such as ropinirole, rarely provide additional benefit. In some individuals the slowness, stiffness, and balance problems of PSP may respond to some degree to antiparkinsonian agents such as levodopa, but the effect is usually minimal and short-lasting. Excessive eye closing can be treated with botulinum injections. Some antidepressant drugs may provide benefit beyond treating depression, such as pain relief and decreasing drooling.

Recent approaches to therapeutic development for PSP have focused primarily on the clearance of abnormally accumulated tau in the brain. One ongoing clinical trial will determine the safety and tolerability of a compound that prevents accumulation of tau in preclinical models. Other studies are exploring improved tau imaging agents that will be used to assess disease progression and improvement in response to treatment.

Nondrug treatment for PSP can take many forms. Individuals frequently use weighted walking aids because of their tendency to fall backward. Bifocals or special glasses called prisms are sometimes prescribed for people with PSP to remedy the difficulty of looking down. Formal physical therapy is of no proven benefit in PSP, but certain exercises can be done to keep the joints limber.

A gastrostomy (a minimally invasive surgical procedure that involves the placement of a tube through the skin of the abdomen into the stomach for feeding purposes) may be necessary when there are swallowing disturbances or the definite risk of severe choking. Deep brain stimulation (DBS) (which uses a surgically implanted electrode and pulse generator to stimulate the brain in a way that helps to block signals that cause many of the motor symptoms) and other surgical procedures used in individuals with PD have not been proven effective in PSP.

What Is the Prognosis?

The disease gets progressively worse, with people becoming severely disabled within three to five years of onset. Affected individuals are predisposed to serious complications such as pneumonia, choking, head injury, and fractures. The most common cause of death is pneumonia. With good attention to medical and nutritional needs, it is possible for individuals with PSP to live a decade or more after the first symptoms of the disease.

Part Eight

Seizures and Neurological Disorders of Sleep

Chapter 52

Epilepsy

Chapter Contents

Section 52.1

What Is Epilepsy?

This section contains text excerpted from the following sources: Text in this section begins with excerpts from "About Epilepsy: Frequently Asked Questions," Centers for Disease Control and Prevention (CDC), August 16, 2017; Text beginning with the heading "What Are the Different Kinds of Seizures?" is excerpted from "The Epilepsies and Seizures: Hope through Research," National Institute of Neurological Disorders and Stroke (NINDS), April 2015.

Epilepsy, which is sometimes called a seizure disorder, is a disorder of the brain. A person is diagnosed with epilepsy when they have had two or more seizures.

A seizure is a short change in normal brain activity.

Seizures are the main sign of epilepsy. Some seizures can look like staring spells. Other seizures cause a person to fall, shake, and lose awareness of what's going on around them.

What Causes Epilepsies?

Epilepsy can be caused by different conditions that affect a person's brain. Some known causes include:

- Stroke.

- Brain tumor.

- Brain infection, like neurocysticercosis.

- Traumatic brain injury or head injury.

- Loss of oxygen to the brain (for example, during birth).

- Some genetic disorders (such as Down syndrome).

- Other neurologic diseases (such as Alzheimer disease).

For 2 in 3 people, the cause of epilepsy is unknown. This type of epilepsy is called cryptogenic or idiopathic

536

What Are the Different Kinds of Seizures?

Seizures are divided into two major categories—focal seizures and generalized seizures. However, there are many different types of seizures in each of these categories. In fact, doctors have described more than 30 different types of seizures.

Focal Seizures

Focal seizures originate in just one part of the brain. About 60 percent of people with epilepsy have focal seizures. These seizures are frequently described by the area of the brain in which they originate. Many people are diagnosed with focal frontal lobe or medial temporal lobe seizures.

In some focal seizures, the person remains conscious but may experience motor, sensory, or psychic feelings (for example, intense dejà vu or memories) or sensations that can take many forms. The person may experience sudden and unexplainable feelings of joy, anger, sadness, or nausea. He or she also may hear, smell, taste, see, or feel things that are not real and may have movements of just one part of the body, for example, just one hand.

In other focal seizures, the person has a change in consciousness, which can produce a dreamlike experience. The person may display strange, repetitious behaviors such as blinks, twitches, mouth movements (often like chewing or swallowing, or even walking in a circle). These repetitious movements are called automatisms. More complicated actions, which may seem purposeful, can also occur involuntarily. Individuals may also continue activities they started before the seizure began, such as washing dishes in a repetitive, unproductive fashion. These seizures usually last just a minute or two.

Some people with focal seizures may experience auras—unusual sensations that warn of an impending seizure. Auras are usually focal seizures without interruption of awareness (e.g., dejà vu, or an unusual abdominal sensation) but some people experience a true warning before an actual seizure. An individual's symptoms, and the progression of those symptoms, tend to be similar every time. Other people with epilepsy report experiencing a prodrome, a feeling that a seizure is imminent lasting hours or days.

The symptoms of focal seizures can easily be confused with other disorders. The strange behavior and sensations caused by focal seizures also can be mistaken for symptoms of narcolepsy, fainting, or even mental illness. Several tests and careful monitoring may be needed to make the distinction between epilepsy and these other disorders.

Generalized Seizures

Generalized seizures are a result of abnormal neuronal activity that rapidly emerges on both sides of the brain. These seizures may cause loss of consciousness, falls, or a muscle's massive contractions. The many kinds of generalized seizures include:

- Absence seizures may cause the person to appear to be staring into space with or without slight twitching of the muscles.

- Tonic seizures cause stiffening of muscles of the body, generally those in the back, legs, and arms.

- Clonic seizures cause repeated jerking movements of muscles on both sides of the body.

- Myoclonic seizures cause jerks or twitches of the upper body, arms, or legs.

- Atonic seizures cause a loss of normal muscle tone, which often leads the affected person to fall down or drop the head involuntarily.

- Tonic-clonic seizures cause a combination of symptoms, including stiffening of the body and repeated jerks of the arms and/or legs as well as loss of consciousness.

- Secondary generalized seizures.

Not all seizures can be easily defined as either focal or generalized. Some people have seizures that begin as focal seizures but then spread to the entire brain. Other people may have both types of seizures but with no clear pattern. Some people recover immediately after a seizure, while others may take minutes to hours to feel as they did before the seizure. During this time, they may feel tired, sleepy, weak, or confused. Following focal seizures or seizures that started from a focus, there may be local symptoms related to the function of that focus. Certain characteristics of the postseizure (or postictal) state may help locate the region of the brain where the seizure occurred. A classic example is called Todd's paralysis, a temporary weakness in the part of the body that was affected depending on where in the brain the focal seizure occurred. If the focus is in the temporal lobe, postictal symptoms may include language or behavioral disturbances, even psychosis. After a seizure, some people may experience headache or pain in muscles that contracted.

What Are the Different Kinds of Epilepsy?

Just as there are many different kinds of seizures, there are many different kinds of epilepsy. Hundreds of different epilepsy syndromes—disorders characterized by a specific set of symptoms that include epilepsy as a prominent symptom—have been identified. Some of these syndromes appear to be either hereditary or caused by de novo mutations. For other syndromes, the cause is unknown. Epilepsy syndromes are frequently described by their symptoms or by where in the brain they originate.

Absence epilepsy is characterized by repeated seizures that cause momentary lapses of consciousness. These seizures almost always begin in childhood or adolescence and tend to run in families, suggesting that they may be at least partially due to genetic factors. Individuals may show purposeless movements during their seizures, such as a jerking arm or rapidly blinking eyes, while others may have no noticeable symptoms except for brief times when they appear to be staring off into space. Immediately after a seizure, the person can resume whatever he or she was doing. However, these seizures may occur so frequently (in some cases up to 100 or more a day) that the person cannot concentrate in school or other situations. Childhood absence epilepsy usually stops when the child reaches puberty. Although most children with childhood absence epilepsy have a good prognosis, there may be long-lasting negative consequences and some children will continue to have absence seizures into adulthood and/or go on to develop other seizure types.

Frontal lobe epilepsy is a common epilepsy syndrome that features brief focal seizures that may occur in clusters. It can affect the part of the brain that controls movement and involves seizures that can cause muscle weakness or abnormal, uncontrolled movement such as twisting, waving the arms or legs, eye deviation to one side, or grimacing, and are usually associated with some loss of awareness. Seizures usually occur when the person is asleep but also may occur while awake.

Temporal lobe epilepsy, or TLE, is the most common epilepsy syndrome with focal seizures. These seizures are often associated with auras of nausea, emotions (such as déjà vu or fear), or unusual smell or taste. The seizure itself is a brief period of impaired consciousness which may appear as a staring spell, dream-like state, or repeated automatisms. TLE often begins in childhood or teenage years. Research has shown that repeated temporal lobe seizures are often associated with shrinkage and scarring (sclerosis) of the hippocampus. The hippocampus is important for memory and learning. It is not clear whether localized asymptomatic seizure activity over years causes the hippocampal sclerosis.

Neocortical epilepsy is characterized by seizures that originate from the brain's cortex, or outer layer. The seizures can be either focal or generalized. Symptoms may include unusual sensations, visual hallucinations, emotional changes, muscle contractions, convulsions, and a variety of other symptoms, depending on where in the brain the seizures originate.

There are many other types of epilepsy that begin in infancy or childhood. For example, infantile spasms are clusters of seizures that usually begin before the age of 6 months. During these seizures the infant may drop their head, jerk an arm, bend at the waist and/or cry out. Children with Lennox-Gastaut syndrome (LGS) have several different types of seizures, including atonic seizures, which cause sudden falls and are also called drop attacks. Seizure onset is usually before age four years. This severe form of epilepsy can be very difficult to treat effectively. Rasmussen's encephalitis is a progressive form of epilepsy in which half the brain shows chronic inflammation. Some childhood epilepsy syndromes, such as childhood absence epilepsy, tend to go into remission or stop entirely during adolescence, whereas other syndromes such as juvenile myoclonic epilepsy (which features jerk-like motions upon waking) and Lennox-Gastaut syndrome are usually present for life once they develop. Children with Dravet syndrome have seizures that start before age one and later in infancy develop into other seizure types.

Hypothalamic hamartoma is a rare form of epilepsy that first occurs during childhood and is associated with malformations of the hypothalamus at the base of the brain. People with hypothalamic hamartoma have seizures that resemble laughing or crying. Such seizures frequently go unrecognized and are difficult to diagnose.

When Are Seizures Not Epilepsy?

While any seizure is cause for concern, having a seizure does not by itself mean a person has epilepsy. First seizures, febrile seizures, nonepileptic events, and eclampsia (a life-threatening condition that can occur in pregnant women) are examples of conditions involving seizures that may not be associated with epilepsy. Regardless of the type of seizure, it's important to inform your doctor when one occurs.

First Seizures

Many people have a single seizure at some point in their lives, and it can be provoked or unprovoked, meaning that they can occur with or without any obvious triggering factor. Unless the person has suffered brain damage or there is a family history of epilepsy or other neurological abnormalities, the majority of single seizures usually are not followed by additional seizures. Medical disorders which can provoke a seizure include low blood sugar, very high blood sugar in diabetics, disturbances in salt levels in the blood (sodium, calcium, magnesium), eclampsia during or after pregnancy, impaired function of the kidneys, or impaired function of the liver. Sleep deprivation, missing meals, or stress may serve as seizure triggers in susceptible people.

Many people with a first seizure will never have a second seizure, and physicians often counsel against starting antiseizure drugs at this point. In some cases where additional epilepsy risk factors are present, drug treatment after the first seizure may help prevent future seizures. Evidence suggests that it may be beneficial to begin antiseizure medication once a person has had a second unprovoked seizure, as the chance of future seizures increases significantly after this occurs. A person with a pre-existing brain problem, for example, a prior stroke or traumatic brain injury, will have a higher risk of experiencing a second seizure. In general, the decision to start antiseizure medication is based on the doctor's assessment of many factors that influence how likely it is that another seizure will occur in that person.

In one study that followed individuals for an average of 8 years, 33 percent of people had a second seizure within 4 years after an initial seizure. People who did not have a second seizure within that time remained seizure-free for the rest of the study. For people who did have a second seizure, the risk of a third seizure was about 73 percent by the end of 4 years. Among those with a third unprovoked seizure, the risk of a fourth was 76 percent.

Febrile Seizures

Not infrequently a child will have a seizure during the course of an illness with a high fever. These seizures are called febrile seizures. Antiseizure medications following a febrile seizure are generally not warranted unless certain other conditions are present: a family history

541

of epilepsy, signs of nervous system impairment prior to the seizure, or a relatively prolonged or complicated seizure. The risk of subsequent nonfebrile seizures is low unless one of these factors is present.

Results from a study funded by the National Institute of Neurological Disorders and Stroke (NINDS) suggested that certain findings using diagnostic imaging of the hippocampus may help identify which children with prolonged febrile seizures are subsequently at increased risk of developing epilepsy.

Researchers also have identified several different genes that influence the risks associated with febrile seizures in certain families. Studying these genes may lead to new understandings of how febrile seizures occur and perhaps point to ways of preventing them.

Nonepileptic Events

An estimated 5–20 percent of people diagnosed with epilepsy actually have nonepileptic seizures (NES), which outwardly resemble epileptic seizures, but are not associated with seizure-like electrical discharge in the brain. Nonepileptic events may be referred to as psychogenic nonepileptic seizures or PNES, which do not respond to antiseizure drugs. Instead, PNES are often treated by cognitive behavioral therapy to decrease stress and improve self-awareness.

A history of traumatic events is among the known risk factors for PNES. People with PNES should be evaluated for underlying psychiatric illness and treated appropriately. Two studies together showed a reduction in seizures and fewer coexisting symptoms following treatment with cognitive behavioral therapy. Some people with epilepsy have psychogenic seizures in addition to their epileptic seizures.

Other nonepileptic events may be caused by narcolepsy (sudden attacks of sleep), Tourette syndrome (repetitive involuntary movements called tics), cardiac arrhythmia (irregular heartbeat), and other medical conditions with symptoms that resemble seizures. Because symptoms of these disorders can look very much like epileptic seizures, they are often mistaken for epilepsy.

Are There Special Risks Associated with Epilepsy?

Although most people with epilepsy lead full, active lives, there is an increased risk of death or serious disability associated with epilepsy. There may be an increased risk of suicidal thoughts or actions related to some antiseizure medications that are also used to treat mania and bipolar disorder. Two life-threatening conditions associated with the epilepsies are status epilepticus and sudden unexpected death in epilepsy (SUDEP).

Status Epilepticus

Status epilepticus is a potentially life-threatening condition in which a person either has an abnormally prolonged seizure or does not fully regain consciousness between recurring seizures. Status epilepticus can be convulsive (in which outward signs of a seizure are observed) or nonconvulsive (which has no outward signs and is diagnosed by an abnormal electroencephalography (EEG)). Nonconvulsive status epilepticus may appear as a sustained episode of confusion, agitation, loss of consciousness, or even coma.

Any seizure lasting longer than 5 minutes should be treated as though it was status epilepticus. There is some evidence that 5 minutes is sufficient to damage neurons and that seizures are unlikely to end on their own, making it necessary to seek medical care immediately. One study showed that 80 percent of people in status epilepticus who received medication within 30 minutes of seizure onset eventually stopped having seizures, whereas only 40 percent recovered if 2 hours had passed before they received medication. The mortality rate can be as high as 20 percent if treatment is not initiated immediately.

Researchers are trying to shorten the time it takes for antiseizure medications to be administered. A key challenge has been establishing an intravenous (IV) line to deliver injectable antiseizure drugs in a person having convulsions. An NINDS-funded study on status epilepticus found that when paramedics delivered the medication midazolam to the muscles using an autoinjector, similar to the EpiPen drug delivery system used to treat serious allergic reactions, seizures could be stopped significantly earlier compared to when paramedics took the time to give lorazepam intravenously. In addition, drug delivery by autoinjector was associated with a lower rate of hospitalization compared with IV delivery.

Sudden Unexplained Death in Epilepsy (SUDEP)

For reasons that are poorly understood, people with epilepsy have an increased risk of dying suddenly for no discernible reason. Some studies suggest that each year approximately one case of SUDEP occurs for every 1,000 people with the epilepsies. For some, this risk can be higher, depending on several factors. People with more difficult to control seizures tend to have a higher incidence of SUDEP.

SUDEP can occur at any age. Researchers are still unsure why SUDEP occurs, although some research points to abnormal heart and respiratory function due to gene abnormalities (ones which cause epilepsy and also affect heart function). People with epilepsy may be able to reduce the risk of SUDEP by carefully taking all antiseizure medication as prescribed. Not taking the prescribed dosage of medication on a regular basis may increase the risk of SUDEP in individuals with epilepsy, especially those who are taking more than one medication for their epilepsy.

How Are the Epilepsies Diagnosed?

A number of tests are used to determine whether a person has a form of epilepsy and, if so, what kind of seizures the person has. The following tests are used to diagnose epilepsies:

- Imaging and monitoring
- Medical history
- Blood tests
- Developmental, neurological, and behavioral tests

Can the Epilepsies Be Prevented?

At this time there are no medications or other therapies that have been shown to prevent epilepsy. In some cases, the risk factors that lead to epilepsy can be modified. Good prenatal care, including treatment of high blood pressure and infections during pregnancy, may prevent brain injury in the developing fetus that may lead to epilepsy and other neurological problems later. Treating cardiovascular disease, high blood pressure, and other disorders that can affect the brain during adulthood and aging also may prevent some cases of epilepsy. Prevention or early treatment of infections such as meningitis in high-risk populations may also prevent cases of epilepsy. Also, the wearing of seatbelts and bicycle helmets, and correctly securing children in car seats, may avert some cases of epilepsy associated with head trauma.

Section 52.2

Diagnosing Epilepsy

This section includes text excerpted from "About
Epilepsy—Epilepsy Centers of Excellence," U.S. Department
of Veterans Affairs (VA), May 22, 2017.

How Is Epilepsy Diagnosed?

Epilepsy is diagnosed by meeting with your neurologist and undergoing a series of basic tests. The first step is to review your medical history (including a detailed recounting of the seizures) with your physician. This physician will also conduct a thorough neurological examination. In most cases, an EEG (electroencephalogram) and MRI (magnetic resonance imaging) test will be performed as well. You will meet with the physician after these tests to discuss your overall personal health situation.

What Is an Electroencephalography (EEG)?

An electroencephalogram (EEG) is a test to detect abnormalities in the electrical activity of the brain. Brain cells (or neurons) communicate by producing electrical signals. To perform an EEG test, electrodes are placed on the scalp to detect and record patterns of this electrical activity and check for abnormalities.

The test is performed by an EEG technician in a specially designed room that is located in the hospital. At the beginning of the test, you will lie on your back on a table or in a reclining chair. The technician will apply between 16 and 25 flat metal discs (the electrodes) in different positions on your scalp. The electrodes are affixed to your scalp with a paste and are connected by wires to an amplifier and a recording machine. There is no invasive part of this test, and you should feel no discomfort.

As the test begins, the recording machine converts the electrical signals into a series of wavy lines that are recorded on a computer. You will need to lie still with your eyes closed because any movement can alter these results. You may be asked to do certain things during the recording, such as breathe deeply for several minutes or look at a flickering light.

Your healthcare provider may want you to discontinue some medications before the test. Do not change or stop medications without first consulting your physician.

You should avoid all foods containing caffeine for 8 hours before the test. Sometimes it is necessary to sleep during the test, so you may be asked to reduce your sleep time the night before. Please discuss this possibility with your physician. The EEG test is used to help diagnose the presence and type of seizure disorders, to look for causes of confusion, and to evaluate head injuries, tumors, infections, degenerative diseases, and metabolic disturbances that affect the brain. It is also used to partly evaluate sleep disorders and to investigate periods of unconsciousness.

What Is Magnetic Resonance Imaging (MRI)?

An MRI scan is a noninvasive procedure that uses powerful magnets to construct pictures of the body. Unlike conventional radiography, which uses potentially harmful radiation (X-rays), MRI imaging is based on the magnetic properties of atoms. A powerful magnet in the machine generates an intense magnetic field around the body, and some hydrogen atoms within the human tissue will align with this field. When radio wave pulses are directed at this tissue, the hydrogen atoms that have been affected by the magnet will return a signal. These signals are used to construct pictures of the part of the body being examined. In the case of epilepsy, the brain is the subject of interest.

The MRI scanner must be located within a specially shielded room to avoid outside interference. The patient will be asked to lie on a narrow table which slides into a large tunnel-like tube. If contrast is to be administered, an IV (intravenous) will be placed, usually in a small vein of the hand or forearm. A technologist will operate the machine and observe you during the entire study from an adjacent room. Several sets of images are usually obtained, each taking from 2–15 minutes. A complete scan may take up to one hour or more.

No preparatory tests, diets, or medications are usually needed before having an MRI performed. An MRI can be completed immediately after other imaging studies. Because of the strong magnets, certain metallic objects are not allowed into the room. Items such as jewelry, watches, credit cards, and hearing aids can be damaged, and must be removed prior to taking the test. Removable dental work should be taken out just prior to the scan. Pens, pocket knives, and eyeglasses can become dangerous projectiles when the magnet is activated and should not accompany the patient into the scanner area.

Because the strong magnetic fields can displace or disrupt the action of implanted metallic objects, people with cardiac pacemakers cannot be scanned and should not enter the MRI area. MRI also should not be used for people with metallic objects in their bodies, such as: inner ear (cochlear) implants, brain aneurysm clips, some artificial heart valves, older vascular stents, and recently placed artificial joints. Sheet metal workers, or persons with similar potential exposure to small metal fragments, will first be screened for metal shards within the eyes with X-rays of the skull.

The patient will be asked to sign a consent form confirming that none of the above issues apply before the study will be performed. A hospital gown may be recommended, or the patient may be allowed to wear "sweats" or similar clothing without metal fasteners. There is no pain experienced during the scanning procedure. However, some people do have a claustrophobic. The table may be hard or cold, but you can request a blanket or pillow. The machine produces loud thumping and humming noises during normal operation. Ear plugs are given to the patient to reduce the noise. For people that have trouble with small spaces, a mild sedative may be used during the scan. If this is done, someone needs to be available to help get the patient home. A technologist observes the patient during the entire procedure and may speak through an intercom in the scanner. Some MRI scanners are equipped with televisions and special headphones to help the examination time pass.

What Is a Positron Emission Tomography (PET) Scan?

A positron emission tomography (PET) scan is a diagnostic exam that evaluates the energy activity of the brain. Positrons are tiny particles released from a low dose of radioactive substance administered to the patient prior to the exam. The PET scan measures how intensely different parts of the brain use up glucose, oxygen, or other substances. A small amount of a radioactive substance is injected into one of the patient's veins prior to the test. This substance attaches itself to glucose. Small objects (positrons) are released from the tagged glucose, which is detected by the PET scanner. The images that result are helpful in diagnosing a variety of conditions and diseases, including epilepsy.

The PET images are programmed to show different colors or levels of brightness. The possible area where a seizure occurs may appear darker in the brain tissue in comparison to other areas. The actual PET scanner looks like a large doughnut. Around the central hole of the machine are rings of detectors that record the emission of positrons. As the patient lies on a cushioned table, the patient will be moved into the central hole of the machine. The test will take about 90 minutes. The patient should not eat for at least 6 hours before the PET scan. The patient will be encouraged to drink several glasses of water before the test.

The PET scan itself will cause no discomfort. The patient will lie in a cushioned examination table and be asked to remain still during the exam. Some patients who are claustrophobic may feel anxious while positioned in the PET scanner. Patients should talk with their physicians if they have a history of claustrophobia.

The PET scan allows physicians to better evaluate the functioning of different regions of the brain. It can show where seizures potentially start and help determine if a patient is a candidate for surgery.

For pregnant and nursing women, the radioactive substance may expose the fetus or infants who are breastfeeding to a small amount of radiation. The risk to the fetus or infant should be considered in relation to the potential information gained from the result of the PET examination. If the patient is pregnant or may be pregnant, the patient should inform the PET imaging staff before the examination is performed.

What Is Video EEG Telemetry?

Inpatient video EEG monitoring enables the physicians to gather additional information about the specific types of seizures patients are having. The more accurately we are able to classify the seizure type, the better the chances are to achieve seizure control with medications.

Additionally, for people who are having spells without a clear diagnosis, video EEG telemetry can often be useful in characterizing such episodes. These spells may be diagnosed as epileptic seizures, but may also be determined to be psychogenic nonepileptic events, syncope, or cardiac-related spells.

Video EEG telemetry also assists physicians in localizing the seizure focus in the brain. This is critical if patients wish to know if they have the type of seizures that may be treated surgically. Seizure surgery is most successful when physicians are able to localize the precise area in the brain where seizures originate. Prolonged video

EEG monitoring allows physicians to record a number of seizures, providing the best video and EEG data possible.

The video EEG telemetry procedure has two parts:

1. **EEG telemetry:** As during a routine EEG, electrodes are glued to the patient's scalp. The electrodes then record for 24 hours per day. A computer monitors the EEG recording continuously so that seizure activity can be marked. This recording gives physicians an accurate count of seizures and allows the doctors to compare what is physically happening to the patient during a seizure with what is seen on the brainwave recordings.

2. **Video:** A camera is used to continuously film the patient while you are connected to EEG electrodes. By using the video, the physicians can see what happens to patients physically while they are having a seizure. Seeing what happens physically allows the physicians to better determine what type of seizures the patient is experiencing and where the seizure might be starting in the brain.

What Is Magnetoencephalography (MEG)?

A magnetoencephalogram (MEG) is a test that identifies brain activity by measuring small electrical currents arising from the neurons of the brain. These currents produce magnetic fields. The MEG generates an accurate location of the magnetic fields produced by the neurons. The MEG test is somewhat related to the electroencephalography (EEG) test except that it is using magnetic fields as the primary information for determining where seizures might be originating.

The MEG test takes approximately two hours. An EEG is done at the same time as the MEG. Electrodes will be placed on the patient's scalp using paste. All electronic items or items with a magnetic strip (cell phones, credit cards) will be removed. Also, all metal above the waist should be removed, such as underwire bra, shirts with zippers or snaps, jewelry, and wrist watches. The patient will be in a specially shielded room during the test, and will lay in a bed with the head resting in the helmet-like MEG scanner. The MEG scanner does not emit radiation or magnetic fields. It only detects and amplifies magnetic signals produced by the brain.

There are video and intercom systems in the room. The technician can see, hear, and communicate with the patient at all times. During the scan, the patient must keep his/her head still. The head is immobilized by using cushions that are placed on both sides of the head. The patient may be asked to arrive sleep-deprived in the hopes of recording brain activity in the awake, drowsy, and sleep states. The MEG test causes no discomfort. The scanner does not make noise. The patient will be able to have someone in the room with you during the test, but they must also remove electronic and metallic objects.

Section 52.3

Treating Epilepsy

This section contains text excerpted from the following sources: Text beginning with the heading "Seizure First Aid" is excerpted from "Seizure First Aid," Center for Disease Control and Prevention (CDC), January 8, 2018; Text beginning with the heading "How Is Epilepsy Treated?" is excerpted from "About Epilepsy," Center for Disease Control and Prevention (CDC), August 16, 2017.

Seizure First Aid

About 1 out of 10 people has had a seizure. That means seizures are common, and one day you might need to help someone during or after a seizure.

First Aid for Any Type of Seizure

There are many types of seizures. Most seizures end in a few minutes.

These are general steps to help someone who is having any type seizure:

- Stay with the person until the seizure ends and he or she is fully awake. After it ends, help the person sit in a safe place. Once they are alert and able to communicate, tell them what happened in very simple terms.

- Comfort the person and speak calmly.

- Check to see if the person is wearing a medical bracelet or other emergency information.

- Keep yourself and other people calm.

- Offer to call a taxi or another person to make sure the person gets home safely.

First Aid for Generalized Tonic-Clonic (Grand Mal) Seizures

When most people think of a seizure, they think of a generalized tonic-clonic seizure, also called a grand mal seizure. In this type of seizure, the person may cry out, fall, shake or jerk, and become unaware of what's going on around them.

Here are things you can do to help someone who is having this type of seizure:

- Ease the person to the floor.

- Turn the person gently onto one side. This will help the person breathe.

- Clear the area around the person of anything hard or sharp. This can prevent injury.

- Put something soft and flat, like a folded jacket, under his or her head.

- Remove eyeglasses.

- Loosen ties or anything around the neck that may make it hard to breathe.

- Time the seizure. Call 911 if the seizure lasts longer than 5 minutes.

How Is Epilepsy Treated?

There are many things a provider and person with epilepsy can do to stop or lessen seizures.

The most common treatments for epilepsy are:

- Medicine. Anti-seizure drugs are medicines that limit the spread of seizures in the brain. A healthcare provider will change the amount of the medicine or prescribe a new drug if needed to find the best treatment plan. Medicines work for about 2 in 3 people with epilepsy.

- Surgery. When seizures come from a single area of the brain (focal seizures), surgery to remove that area may stop future seizures or make them easier to control with medicine. Epilepsy surgery is mostly used when the seizure focus is located in the temporal lobe of the brain.

- Other treatments. When medicines do not work and surgery is not possible, other treatments can help. These include vagus nerve stimulation, where an electrical device is placed, or implanted, under the skin on the upper chest to send signals to a large nerve in the neck. Another option is the ketogenic diet, a high fat, low carbohydrate diet with limited calories.

Who Treats Epilepsy?

Many kinds of health providers treat people with epilepsy. Primary care providers such as family physicians, pediatricians, and nurse practitioners are often the first people to see a person with epilepsy who has new seizures. These providers may make the diagnosis of epilepsy or they may talk with a neurologist or epileptologist.

A neurologist is a doctor who specializes in the brain and nervous system. An epileptologist is a neurologist who specializes in epilepsy. When problems occur such as seizures or medication side effects, the primary health provider may send the patient to a neurologist or epileptologists for specialized care.

People who have seizures that are difficult to control or who need advanced care for epilepsy may be referred to an epilepsy centers. Epilepsy centers are staffed by providers who specialize in epilepsy care, such as

- Epileptologists and neurologists.

- Nurses.

- Psychologists.

- Technicians.

Many epilepsy centers work with university hospitals and researchers.

How Do I Find an Epilepsy Specialist?

There are several ways you can find a neurologist or an epileptologist near you. Your primary care or family provider can tell you about types of specialists. The American Academy of Neurology and the

American Epilepsy Society provide a listing of its member neurologists and epilepsy specialists, including epileptologists. The National Association of Epilepsy Centers (NAEC) also provides a list of its member centers, organized by state.

What Can I Do to Manage My Epilepsy?

Self-management is what you do to take care of yourself. You can learn how to manage seizures and keep an active and full life. Begin with these tips:

- Take your medicine.
- Talk with your doctor or nurse when you have questions.
- Recognize seizure triggers (such as flashing or bright lights).
- Keep a record of your seizures.
- Get enough sleep.
- Lower stress.

Section 52.4

Living with Epilepsy

This section includes text excerpted from "The Epilepsies and Seizures: Hope through Research," National Institute of Neurological Disorders and Stroke (NINDS), April 2015.

The majority of people with epilepsy can do the same things as people without the disorder and have successful and productive lives. In most cases it does not affect job choice or performance. One-third or more of people with epilepsy, however, may have cognitive or neuropsychiatric co-concurring symptoms that can negatively impact their quality of life. Many people with epilepsy are significantly helped by available therapies, and some may go months or years without having a seizure.

However, people with treatment-resistant epilepsy can have as many as hundreds of seizures a day or they can have one seizure a year with sometimes disabling consequences. On average, having treatment-resistant epilepsy is associated with an increased risk of cognitive impairment, particularly if the seizures developed in early childhood. These impairments may be related to the underlying conditions associated with the epilepsy rather than to the epilepsy itself.

Mental Health and Stigmatization

Depression is common among people with epilepsy. It is estimated that one of every three persons with epilepsy will have depression in the course of his or her lifetime, often with accompanying symptoms of anxiety disorder. In adults, depression and anxiety are the two most frequent mental health-related diagnoses. In adults, a depression screening questionnaire specifically designed for epilepsy helps healthcare professions identify people who need treatment. Depression or anxiety in people with epilepsy can be treated with counseling or most of the same medications used in people who don't have epilepsy. People with epilepsy should not simply accept that depression is part of having epilepsy and should discuss symptoms and feelings with healthcare professionals.

Children with epilepsy also have a higher risk of developing depression and/or attention deficit hyperactivity disorder compared with their peers. Behavioral problems may precede the onset of seizures in some children.

Children are especially vulnerable to the emotional problems caused by ignorance or the lack of knowledge among others about epilepsy. This often results in stigmatization, bullying, or teasing of a child who has epilepsy. Such experiences can lead to behaviors of avoidance in school and other social settings. Counseling services and support groups can help families cope with epilepsy in a positive manner.

Driving and Recreation

Most states and the District of Columbia will not issue a driver's license to someone with epilepsy unless the person can document that she/he has been seizure-free for a specific amount of time (the waiting period varies from a few months to several years). Some states make exceptions for this policy when seizures don't impair consciousness, occur only during sleep, or have long auras or other warning signs that allow the person to avoid driving when a seizure is likely to occur. Studies show that the risk of having a seizure-related accident decreases as the length of time since the last seizure increases. Commercial drivers' licenses have additional restrictions. In addition, people with epilepsy should take extra care if a job involves operation of machinery or vehicles.

The risk of seizures also limits people's recreational choices. Individuals may need to take precautions with activities such as climbing, sailing, swimming, or working on ladders. Studies have not shown any increase in seizures due to sports, although these studies have not focused on any activity in particular. There is some evidence that regular exercise may improve seizure control in some people, but this should be done under a doctor's supervision. The benefits of sports participation may outweigh the risks and coaches or other leaders can take appropriate safety precautions. Steps should be taken to avoid dehydration, overexertion, and hypoglycemia, as these problems can increase the risk of seizures.

Education and Employment

By law, people with epilepsy (or disabilities) in the United States cannot be denied employment or access to any educational, recreational, or other activity because of their epilepsy. However, significant barriers still exist for people with epilepsy in school and work. Antiseizure drugs may cause side effects that interfere with concentration and memory. Children with epilepsy may need extra time to complete schoolwork, and they sometimes may need to have instructions or other information repeated for them. Teachers should be told what to do if a child in their classroom has a seizure, and parents should work with the school system to find reasonable ways to accommodate any special needs their child may have.

Pregnancy and Motherhood

Women with epilepsy are often concerned about whether they can become pregnant and have a healthy child. Epilepsy itself does not interfere with the ability to become pregnant. With the right planning, supplemental vitamin use, and medication adjustments prior to pregnancy, the odds of a woman with epilepsy having a healthy pregnancy and a healthy child are similar to a woman without a chronic medical condition.

Children of parents with epilepsy have about 5 percent risk of developing the condition at some point during life, in comparison to about a 1 percent risk in a child in the general population. However, the risk of developing epilepsy increases if a parent has a clearly hereditary form of the disorder. Parents who are worried that their epilepsy may be hereditary may wish to consult a genetic counselor to determine their risk of passing on the disorder.

Other potential risks to the developing child of a woman with epilepsy or on antiseizure medication include increased risk for major congenital malformations (also known as birth defects) and adverse effects on the developing brain. The types of birth defects that have been most commonly reported with antiseizure medications include cleft lip or cleft palate, heart problems, abnormal spinal cord development (spina bifida), urogenital defects, and limb-skeletal defects. Some antiseizure medications, particularly valproate, are known to increase the risk of having a child with birth defects and/or neurodevelopmental problems, including learning disabilities, general intellectual disabilities, and autism spectrum disorder. It is important that a woman work with a team of providers that includes her neurologist and her obstetrician to learn about any special risks associated with her epilepsy and the medications she may be taking.

Although planned pregnancies are essential to ensuring a healthy pregnancy, effective birth control is also essential. Some antiseizure medications that induce the liver's metabolic capacity can interfere with the effectiveness of hormonal contraceptives (e.g., birth control pills, vaginal ring). Women who are on these enzyme-inducing antiseizure medications and using hormonal contraceptives may need to switch to a different kind of birth control that is more effective (such as different intrauterine devices, progestin implants, or long-lasting injections).

Prior to a planned pregnancy, a woman with epilepsy should meet with her healthcare team to reassess the current need for antiseizure medications and to determine:

1. the optimal medication to balance seizure control and avoid birth defects and

2. the lowest dose for going into a planned pregnancy.

Any transitions to either a new medication or dosage should be phased in prior to the pregnancy, if possible. If a woman's seizures are controlled for the 9 months prior to pregnancy, she is more likely to continue to have seizure control during pregnancy. For all women with epilepsy during pregnancy, approximately 15–25 percent will have seizure worsening, but another 15–25 percent will have seizure improvement. As a woman's body changes during pregnancy, the dose of seizure medication may need to be increased. For most medicines, monthly monitoring of blood levels of the antiseizure medicines can help to assure continued seizure control. Many of the birth defects seen with antiseizure medications occur in the first six weeks of pregnancy, often before a woman is aware she is pregnant. In addition, up to 50 percent of pregnancies in the United States are unplanned. For these reasons, the discussion about the medications should occur early between the healthcare professional and any woman with epilepsy who is in her childbearing years.

For all women thinking of becoming pregnant, using supplemental folic acid beginning prior to conception and continuing the supplement during pregnancy is an important way to lower the risk for birth defects and developmental delays. Prenatal multivitamins should also be used prior to the beginning of pregnancy. Pregnant women with epilepsy should get plenty of sleep and avoid other triggers or missed medications to avoid worsening of seizures.

Most pregnant women with epilepsy can deliver with the same choices as women without any medical complications. During the labor and delivery, it is important that the woman be allowed to take her same formulations and doses of antiseizure drugs at her usual times; it is often helpful for her to bring her medications from home. If a seizure does occur during labor and delivery, intravenous short-acting medications can be given if necessary. It is unusual for the newborns of women with epilepsy to experience symptoms of withdrawal from the mother's antiseizure medication (unless she is on phenobarbital or a standing dose of benzodiazepines), but the symptoms resolve quickly and there are usually no serious or long-term effects.

The use of antiseizure medications is considered safe for women who choose to breastfeed their child. On very rare occasions, the baby may become excessively drowsy or feed poorly, and these problems should be closely monitored. However, experts believe the benefits of breastfeeding outweigh the risks except in rare circumstances. One large study showed that the children who were breastfed by mothers with epilepsy on antiseizure medications performed better on learning and developmental scales than the babies who were not breastfed. It is common for the antiseizure medication dosing to be adjusted again in the postpartum setting, especially if the dose was altered during pregnancy. With the appropriate selection of safe antiseizure medicines during pregnancy, use of supplemental folic acid, and ideally, with prepregnancy planning, most women with epilepsy can have a healthy pregnancy with good outcomes for themselves and their developing child.

Chapter 53

Nonepileptic Seizures

Chapter Contents

Section 53.1

Physiologic and Psychogenic Nonepileptic Seizures

"Physiologic and Psychogenic Nonepileptic Seizures,"
© 2018 Omnigraphics. Reviewed February 2018.

What Are Nonepileptic Seizures?

Nonepileptic seizures are episodes that can briefly change an individual's movement, sensation, or behavior. They are quite similar in appearance to epileptic seizures, but they are not triggered by electrical changes in the brain. Epileptic and nonepileptic seizures are hard to differentiate, even by a trained healthcare professional. Patients with nonepileptic seizures are often misdiagnosed and treated for epilepsy.

An epileptic seizure generally starts off abruptly, while a nonepileptic seizure begins slowly and builds in intensity. A person who undergoes a nonepileptic seizure usually takes only a very short period to recover fully, whereas a person who experiences an epileptic seizure may take several hours for recovery, which is often accompanied by extreme headache, severe exhaustion, and mild confusion.

Some of the factors that can cause a nonepileptic seizure include emotional and mental trauma, narcolepsy, migraines, and some physiological conditions that affect blood flow and oxygen levels in the brain, as well as changes in brain sugar levels.

Types of Nonepileptic Seizures

Nonepileptic seizures are classified into two subcategories:

- **Psychogenic Nonepileptic Seizures.** Psychogenic seizures, also known as nonepileptic attack disorders (NEAD), are a direct result of the body's response to severe emotional, mental, or physical trauma, such as sexual abuse, domestic violence, or the death of a loved one. High levels of stress can also trigger psychogenic seizures, along with extreme mood swings and hallucinations.

- **Physiologic Nonepileptic Seizures.** There are several factors that can contribute to physiologic nonepileptic seizures, many of which result in sudden changes in the blood supply to the brain or oxygen and sugar levels in the brain. Such conditions include cardiac arrhythmia (changes in heart rhythm), syncopal episodes (rapid drops in blood pressure), or hypoglycemia (low blood sugar). Other factors that can trigger a physiologic nonepileptic seizure include excessive amounts of alcohol, fainting spells, and abnormal sleep patterns.

Causes of Nonepileptic Seizures

Specific traumatic events, such as sexual or physical abuse, divorce, incest, death of a loved one, and sudden change can trigger nonepileptic seizures. Psychogenic nonepileptic seizures are defined as physical manifestation of a psychological disturbance. There's a type of somatoform disorder known as conversion disorder. It's characterized by physical symptoms caused by psychological conflict that unconsciously manifest as a neurologic disorder. Although it can occur at any age, this condition generally develops during adolescence and is more prevalent among women than men. People suffering from somatoform disorder may appear to have some underlying physical condition, but on examination, no such conditions are found.

Symptoms of Nonepileptic Seizures

Some of the symptoms include:

- Biting the tip or sides of the tongue during a seizure.

- Severe emotional trauma or psychological stress leading to sudden emotional outbursts, such as uncontrollable crying, screaming or shrieking.

- Jerking movements, such as bending the neck, head, and spine backward or thrusting the pelvis.

- Breaking things and thrashing around while convulsing.

The symptoms of a nonepileptic seizure need to be considered carefully since it is an acute condition and can be dangerous.

Diagnosis of Nonepileptic Seizures

Healthcare providers who diagnose nonepileptic seizures include neurologists, psychiatrists, and psychologists. If nonepileptic seizure is suspected, then the healthcare professional will conduct a complete medical history of the patient to confirm the root cause of the condition. Different tests may be done to confirm that the seizure is nonepileptic. These include:

- **Electroencephalogram (EEG).** This traces brain-wave activity.

- **Magnetic resonance imaging (MRI) and computed tomography (CT).** These help capture pictures of the brain and detect brain activity.

- **Video-electroencephalogram.** This test is used to record changes in behavior.

- **Blood tests.** These check the overall condition of the body.

Treatment of Nonepileptic Seizures

Antidepressants and other medications are most often used to treat patients with nonepileptic seizure. Certain therapies and counseling are also recommended to help patients deal with their emotional, physical, and mental reactions. Healthcare providers carefully examine and test for additional or underlying health problems before recommending any treatment for nonepileptic seizures.

References

1. Alsaadi, M. Taoufik, MD, and Anna Vinter Marquez, MD. "Psychogenic Nonepileptic Seizures," American Family Physician, September 1, 2005.

2. "Nonepileptic Seizures," Epilepsy Foundation of Greater Chicago, February 1, 2002.

3. "Non-Epileptic Seizures," iHealth Healthcare Information Directory, February 10, 2012.

4. "Non-Epileptic Seizures," Functional Neurological Disorder— Hope, October 19, 2015.

5. "The Truth about Psychogenic Nonepileptic Seizures," Epilepsy Foundation, November 1, 2007.

Section 53.2

Febrile Seizures

This section includes text excerpted from "Febrile Seizures
Fact Sheet," National Institute of Neurological Disorders
and Stroke (NINDS), September 2015.

What Are Febrile Seizures?

Febrile seizures are seizures or convulsions that occur in young
children and are triggered by fever. Young children between the ages
of about 6 months and 5 years old are the most likely to experience
febrile seizures; this risk peaks during the second year of life. The
fever may accompany common childhood illnesses such as a cold, the
flu, or an ear infection. In some cases, a child may not have a fever at
the time of the seizure but will develop one a few hours later.

The vast majority of febrile seizures are convulsions. Most often
during a febrile seizure, a child will lose consciousness and both arms
and legs will shake uncontrollably. Less common symptoms include eye
rolling, rigid (stiff) limbs, or twitching on only one side or a portion of
the body, such as an arm or a leg. Sometimes during a febrile seizure,
a child may lose consciousness but will not noticeably shake or move.

Most febrile seizures last only a few minutes and are accompanied
by a fever above 101°F (38.3°C). Although they can be frightening for
parents, brief febrile seizures (less than 15 minutes) do not cause any
long-term health problems. Having a febrile seizure does not mean
a child has epilepsy, since that disorder is characterized by reoccurring seizures that are not triggered by fever. Even prolonged seizures
(lasting more 15 minutes) generally have a good outcome but carry an
increased risk of developing epilepsy.

How Common Are Febrile Seizures?

Febrile seizures are the most common type of convulsions in infants
and young children and occur in 2–5 percent of American children
before age 5. Approximately 40 percent of children who experience
one febrile seizure will have a recurrence. Children at highest risk for
recurrence are those who have:

- their first febrile seizure at a young age (younger than 18 months)

- a family history of febrile seizures

- a febrile seizure as the first sign of an illness

- a relatively low temperature increases with their first febrile seizure

A prolonged initial febrile seizure does not substantially boost the risk of reoccurring febrile seizures. However, if another does occur, it is more likely to be prolonged.

What Should Be Done for a Child Having a Febrile Seizure?

It is important that parents and caretakers remain calm, take first aid measures, and carefully observe the child. If a child is having a febrile seizure, parents and caregivers should do the following:

- Note the start time of the seizure. If the seizure lasts longer than 5 minutes, call an ambulance. The child should be taken immediately to the nearest medical facility for diagnosis and treatment.

- Call an ambulance if the seizure is less than 5 minutes but the child does not seem to be recovering quickly.

- Gradually place the child on a protected surface such as the floor or ground to prevent accidental injury. Do not restrain or hold a child during a convulsion.

- Position the child on his or her side or stomach to prevent choking. When possible, gently remove any objects from the child's mouth. Nothing should ever be placed in the child's mouth during a convulsion. These objects can obstruct the child's airway and make breathing difficult.

- Seek immediate medical attention if this is the child's first febrile seizure and take the child to the doctor once the seizure has ended to check for the cause of the fever. This is especially urgent if the child shows symptoms of stiff neck, extreme lethargy, or abundant vomiting, which may be signs of meningitis, an infection over the brain surface.

Are Febrile Seizures Harmful?

The vast majority of febrile seizures are short and do not cause any long-term damage. During a seizure, there is a small chance that the child may be injured by falling or may choke on food or saliva in the mouth. Using proper first aid for seizures can help avoid these hazards.

There is no evidence that short febrile seizures cause brain damage. Large studies have found that even children with prolonged febrile seizures have normal school achievement and perform as well on intellectual tests as their siblings who do not have seizures. Even when the seizures last a long time, most children recover completely.

Multiple or prolonged seizures are a risk factor for epilepsy but most children who experience febrile seizures do not go on to develop the reoccurring seizures that are characteristic of epilepsy. Some children, including those with cerebral palsy, delayed development, or other neurological abnormalities as well as those with a family history of epilepsy are at increased risk of developing epilepsy whether or not they have febrile seizures. Febrile seizures may be more common in these children but do not contribute much to the overall risk of developing epilepsy.

Children who experience a brief, full body febrile seizure are slightly more likely to develop epilepsy than the general population. Children who have a febrile seizure that lasts longer than 10 minutes; a focal seizure (a seizure that starts on one side of the brain); or seizures that reoccur within 24 hours, have a moderately increased risk (about 10 percent) of developing epilepsy as compared to children who do not have febrile seizures.

Of greatest concern is the small group of children with very prolonged febrile seizures lasting longer than 30 minutes. In these children, the risk of epilepsy is as high as 30–40 percent though the condition may not occur for many years. Recent studies suggest that prolonged febrile seizures can injure the hippocampus, a brain structure involved with temporal lobe epilepsy (TLE).

How Are Febrile Seizures Evaluated?

Before diagnosing febrile seizures in infants and children, doctors sometimes perform tests to be sure that the seizures are not caused by an underlying or more serious health condition. For example, meningitis, an infection of the membranes surrounding the brain, can cause both fever and seizures that can look like febrile seizures but are much more serious. If a doctor suspects a child has meningitis a spinal tap may be needed to check for signs of the infection in the cerebrospinal fluid (fluid surrounding the brain and spinal cord). If there has been severe diarrhea or vomiting, dehydration could be responsible for seizures. Also, doctors often perform other tests such as examining the blood and urine to pinpoint the cause of the child's fever. If the seizure is either very prolonged or is accompanied by a serious infection, or if the child is younger than 6 months of age, the clinician may recommend hospitalization. In most cases, however, a child who has a febrile seizure usually will not need to be hospitalized.

Can Subsequent Febrile Seizures Be Prevented?

Experts recommend that children who have experienced a febrile seizure not take any antiseizure medication to prevent future seizures, as the side effects of these daily medications outweigh any benefits. This is especially true since most febrile seizures are brief and harmless.

If a child has a fever, most parents will use fever-lowering drugs such as acetaminophen or ibuprofen to make the child more comfortable. However, available studies show this does not reduce the risk of having another febrile seizure.

Although the majority of children with febrile seizures do not need medication, children especially prone to febrile seizures may be treated with medication, such as diazepam, when they have a fever. This medication may lower the risk of having another febrile seizure. It is usually well tolerated, although it occasionally can cause drowsiness, a lack of coordination, or hyperactivity. Children vary widely in their susceptibility to such side effects.

A child whose first febrile seizure is a prolonged one does not necessarily have a higher risk of having reoccurring prolonged seizures. But if the child has another seizure, it is likely to be prolonged. Because very long febrile seizures are associated with the potential for injury and an increased risk of developing epilepsy, some doctors may prescribe medication to these children to prevent prolonged seizures. The parents of children who have experienced a long febrile may wish to talk to their doctor about this treatment option.

Chapter 54

Myoclonus: Involuntary Muscle Jerking

What Is Myoclonus?

Myoclonus describes a symptom and not a diagnosis of a disease. It refers to sudden, involuntary jerking of a muscle or group of muscles. Myoclonic twitches or jerks usually are caused by sudden muscle contractions, called positive myoclonus, or by muscle relaxation, called negative myoclonus. Myoclonic jerks may occur alone or in sequence, in a pattern or without pattern. They may occur infrequently or many times each minute. Myoclonus sometimes occurs in response to an external event or when a person attempts to make a movement. The twitching cannot be controlled by the person experiencing it.

In its simplest form, myoclonus consists of a muscle twitch followed by relaxation. A hiccup is an example of this type of myoclonus. Other familiar examples of myoclonus are the jerks or "sleep starts" that some people experience while drifting off to sleep. These simple forms of myoclonus occur in normal, healthy persons and cause no difficulties. When more widespread, myoclonus may involve persistent, shock-like contractions in a group of muscles. In some cases, myoclonus begins in one region of the body and spreads to muscles in other areas. More severe cases of myoclonus can distort movement and severely limit a

This chapter includes text excerpted from "Myoclonus Fact Sheet," National Institute of Neurological Disorders and Stroke (NINDS), July 2012. Reviewed February 2018.

person's ability to eat, talk, or walk. These types of myoclonus may indicate an underlying disorder in the brain or nerves.

What Are the Causes of Myoclonus?

Myoclonus may develop in response to infection, head or spinal cord injury, stroke, brain tumors, kidney or liver failure, lipid storage disease, chemical or drug poisoning, or other disorders. Prolonged oxygen deprivation to the brain, called hypoxia, may result in posthypoxic myoclonus. Myoclonus can occur by itself, but most often it is one of several symptoms associated with a wide variety of nervous system disorders. For example, myoclonic jerking may develop in patients with multiple sclerosis, Parkinson disease, Alzheimer disease, or Creutzfeldt–Jakob disease (CJD). Myoclonic jerks commonly occur in persons with epilepsy, a disorder in which the electrical activity in the brain becomes disordered leading to seizures.

What Are the Types of Myoclonus?

Classifying the many different forms of myoclonus is difficult because the causes, effects, and responses to therapy vary widely. Listed below are the types most commonly described.

- **Action myoclonus** is characterized by muscular jerking triggered or intensified by voluntary movement or even the intention to move. It may be made worse by attempts at precise, coordinated movements. Action myoclonus is the most disabling form of myoclonus and can affect the arms, legs, face, and even the voice. This type of myoclonus often is caused by brain damage that results from a lack of oxygen and blood flow to the brain when breathing or heartbeat is temporarily stopped.

- **Cortical reflex myoclonus** is thought to be a type of epilepsy that originates in the cerebral cortex—the outer layer, or "gray matter," of the brain, responsible for much of the information processing that takes place in the brain. In this type of myoclonus, jerks usually involve only a few muscles in one part of the body, but jerks involving many muscles also may occur. Cortical reflex myoclonus can be intensified when individuals attempt to move in a certain way (action myoclonus) or perceive a particular sensation.

- **Essential myoclonus** occurs in the absence of epilepsy or other apparent abnormalities in the brain or nerves. It can occur randomly in people with no family history, but it also can appear among members of the same family, indicating that it sometimes may be an inherited disorder. Essential myoclonus tends to be stable without increasing in severity over time. In some families, there is an association of essential myoclonus, essential tremor, and even a form of dystonia, called myoclonus dystonia. Another form of essential myoclonus may be a type of epilepsy with no known cause.

- **Palatal myoclonus** is a regular, rhythmic contraction of one or both sides of the rear of the roof of the mouth, called the soft palate. These contractions may be accompanied by myoclonus in other muscles, including those in the face, tongue, throat, and diaphragm. The contractions are very rapid, occurring as often as 150 times a minute, and may persist during sleep. The condition usually appears in adults and can last indefinitely. Some people with palatal myoclonus regard it as a minor problem, although some occasionally complain of a "clicking" sound in the ear, a noise made as the muscles in the soft palate contract. The disorder can cause discomfort and severe pain in some individuals.

- **Progressive myoclonus epilepsy (PME)** is a group of diseases characterized by myoclonus, epileptic seizures, and other serious symptoms such as trouble walking or speaking. These rare disorders often get worse over time and sometimes are fatal. Studies have identified many forms of PME. Lafora body disease is inherited as an autosomal recessive disorder, meaning that the disease occurs only when a child inherits two copies of a defective gene, one from each parent. Lafora body disease is characterized by myoclonus, epileptic seizures, and dementia (progressive loss of memory and other intellectual functions). The second group of PME diseases belonging to the class of cerebral storage diseases usually involves myoclonus, visual problems, dementia, and dystonia (sustained muscle contractions that cause twisting movements or abnormal postures). Another group of PME disorders in the class of system degenerations often is accompanied by action myoclonus, seizures, and problems with balance and walking. Many of these PME diseases begin in childhood or adolescence.

- **Reticular reflex myoclonus** is thought to be a type of generalized epilepsy that originates in the brainstem, the part of the brain that connects to the spinal cord and controls vital functions such as breathing and heartbeat. Myoclonic jerks usually affect the whole body, with muscles on both sides of the body affected simultaneously. In some people, myoclonic jerks occur in only a part of the body, such as the legs, with all the muscles in that part being involved in each jerk. Reticular reflex myoclonus can be triggered by either a voluntary movement or an external stimulus.

- **Stimulus-sensitive myoclonus** is triggered by a variety of external events, including noise, movement, and light. Surprise may increase the sensitivity of the individual.

- **Sleep myoclonus** occurs during the initial phases of sleep, especially at the moment of dropping off to sleep. Some forms appear to be stimulus-sensitive. Some persons with sleep myoclonus are rarely troubled by, or need treatment for, the condition. However, myoclonus may be a symptom in more complex and disturbing sleep disorders, such as restless legs syndrome, and may require treatment by a doctor.

What Do Scientists Know about Myoclonus?

Although rare cases of myoclonus are caused by an injury to the peripheral nerves (defined as the nerves outside the brain and spinal cord, or the central nervous system), most myoclonus is caused by a disturbance of the central nervous system (CNS). Studies suggest that several locations in the brain are involved in myoclonus. One such location, for example, is in the brainstem close to structures that are responsible for the startle response, an automatic reaction to an unexpected stimulus involving rapid muscle contraction.

The specific mechanisms underlying myoclonus are not yet fully understood. Scientists believe that some types of stimulus-sensitive myoclonus may involve overexcitability of the parts of the brain that control movement. These parts are interconnected in a series of feedback loops called motor pathways. These pathways facilitate and modulate communication between the brain and muscles. Key elements of this communication are chemicals known as neurotransmitters, which carry messages from one nerve cell, or neuron, to another. Neurotransmitters are released by neurons and attach themselves to receptors on parts of neighboring cells. Some neurotransmitters may make the receiving cell more sensitive, while others tend to make the receiving cell less sensitive. Laboratory studies suggest that an imbalance between these chemicals may underlie myoclonus.

Some researchers speculate that abnormalities or deficiencies in the receptors for certain neurotransmitters may contribute to some forms of myoclonus. Receptors that appear to be related to myoclonus include those for two important inhibitory neurotransmitters: serotonin and gamma-aminobutyric acid (GABA). Other receptors with links to myoclonus include those for opiates and glycine, the latter an inhibitory neurotransmitter that is important for the control of motor and sensory functions in the spinal cord. More research is needed to determine how these receptor abnormalities cause or contribute to myoclonus.

How Is Myoclonus Treated?

Treatment of myoclonus focuses on medications that may help reduce symptoms. The drug of first choice to treat myoclonus, especially certain types of action myoclonus, is clonazepam, a type of tranquilizer. Dosages of clonazepam usually are increased gradually until the individual improves or side effects become harmful. Drowsiness and loss of coordination are common side effects. The beneficial effects of clonazepam may diminish over time if the individual develops a tolerance for the drug.

Many of the drugs used for myoclonus, such as barbiturates, levetiracetam, phenytoin, and primidone, are also used to treat epilepsy. Barbiturates slow down the central nervous system and cause tranquilizing or antiseizure effects. Phenytoin, levetiracetam, and primidone are effective antiepileptic drugs, although phenytoin can cause liver failure or have other harmful long-term effects in individuals with PME. Sodium valproate is an alternative therapy for myoclonus and can be used either alone or in combination with clonazepam. Although clonazepam and/or sodium valproate are effective in the majority of people with myoclonus, some people have adverse reactions to these drugs.

Some studies have shown that doses of 5-hydroxytryptophan (5-HTP), a building block of serotonin, leads to improvement in people with some types of action myoclonus and PME. However, other studies indicate that 5-HTP therapy is not effective in all people with myoclonus, and, in fact, may worsen the condition in some individuals. These differences in the effect of 5-HTP on individuals with myoclonus have not yet been explained, but they may offer important clues to underlying abnormalities in serotonin receptors.

The complex origins of myoclonus may require the use of multiple drugs for effective treatment. Although some drugs have a limited effect when used individually, they may have a greater effect when used with drugs that act on different pathways or mechanisms in the brain. By combining several of these drugs, scientists hope to achieve greater control of myoclonic symptoms. Some drugs currently being studied in different combinations include clonazepam, sodium valproate, levetiracetam, and primidone. Hormonal therapy also may improve responses to antimyoclonic drugs in some people.

Chapter 55

Restless Legs Syndrome (RLS)

What Is Restless Legs Syndrome (RLS)?

Restless legs syndrome (RLS), also called Willis-Ekbom disease, causes unpleasant or uncomfortable sensations in the legs and an irresistible urge to move them. Symptoms commonly occur in the late afternoon or evening hours, and are often most severe at night when a person is resting, such as sitting or lying in bed. They also may occur when someone is inactive and sitting for extended periods (for example, when taking a trip by plane or watching a movie). Since symptoms can increase in severity during the night, it could become difficult to fall asleep or return to sleep after waking up. Moving the legs or walking typically relieves the discomfort but the sensations often recur once the movement stops. RLS is classified as a sleep disorder since the symptoms are triggered by resting and attempting to sleep, and as a movement disorder, since people are forced to move their legs in order to relieve symptoms. It is, however, best characterized as a neurological sensory disorder with symptoms that are produced from within the brain itself.

RLS is one of several disorders that can cause exhaustion and daytime sleepiness, which can strongly affect mood, concentration,

This chapter includes text excerpted from "Restless Legs Syndrome Fact Sheet," National Institute of Neurological Disorders and Stroke (NINDS), May 2017.

573

job and school performance, and personal relationships. Many people with RLS report they are often unable to concentrate, have impaired memory, or fail to accomplish daily tasks. Untreated moderate to severe RLS can lead to about a 20 percent decrease in work productivity and can contribute to depression and anxiety. It also can make traveling difficult.

It is estimated that up to 7–10 percent of the U.S. population may have RLS. RLS occurs in both men and women, although women are more likely to have it than men. It may begin at any age. Many individuals who are severely affected are middle-aged or older, and the symptoms typically become more frequent and last longer with age.

More than 80 percent of people with RLS also experience periodic limb movement of sleep (PLMS). PLMS is characterized by involuntary leg (and sometimes arm) twitching or jerking movements during sleep that typically occur every 15–40 seconds, sometimes throughout the night. Although many individuals with RLS also develop PLMS, most people with PLMS do not experience RLS. Fortunately, most cases of RLS can be treated with nondrug therapies and if necessary, medications.

What Are Common Signs and Symptoms of Restless Legs?

People with RLS feel the irresistible urge to move, which is accompanied by uncomfortable sensations in their lower limbs that are unlike normal sensations experienced by people without the disorder. The sensations in their legs are often difficult to define but may be described as aching throbbing, pulling, itching, crawling, or creeping. These sensations less commonly affect the arms, and rarely the chest or head. Although the sensations can occur on just one side of the body, they most often affect both sides. They can also alternate between sides. The sensations range in severity from uncomfortable to irritating to painful.

Because moving the legs (or other affected parts of the body) relieves the discomfort, people with RLS often keep their legs in motion to minimize or prevent the sensations. They may pace the floor, constantly move their legs while sitting, and toss and turn in bed.

A classic feature of RLS is that the symptoms are worse at night with a distinct symptom-free period in the early morning, allowing for more refreshing sleep at that time. Some people with RLS have difficulty falling asleep and staying asleep. They may also note a worsening of symptoms if their sleep is further reduced by events or activity.

RLS symptoms may vary from day to day, in severity and frequency, and from person to person. In moderately severe cases, symptoms occur only once or twice a week but often result in significant delay of sleep onset, with some disruption of daytime function. In severe cases of RLS, the symptoms occur more than twice a week and result in burdensome interruption of sleep and impairment of daytime function.

People with RLS can sometimes experience remissions—spontaneous improvement over a period of weeks or months before symptoms reappear—usually during the early stages of the disorder. In general, however, symptoms become more severe over time.

People who have both RLS and an associated medical condition tend to develop more severe symptoms rapidly. In contrast, those who have RLS that is not related to any other condition show a very slow progression of the disorder, particularly if they experience onset at an early age; many years may pass before symptoms occur regularly.

What Causes Restless Legs Syndrome?

In most cases, the cause of RLS is unknown (called primary RLS). However, RLS has a genetic component and can be found in families where the onset of symptoms is before age 40. Specific gene variants have been associated with RLS. Evidence indicates that low levels of iron in the brain also may be responsible for RLS.

Considerable evidence also suggests that RLS is related to a dysfunction in one of the sections of the brain that control movement (called the basal ganglia) that use the brain chemical dopamine. Dopamine is needed to produce smooth, purposeful muscle activity and movement. Disruption of these pathways frequently results in involuntary movements. Individuals with Parkinson disease, another disorder of the basal ganglia's dopamine pathways, have increased chance of developing RLS.

RLS also appears to be related to or accompany the following factors or underlying conditions:

- end-stage renal disease and hemodialysis
- iron deficiency
- certain medications that may aggravate RLS symptoms, such as antinausea drugs (e.g., prochlorperazine or metoclopramide), antipsychotic drugs (e.g., haloperidol or phenothiazine derivatives), antidepressants that increase serotonin (e.g., fluoxetine or

sertraline), and some cold and allergy medications that contain older antihistamines (e.g., diphenhydramine)

• use of alcohol, nicotine, and caffeine

• pregnancy, especially in the last trimester; in most cases, symptoms usually disappear within 4 weeks after delivery

• neuropathy (nerve damage)

Sleep deprivation and other sleep conditions like sleep apnea also may aggravate or trigger symptoms in some people. Reducing or completely eliminating these factors may relieve symptoms.

How Is Restless Legs Syndrome Diagnosed?

Since there is no specific test for RLS, the condition is diagnosed by a doctor's evaluation. The five basic criteria for clinically diagnosing the disorder are:

• A strong and often overwhelming need or urge to move the legs that is often associated with abnormal, unpleasant, or uncomfortable sensations.

• The urge to move the legs starts or get worse during rest or inactivity.

• The urge to move the legs is at least temporarily and partially or totally relieved by movements.

• The urge to move the legs starts or is aggravated in the evening or night.

• The above four features are not due to any other medical or behavioral condition.

A physician will focus largely on the individual's descriptions of symptoms, their triggers and relieving factors, as well as the presence or absence of symptoms throughout the day. A neurological and physical exam, plus information from the person's medical and family history and list of current medications, may be helpful. Individuals may be asked about frequency, duration, and intensity of symptoms; if movement helps to relieve symptoms; how much time it takes to fall asleep; any pain related to symptoms; and any tendency toward daytime sleep patterns and sleepiness, disturbance of sleep, or daytime function. Laboratory tests may rule out other conditions such as kidney failure, iron deficiency anemia (which is a separate condition related to iron deficiency), or pregnancy that may be causing symptoms of RLS. Blood tests can identify iron deficiencies as well as other medical disorders associated with RLS. In some cases, sleep studies such as polysomnography (a test that records the individual's brainwaves, heartbeat, breathing, and leg movements during an entire night) may identify the presence of other causes of sleep disruption (e.g., sleep apnea), which may impact management of the disorder. Periodic limb movement of sleep during a sleep study can support the diagnosis of RLS but, again, is not exclusively seen in individuals with RLS. Diagnosing RLS in children may be especially difficult, since it may be hard for children to describe what they are experiencing, when and how often the symptoms occur, and how long symptoms last. Pediatric RLS can sometimes be misdiagnosed as "growing pains" or attention deficit disorder.

How Is Restless Legs Syndrome Treated?

RLS can be treated, with care directed toward relieving symptoms. Moving the affected limb(s) may provide temporary relief. Sometimes RLS symptoms can be controlled by finding and treating an associated medical condition, such as peripheral neuropathy, diabetes, or iron deficiency anemia.

Iron supplementation or medications are usually helpful but no single medication effectively manages RLS for all individuals. Trials of different drugs may be necessary. In addition, medications taken regularly may lose their effect over time or even make the condition worse, making it necessary to change medications.

Treatment options for RLS include:

Lifestyle changes. Certain lifestyle changes and activities may provide some relief in persons with mild to moderate symptoms of RLS. These steps include avoiding or decreasing the use of alcohol and tobacco, changing or maintaining a regular sleep pattern, a program of moderate exercise, and massaging the legs, taking a warm bath, or using a heating pad or ice pack. There are new medical devices that have been cleared by the U.S. Food and Drug Administration (FDA), including a foot wrap that puts pressure underneath the foot and another that is a pad that delivers vibration to the back of the legs. Aerobic and leg-stretching exercises of moderate intensity also may provide some relief from mild symptoms.

Iron. For individuals with low or low-normal blood tests called ferritin and transferrin saturation, a trial of iron supplements is recommended as the first treatment. Iron supplements are available over-the-counter (OTC). A common side effect is upset stomach, which may improve with use of a different type of iron supplement. Because iron is not well-absorbed into the body by the gut, it may cause constipation that can be treated with a stool softeners such as polyethylene glycol. In some people, iron supplementation does not improve a person's iron levels. Others may require iron given through an IV (intravenous) line in order to boost the iron levels and relieve symptoms.

Antiseizure drugs. Antiseizure drugs are becoming the first-line prescription drugs for those with RLS. The FDA has approved gabapentin enacarbil for the treatment of moderate to severe RLS, This drug appears to be as effective as dopaminergic treatment (discussed below) and, at least to date, there have been no reports of problems with a progressive worsening of symptoms due to medication (called augmentation). Other medications may be prescribed "off-label" to relieve some of the symptoms of the disorder.

Other antiseizure drugs such as the standard form of gabapentin and pregabalin can decrease such sensory disturbances as creeping and crawling as well as nerve pain. Dizziness, fatigue, and sleepiness are among the possible side effects. Recent studies have shown that pregabalin is as effective for RLS treatment as the dopaminergic drug pramipexole, suggesting this class of drug offers equivalent benefits.

Dopaminergic agents. These drugs, which increase dopamine effect, are largely used to treat Parkinson disease. They have been shown to reduce symptoms of RLS when they are taken at nighttime. The FDA has approved ropinirole, pramipexole, and rotigotine to treat moderate to severe RLS. These drugs are generally well tolerated but can cause nausea, dizziness, or other short-term side effects. Levodopa plus carbidopa may be effective when used intermittently, but not daily.

Although dopamine-related medications are effective in managing RLS symptoms, long-term use can lead to worsening of the symptoms in many individuals. With chronic use, a person may begin to experience symptoms earlier in the evening or even earlier until the symptoms are present around the clock. Over time, the initial evening or bedtime dose can become less effective, the symptoms at night become more intense, and symptoms could begin to affect the arms or trunk. Fortunately, this apparent progression can be reversed by removing the person from all dopamine-related medications.

Another important adverse effect of dopamine medications that occurs in some people is the development of impulsive or obsessive behaviors such as obsessive gambling or shopping. Should they occur, these behaviors can be improved or reversed by stopping the medication.

Opioids. Drugs such as methadone, codeine, hydrocodone, or oxycodone are sometimes prescribed to treat individuals with more severe symptoms of RLS who did not respond well to other medications. Side effects include constipation, dizziness, nausea, exacerbation of sleep apnea, and the risk of addiction; however, very low doses are often effective in controlling symptoms of RLS.

Benzodiazepines. These drugs can help individuals obtain a more restful sleep. However, even if taken only at bedtime they can sometimes cause daytime sleepiness, reduce energy, and affect concentration. Benzodiazepines such as clonazepam and lorazepam are generally prescribed to treat anxiety, muscle spasms, and insomnia. Because these drugs also may induce or aggravate sleep apnea in some cases, they should not be used in people with this condition. These are last-line drugs due to their side effects.

What Is the Prognosis for People with Restless Legs Syndrome?

RLS is generally a lifelong condition for which there is no cure. However, current therapies can control the disorder, minimize symptoms, and increase periods of restful sleep. Symptoms may gradually worsen with age, although the decline may be somewhat faster for individuals who also suffer from an associated medical condition. A diagnosis of RLS does not indicate the onset of another neurological disease, such as Parkinson disease. In addition, some individuals have remissions—periods in which symptoms decrease or disappear for days, weeks, months, or years—although symptoms often eventually reappear. If RLS symptoms are mild, do not produce significant daytime discomfort, or do not affect an individual's ability to fall asleep, the condition does not have to be treated.

Chapter 56

Narcolepsy

Narcolepsy is a chronic neurological disorder caused by the brain's inability to regulate sleep-wake cycles. Many people with narcolepsy also experience uneven and interrupted sleep that can involve waking up frequently during the night. At various times throughout the day, people with narcolepsy experience irresistible bouts of sleep. If the urge becomes overwhelming, individuals will fall asleep for periods lasting from a few seconds to several minutes. In rare cases, some people may remain asleep for an hour or longer. In addition to excessive daytime sleepiness (EDS), people with narcolepsy experience some or all of the typical symptoms of cataplexy (the sudden loss of voluntary muscle tone), vivid hallucinations during sleep onset or upon awakening, and brief episodes of total paralysis at the beginning or end of sleep called sleep paralysis). Because narcolepsy is often misdiagnosed as other conditions, it may take years to get the proper diagnosis.

Cause

The cause of narcolepsy remains unknown. It is likely that narcolepsy involves multiple factors interacting to cause neurological dysfunction and sleep disturbances.

This chapter includes text excerpted from "Narcolepsy Information Page," National Institute of Neurological Disorders and Stroke (NINDS), December 7, 2017.

Treatment

There is no cure for narcolepsy. The U.S. Food and Drug Administration (FDA) approved the drug modafinil (a central nervous system stimulant) to treat EDS. In cases where modafinil is not effective, doctors may prescribe amphetamine-like stimulants such as methylphenidate to alleviate excessive daytime sleepiness. Two classes of antidepressant drugs have proved effective in controlling cataplexy in many individuals: tricyclics (including imipramine, desipramine, clomipramine, and protriptyline) and selective serotonin reuptake inhibitors (including venlafaxine, fluoxetine, and sertraline). The FDA also has approved sodium oxybate (also known as gamma hydroxybutyrate or GHB) to treat cataplexy and EDS in individuals with narcolepsy. Drug therapy should accompany various behavioral strategies. For example, many people with narcolepsy take short, regularly scheduled naps at times when they tend to feel sleepiest. Improving the quality of nighttime sleep can combat EDS and help relieve persistent feelings of fatigue. Among the most important common-sense measures people with narcolepsy can take to enhance sleep quality are actions such as maintaining a regular sleep schedule, relaxing before bed, and avoiding large meals, alcohol, and caffeine-containing beverages before bedtime.

Prognosis

None of the currently available medications enables people with narcolepsy to consistently maintain a fully normal state of alertness. But EDS and cataplexy, the most disabling symptoms of the disorder, can be controlled in most patients with drug treatment. Often the treatment regimen is modified as symptoms change. Whatever the age of onset, patients find that the symptoms tend to get worse over the two to three decades after the first symptoms appear. Many older patients find that some daytime symptoms decrease in severity after age 60.

Part Nine

Additional Help
and Information

Chapter 57

Glossary of Terms Related to Brain Disorders

abdominal migraine: A type of migraine that mostly affects young children and involves moderate to severe abdominal pain, with little or no headache.

acetylcholine: A neurotransmitter that plays an important role in many neurological functions, including learning and memory.

acyclovir: One of three available antiviral drugs that can reduce the severity and duration of a shingles attack if given soon after onset.

agnosia: A cognitive disability characterized by ignorance of or inability to acknowledge one side of the body or one side of the visual field.

alpha-synuclein: A protein that is implicated in abnormal clumps called Lewy bodies, which are seen in the brains of people with Parkinson disease and some dementias. Disorders in which alpha-synuclein accumulates inside nerve cells are called synucleinopathies.

Alzheimer disease: The most common cause of dementia in people aged 65 and older. Nearly all brain functions, including memory, movement, language, judgment, and behavior, are eventually affected.

amygdala: An almond-shaped structure involved in processing and remembering strong emotions such as fear. It is part of the limbic system and located deep inside the brain.

This glossary contains terms excerpted from documents produced by several sources deemed reliable.

amyloid: A protein found in the characteristic clumps of tissue (called plaques) that appear in the brains of people with Alzheimer disease.

aneurysm: A weak or thin spot on an artery wall that has stretched or ballooned out from the wall and filled with blood, or damage to an artery leading to pooling of blood between the layers of the blood vessel walls.

antibodies: Proteins made by the immune system that bind to structures (antigens) they recognize as foreign to the body.

aphasia: Difficulty understanding and/or producing spoken and written language.

apolipoprotein E (APOE): A protein that carries cholesterol in blood and that appears to play some role in brain function. The gene that produces this protein comes in several forms, or alleles: ε2, ε3, and ε4. The APOE ε2 allele is relatively rare and may provide some protection against AD (but it may increase risk of early heart disease). APOE ε3 is the most common allele and appears to play a neutral role in AD. APOE ε4 occurs in about 40 percent of all people with AD who develop the disease in later life; it increases the risk of developing AD.

arteriovenous malformation (AVM): A congenital disorder characterized by a complex tangled web of arteries and veins.

ataxia: A condition in which the muscles fail to function in a coordinated manner.

atherosclerosis: A blood vessel disease characterized by deposits of lipid material on the inside of the walls of large to medium-sized arteries which make the artery walls thick, hard, brittle, and prone to breaking.

atrial fibrillation: Irregular beating of the left atrium, or left upper chamber, of the heart.

aura: A warning of a migraine headache. Usually visual, it may appear as flashing lights, zigzag lines, or a temporary loss of vision, along with numbness or trouble speaking.

autoimmune disease: A disease in which the body's defense system malfunctions and attacks a part of the body itself rather than foreign matter.

autonomic: Occurring involuntary. Autonomic nervous system dysfunction is frequently associated with various types of migraine.

axon: The long extension from a neuron that transmits outgoing signals to other cells.

basal ganglia: A region located at the base of the brain composed of four clusters of neurons, or nerve cells. This area is responsible for body movement and coordination. The neuron groups most prominently and consistently affected by Huntington disease (HD)—the pallidum and striatum—are located here.

benign intracranial hypertension: Increased pressure within the brain that causes severe headaches. It can be caused by clotting in the major cerebral veins or from certain medications (including some antibiotics, human growth hormone replacement, and vitamin A and related compounds).

biofeedback: A process that increases an individual's voluntary control of physiologic states such as blood pressure and pain response.

blood-brain barrier: A network of blood vessels with closely spaced cells that controls the passage of substances from the blood into the central nervous system.

brain death: An irreversible cessation of measurable brain function.

brainstem: The portion of the brain that connects to the spinal cord and controls automatic body functions, such as breathing, heart rate, and blood pressure.

capillary: A tiny blood vessel. The brain has billions of capillaries that carry oxygen, glucose (the brain's principal source of energy), nutrients, and hormones to brain cells so they can do their work. Capillaries also carry away carbon dioxide and cell waste products.

carbamazepine: A drug that works both as an anticonvulsant and a pain reliever.

carotid artery: An artery, located on either side of the neck, that supplies the brain with blood.

cerebellum: The part of the brain responsible for maintaining the body's balance and coordination.

cerebral: Relating to the two hemispheres of the human brain.

cerebral cortex: The outer layer of nerve cells surrounding the cerebral hemispheres.

cerebral hemispheres: The largest portion of the brain, composed of billions of nerve cells in two structures connected by the corpus callosum. The cerebral hemispheres control conscious thought, language, decision making, emotions, movement, and sensory functions.

cerebrospinal fluid: The fluid found in and around the brain and spinal cord. It protects these organs by acting like a liquid cushion and by providing nutrients.

cerebrovascular disease: A reduction in the supply of blood to the brain either by narrowing of the arteries through the buildup of plaque on the inside walls of the arteries, called stenosis, or through blockage of an artery due to a blood clot.

cerebrum: The portion of the forebrain involved in conscious thought, memory and analysis of sensory signals.

cholesterol: A waxy substance, produced naturally by the liver and also found in foods, that circulates in the blood and helps maintain tissues and cell membranes. Excess cholesterol in the body can contribute to atherosclerosis and high blood pressure.

chromosome: The structures in cells that contain genes. They are composed of deoxyribonucleic acid (DNA) and proteins and, under a microscope, appear as rod-like structures.

chronic headache: Headache that occurs 15 or more days a month over a 3-month period.

clinical trial: A research study involving humans that rigorously tests safety, side effects, and how well a medication or behavioral treatment works.

clipping: Surgical procedure for treatment of brain aneurysms, involving clamping an aneurysm from a blood vessel, surgically removing this ballooned part of the blood vessel, and closing the opening in the artery wall.

cluster headache: Sudden, extremely painful headaches that occur in a closely grouped pattern several times a day and at the same times over a period of weeks.

cognitive functions: All aspects of conscious thought and mental activity, including learning, perceiving, making decisions, and remembering.

coma: a state of profound unconsciousness caused by disease, injury, or poison.

computed tomography (CT): A type of diagnostic imaging that uses X-rays and computer technology to produce two-dimensional images of organs, bones, and tissues.

concussion: Injury to the brain caused by a hard blow or violent shaking, causing a sudden and temporary impairment of brain function, such as a short loss of consciousness or disturbance of vision and equilibrium.

contracture: A condition in which muscles become fixed in a rigid, abnormal position, which causes distortion or deformity.

cortex: Part of the brain responsible for thought, perception, and memory. Huntington disease (HD) affects the basal ganglia and cortex.

cytokines: Small, hormone-like proteins released by leukocytes, endothelial cells, and other cells to promote an inflammatory immune response to an injury.

deep brain stimulation: Therapy that uses a surgically implanted, battery-operated medical device called a neurostimulator to deliver electrical stimulation to targeted areas in the brain that control movement, blocking the abnormal nerve signals that cause tremor and other movement symptoms.

dementia: A broad term referring to a decline in cognitive function to the extent that it interferes with daily life and activities.

deoxyribonucleic acid (DNA): The substance of heredity containing the genetic information necessary for cells to divide and produce proteins. DNA carries the code for every inherited characteristic of an organism.

developmental delay: Behind schedule in reaching the milestones of early childhood development.

dominant: A trait that is apparent even when the gene for that disorder is inherited from only one parent.

dopamine: A neurotransmitter that affects mood and helps control complex movements.

dura: A tough, fibrous membrane lining the brain; the outermost of the three membranes collectively called the meninges.

dysarthria: Inability or difficulty articulating words due to emotional stress, brain injury, paralysis, or spasticity of the muscles needed for speech.

dysphagia: Trouble swallowing.

early-onset Alzheimer disease (AD): A rare form of AD that usually affects people between ages 30 and 60. It is called familial AD (FAD) if it runs in the family.

enzyme: A protein that causes or speeds up a biochemical reaction.

exacerbation: A sudden worsening of symptoms or the appearance of new symptoms that lasts for at least 24 hours.

fatigue: Tiredness that may accompany activity or may persist even without exertion.

forebrain: The largest part of the human brain, composed primarily of the cerebrum.

frontotemporal disorders: A group of dementias characterized by degeneration of nerve cells, especially those in the frontal and temporal lobes of the brain.

functional magnetic resonance imaging (fMRI): A type of imaging that measures increases in blood flow within the brain.

gabapentin: An anti-seizure medicine that is also used as a pain reliever.

gene: The basic unit of heredity, composed of a segment of deoxyribonucleic acid (DNA) containing the code for a specific trait.

Glasgow Coma Scale (GCS): A clinical tool used to assess the degree of consciousness and neurological functioning—and therefore severity of brain injury—by testing motor responsiveness, verbal acuity, and eye opening.

glia: Also called neuroglia; supportive cells of the nervous system that make up the blood-brain barrier, provide nutrients and oxygen to the vital neurons, and protect the neurons from infection, toxicity, and trauma. Some examples of glia are oligodendroglia, astrocytes, and microglia.

glutamate: Also known as glutamic acid, an amino acid that acts as an excitatory neurotransmitter in the brain.

gray matter: Part of the brain that contains nerve cells and has a gray color.

hematoma: Heavy bleeding into or around the brain caused by damage to a major blood vessel in the head.

hemicrania continua: One-sided headaches that are chronic or continuous and respond to indomethacin treatment.

hemiplegic migraine: A type of migraine causing temporary paralysis on one side of the body.

hemorrhagic stroke: Stroke caused by bleeding out of one of the major arteries leading to the brain.

hindbrain: The most primitive part of the brain, which controls the body's most basic functions such as respiration and heart rate.

hippocampus: A structure in the brain that plays a major role in learning and memory and is involved in converting short-term to long-term memory.

HIV-associated dementia: A dementia that results from infection with the human immunodeficiency virus (HIV) that causes acquired immune deficiency syndrome (AIDS).

hormone: A chemical message produced by an endocrine gland which travels through the bloodstream to a target organ.

huntingtin: The protein encoded by the gene that carries the Huntington disease (HD) defect. The repeated CAG sequence in the gene causes an abnormal form of huntingtin to be formed. The function of the normal form of huntingtin is not yet known.

hypermetabolism: A condition in which the body produces too much heat energy.

hypertension (high blood pressure): Characterized by persistently high arterial blood pressure defined as a measurement greater than or equal to 140 mm/Hg systolic pressure over 90 mm/Hg diastolic pressure.

hypothalamus: A structure in the brain under the thalamus that monitors activities such as body temperature and food intake.

hypotonia: Decreased muscle tone.

hypoxia: A state of decreased oxygen delivery to a cell so that the oxygen falls below normal levels.

ice cream headache: A painful headache brought on by changes in blood flow that result from a sudden chilling of the roof of the mouth.

incidence: The extent or frequency of an occurrence; the number of specific new events in a given period of time.

infarct: An area of tissue that is dead or dying because of a loss of blood supply.

intracerebral hematoma: Bleeding within the brain caused by damage to a major blood vessel.

intracerebral hemorrhage (ICH): Occurs when a vessel within the brain leaks blood into the brain.

ischemia: A loss of blood flow to tissue, caused by an obstruction of the blood vessel, usually in the form of plaque stenosis or a blood clot.

ischemic stroke: Stroke caused by the formation of a clot that blocks blood flow through an artery to the brain.

late-onset Alzheimer disease (AD): The most common form of AD. It occurs in people aged 60 and older.

lesion: An abnormal change in the structure of an organ due to disease or injury.

Lewy body dementia (LBD): One of the most common types of progressive dementia, characterized by the presence of abnormal structures called Lewy bodies in the brain.

limbic system: A brain region that links the brainstem with the higher reasoning elements of the cerebral cortex. It controls emotions, instinctive behavior, and the sense of smell.

locked-in syndrome: A condition in which a patient is aware and awake, but cannot move or communicate due to complete paralysis of the body.

magnetic resonance angiography (MRA): An imaging technique involving injection of a contrast dye into a blood vessel and using magnetic resonance techniques to create an image of the flowing blood through the vessel; often used to detect stenosis of the brain arteries inside the skull.

magnetic resonance imaging (MRI): An imaging technique that uses radio waves, magnetic fields, and computer analysis to create a picture of body tissues and structures.

marker: A piece of deoxyribonucleic acid (DNA) that lies on the chromosome so close to a gene that the two are inherited together. Like a signpost, markers are used during genetic testing and research to locate the nearby presence of a gene.

meninges: The three layers of membrane that cover the brain and spinal cord.

meningitis: Inflammation of the three membranes that envelop the brain and spinal cord, collectively known as the meninges; the meninges include the dura, pia mater, and arachnoid.

metabolism: All of the chemical processes that take place inside the body. In some metabolic reactions, complex molecules are broken down to release energy. In others, the cells use energy to make complex compounds out of simpler ones (like making proteins from amino acids).

microtubule: An internal support structure for a neuron that guides nutrients and molecules from the body of the cell to the end of the axon.

midbrain: The upper part of the brainstem, which controls some reflexes and eye movements.

migraine: headaches that are usually pulsing or throbbing and occur on one or both sides of the head. They are moderate to severe in intensity, associated with nausea, vomiting, sensitivity to light and noise, and worsen with routine physical activity.

mild cognitive impairment (MCI): A condition in which a person has memory problems greater than those expected for his or her age, but not the personality or cognitive problems that characterize Alzheimer disease (AD).

mitochondria: Microscopic, energy-producing bodies within cells that are the cells' "power plants."

mixed dementia: Dementia in which one form of dementia and another condition or dementia cause damage to the brain, for example, Alzheimer disease and small vessel disease or vascular dementia.

motor neuron: A nerve that causes a muscle to contract.

multi-infarct dementia: A type of vascular dementia caused by numerous small strokes in the brain.

mutation: A permanent change in a cell's deoxyribonucleic acid (DNA) that can cause a disease.

myelin: A whitish, fatty layer surrounding an axon that helps the axon rapidly transmit electrical messages from the cell body to the synapse.

myoclonus: A condition in which muscles or portions of muscles contract involuntarily in a jerky fashion.

necrosis: A form of cell death resulting from anoxia, trauma, or any other form of irreversible damage to the cell; involves the release of toxic cellular material into the intercellular space, poisoning surrounding cells.

nerve: A bundle of axons in the nervous system.

nervous system: The system that coordinates an organism's response to the environment.

neurodegenerative disease: A disease characterized by a progressive decline in the structure, activity, and function of brain tissue. These diseases include Alzheimer disease (AD), Parkinson disease (PD), frontotemporal lobar degeneration, and dementia with Lewy bodies. They are usually more common in older people.

neuron: The main functional cell of the brain and nervous system, consisting of a cell body, an axon, and dendrites.

neurotransmitters: Special chemicals that transmit nerve impulses from one cell to another.

norepinephrine: A neurotransmitter that increases the rate of metabolism and helps an organism respond to threats.

nucleus: The structure within a cell that contains the chromosomes and controls many of its activities.

occipital lobe: Part of the cerebral cortex at the back of the brain, which processes images from the eyes and links it to memory.

oligodendrocytes: A type of support cell in the brain that produces myelin, the fatty sheath that surrounds and insulates axons.

optic neuritis: An inflammatory disorder of the optic nerve that usually occurs in only one eye and causes visual loss and sometimes blindness. It is generally temporary.

palsy: Paralysis, or the lack of control over voluntary movement.

parietal lobe: The topmost part of the cerebral cortex behind the frontal lobes which receives information about temperature, taste, touch, and movement.

Parkinson disease dementia: A secondary dementia that sometimes occurs in people with advanced Parkinson disease. Many people with Parkinson disease have the amyloid plaques and neurofibrillary tangles found in Alzheimer disease, but it is not clear if the diseases are linked.

placenta: An organ that joins a mother with her unborn baby and provides nourishment and sustenance.

plaque: Fatty cholesterol deposits found along the inside of artery walls that lead to atherosclerosis and stenosis of the arteries.

plasma: The liquid portion of the blood that is involved in controlling infection.

plasticity: The ability to be formed or molded; in reference to the brain, the ability to adapt to deficits and injury.

platelets: Structures found in blood that are known primarily for their role in blood coagulation.

positron emission tomography (PET): A tool used to diagnose brain functions and disorders. PET produces three-dimensional, colored images of chemicals or substances functioning within the body. These images are called PET scans. PET shows brain function, in contrast to computed tomography (CT) or magnetic resonance imaging (MRI), which show brain structure.

potential: A voltage or difference in electrical charge.

prednisone: An anti-inflammatory corticosteroid drug routinely given to shingles patients when an eye or other facial nerve is involved.

prevalence: The number of cases of a disease that are present in a particular population at a given time.

prompt: A verbal or physical support that helps a child get through an action.

pruning: Process whereby an injury destroys an important neural network in children, and another less useful neural network that would have eventually died takes over the responsibilities of the damaged network.

quadriplegia: Paralysis of both the arms and legs.

receptor: Proteins that serve as recognition sites on cells and cause a response in the body when stimulated by chemicals called neurotransmitters. They act as on-and-off switches for the next nerve cell.

recessive: A trait that is apparent only when the gene or genes for it are inherited from both parents.

relapsing-remitting multiple sclerosis (MS): A form of MS in which an episode of symptoms occurs and is followed by a recovery period before another attack occurs.

schizophrenia: A brain disease caused by defects in neurotransmitters (especially dopamine), characterized by delusions and severe behavioral changes.

scoliosis: A disease of the spine in which the spinal column tilts or curves to one side of the body.

secondary headaches: Headaches that are caused by an underlying condition or disease.

seizure: Abnormal activity of nerve cells in the brain causing strange sensations, emotions, and behavior, or sometimes convulsions, muscle spasms, and loss of consciousness.

serotonin: A neurotransmitter present throughout the body and brain that plays an important role in headache and migraine, mood disorders, regulating body temperature, sleep, vomiting, sexuality, and appetite.

spastic (or spasticity): Describes stiff muscles and awkward movements.

spasticity: Involuntary muscle contractions leading to spasms and stiffness or rigidity. In multiple sclerosis (MS), this condition primarily affects the lower limbs.

spinal cord: The mass of nervous tissue along the axis of an animal (within the backbone of vertebrates).

stenosis: Narrowing of an artery due to the buildup of plaque on the inside wall of the artery.

subarachnoid hemorrhage (SCH): Bleeding within the meninges, or outer membranes, of the brain into the clear fluid that surrounds the brain.

subdural hematoma: Bleeding confined to the area between the dura and the arachnoid membranes.

synapse: The tiny gap between nerve cells across which neurotransmitters pass.

tau: A protein that helps to maintain the structure of microtubules in normal nerve cells. Abnormal tau is a principal component of the paired helical filaments in neurofibrillary tangles.

thalamus: A small structure in the front of the cerebral hemispheres that serves as a way station that receives sensory information of all kinds and relays it to the cortex; it also receives information from the cortex.

thrombosis: The formation of a blood clot in one of the cerebral arteries of the head or neck that stays attached to the artery wall until it grows large enough to block blood flow.

trait: Any genetically determined characteristic.

transverse myelitis: An acute spinal cord disorder causing sudden low back pain and muscle weakness and abnormal sensory sensations in the lower extremities. Transverse myelitis often remits spontaneously; however, severe or long-lasting cases may lead to permanent disability.

tremor: An involuntary trembling or quivering.

trigger: Something that brings about a disease or condition.

vascular: Refers to blood vessels or the flow of blood.

vascular dementia: A type of dementia caused by brain damage from cerebrovascular or cardiovascular problems, usually strokes.

vasospasm: A dangerous side effect of subarachnoid hemorrhage in which the blood vessels in the subarachnoid space constrict erratically, cutting off blood flow.

vegetative state: A condition in which patients are unconscious and unaware of their surroundings, but continue to have a sleep/wake cycle and can have periods of alertness.

ventricles: cavities Within the brain that are filled with cerebrospinal fluid. In Huntington disease (HD), tissue loss causes enlargement of the ventricles.

ventriculostomy: A surgical procedure that drains cerebrospinal fluid from the brain by creating an opening in one of the small cavities called ventricles.

white matter: Nerve fibers that are the site of many multiple sclerosis (MS) lesions and that connect areas of gray matter in the brain and spinal cord.

Chapter 58

Directory of Organizations with Information about Brain Disorders

Government Agencies That Provide Information about Brain Disorders

Administration for Community Living (ACL)
National Institute on Disability, Independent Living, and Rehabilitation Research (NIDILRR)
330 C St. S.W.
Washington, DC 20201
Toll-Free: 800-677-1116
Phone: 202-401-4634
Website: www.acl.gov

Agency for Healthcare Research and Quality (AHRQ)
U.S. Department of Health and Human Services (HHS)
5600 Fishers Ln.
Rockville, MD 20857
Phone: 301-427-1364
Website: www.ahrq.gov

Resources in this chapter were compiled from several sources deemed reliable; all contact information was verified and updated in February 2018.

Agency for Toxic Substances and Disease Registry (ATSDR)
4770 Buford Hwy. N.E.
Atlanta, GA 30341
Toll-Free: 800-CDC-INFO
(800-232-4636)
Toll-Free TTY: 888-232-6348
Website: www.atsdr.cdc.gov

AIDSinfo (AIDS Information Service)
U.S. Department of Health and Human Services (HHS)
P.O. Box 4780
Rockville, MD 20849-6303
Toll-Free: 800-HIV-0440
(800-448-0440)
Fax: 301-315-2818
Website: aidsinfo.nih.gov
E-mail: contactus@aidsinfo.nih.gov

Alzheimer's Disease Education and Referral Center (ADEAR)
P.O. Box 8250
Silver Spring, MD 20907-8250
Toll-Free: 800-438-4380
Phone: 301-495-3311
Website: www.nia.nih.gov/alzheimers
E-mail: adear@nia.nih.gov

Brain Resources and Information Network (BRAIN)
National Institute of Neurological Disorders and Stroke (NINDS)
P.O. Box 5801
Bethesda, MD 20824
Toll-Free: 800-352-9424
Phone: 301-496-5751
Fax: 301-402-2186
Website: www.ninds.nih.gov
E-mail: braininfo@ninds.nih.gov

Centers for Disease Control and Prevention (CDC)
U.S. Department of Health and Human Services (HHS)
1600 Clifton Rd. N.E.
Atlanta, GA 30333-4027
Toll-Free: 800-CDC-INFO
(800-232-4636)
Toll-Free TTY: 888-232-6348
Website: www.cdc.gov

Eldercare Locator
U.S. Department of Health and Human Services (HHS):
Administration on Aging (AOA)
330 C St. S.W.
Washington, DC 20201
Toll-Free: 800-677-1116
Phone: 202-619-0724
Toll-Free TTY/TDD:
800-877-8339
Fax: 202-357-3555
Website: www.eldercare.gov
E-mail: eldercarelocator@n4a.org

Eunice Kennedy Shriver
National Institute of
Child Health and Human
Development (NICHD)
Information Resource Center
P.O. Box 3006
Rockville, MD 20847
Toll-Free: 800-370-2943
Toll-Free TTY: 888-320-6942
Toll-Free Fax: 866-760-5947
Website: www.nichd.nih.gov
E-mail:
NICHDInformationResource
Center@mail.nih.gov

National Cancer Institute
(NCI)
NCI Public Inquiries Office
9609 Medical Center Dr.
Bethesda, MD 20892-9760
Toll-Free: 800-4-CANCER
(800-422-6237)
Website: www.cancer.gov

National Center for
Advancing Translational
Sciences (NCATS)
Office of Rare Diseases Research
6701 Democracy Blvd.
MSC 4874
Bethesda, MD 20892-4874
Website: www.ncats.nih.gov
E-mail: info@ncats.nih.gov

National Eye Institute (NEI)
Information Office
31 Center Dr. MSC 2510
Bethesda, MD 20892-2510
Phone: 301-496-5248
Website: www.nei.nih.gov
E-mail: 2020@nei.nih.gov

National Heart, Lung, and
Blood Institute (NHLBI)
31 Center Dr.
Bethesda, MD 20892
Phone: 301-592-8573
Website: www.nhlbi.nih.gov
E-mail: nhlbiinfo@nhlbi.nih.gov

National Institute of Allergy
and Infectious Diseases
(NIAID)
Office of Communications and
Government Relations
5601 Fishers Ln. MSC 9806
Bethesda, MD 20892-9806
Toll-Free: 866-284-4107
Fax: 301-402-3573
Website: www.niaid.nih.gov
E-mail: ocpostoffice@niaid.nih.
gov

National Institute of
Diabetes and Digestive and
Kidney Diseases (NIDDK)
National Institutes of Health
(NIH)
9000 Rockville Pike
Bethesda, MD 20892
Toll-Free: 800-860-8747
Toll-Free TTY: 866-569-1162
Website: www.niddk.nih.gov
E-mail: healthinfo@niddk.nih.
gov

National Institute of Mental Health (NIMH)
Science Writing, Press, and Dissemination Branch
6001 Executive Blvd.
Rm. 6200 MSC 9663
Bethesda, MD 20892-9663
Toll-Free: 866-615-6464
Toll-Free TTY: 866-415-8051
TTY: 301-443-8431
Fax: 301-443-4279
Website: www.nimh.nih.gov
E-mail: nimhinfo@nih.gov

National Institute of Neurological Disorders and Stroke (NINDS)
P.O. Box 5801
Bethesda, MD 20824
Toll-Free: 800-352-9424
Phone: 301-496-5751
Website: www.ninds.nih.gov

National Institute on Aging (NIA)
31 Center Dr MSC 2292
Bldg. 31 Rm. 5C27
Bethesda, MD 20892
Toll-Free: 800-222-2225
Toll-Free TTY: 800-222-4225
Website: www.nia.nih.gov
E-mail: niaic@nia.nih.gov

National Kidney & Urologic Diseases Information Clearinghouse (NKUDIC)
3 Information Way
Bethesda, MD 20892-3580
Toll-Free: 800-891-5390
Phone: 301-654-4415
Website: www.ninds.nih.gov/node/6854
E-mail: nkudic@info.niddk.nih.gov

National Library of Medicine (NLM)
8600 Rockville Pike
Bethesda, MD 20894
Toll-Free: 888-FIND-NLM
(888-346-3656)
Phone: 301-594-5983
Website: www.nlm.nih.gov

National Prevention Information Network (NPIN)
Centers for Disease Control and Prevention (CDC)
Website: www.npin.cdc.gov
E-mail: NPIN-info@cdc.gov

NIH Clinical Center
10 Center Dr.
Bethesda, MD 20892
Toll-Free: 800-411-1222
Toll-Free Fax: 866-411-1010
Website: clinicalcenter.nih.gov
E-mail: prpl@mail.cc.nih.gov

Office of Special Education and Rehabilitative Services (OSERS)
U.S. Department of Education (ED)
400 Maryland Ave. S.W.
Washington, DC 20202-7100
Phone: 202-245-7468
Website: www2.ed.gov/about/offices/list/osers/index.html

U.S. Food and Drug Administration (FDA)
10903 New Hampshire Ave.
Silver Spring, MD 20993-0002
Toll-Free: 888-INFO-FDA (888-463-6332)
Phone: 301-796-8240
Website: www.fda.gov

Private Agencies That Provide Information about Brain Disorders

Acoustic Neuroma Association (ANA)
600 Peachtree Pkwy.
Ste. 108
Cumming, GA 30041
Phone: 770-205-8211
Website: www.anausa.org
E-mail: info@anausa.org

ALS Therapy Development Institute (TDI)
300 Technology Sq.
Ste. 400
Cambridge, MA 02139
Phone: 617-441-7200
Website: www.als.net
E-mail: info@als.net

Alzheimer's Association
225 N. Michigan Ave.
17th Fl.
Chicago, IL 60601
Toll-Free: 800-272-3900
Phone: 312-335-8700
TDD: 312-335-5886
Toll-Free Fax: 866-699-1246
Website: www.alz.org

Alzheimer's Drug Discovery Foundation (ADDF)
57 W. 57th St.
Ste. 904
New York, NY 10019
Phone: 212-901-8000
Website: www.alzdiscovery.org

Alzheimer's Foundation of America (AFA)
322 Eighth Ave.
Seventh Fl.
New York, NY 10001
Toll-Free: 866-232-8484
Website: www.alzfdn.org

American Association of Neurological Surgeons (AANS)
5550 Meadowbrook Dr.
Rolling Meadows, IL 60008-3852
Toll-Free: 888-566-AANS (888-566-2267)
Phone: 847-378-0500
Fax: 847-378-0600
Website: www.aans.org

American Autoimmune Related Diseases Association (AARDA)
22100 Gratiot Ave.
Eastpointe, MI 48021
Phone: 586-776-3900
Website: www.aarda.org

American Brain Tumor Association (ABTA)
8550 W. Bryn Mawr Ave.
Ste. 550
Chicago, IL 60631
Toll-Free: 800-886-2282
Phone: 773-577-8750
Fax: 773-577-8738
Website: www.abta.org

American Chronic Pain Association (ACPA)
P.O. Box 850
Rocklin, CA 95677
Toll-Free: 800-533-3231
Fax: 916-652-8190
Website: www.theacpa.org

American College of Radiology (ACR)
1891 Preston White Dr.
Reston, VA 20191
Toll-Free: 800-227-5463
Phone: 703-648-8900
Website: www.acr.org

American Diabetes Association (ADA)
2451 Crystal Dr.
Ste. 900
Arlington, VA 22202
Toll-Free: 800-DIABETES
(800-342-2383)
Website: www.diabetes.org

American Heart Association (AHA)
7272 Greenville Ave.
Dallas, TX 75231
Toll-Free: 800-AHA-USA-1
(800-242-8721)
Website: www.heart.org

American Migraine Foundation (AMF)
19 Mantua Rd.
Mt. Royal, NJ 08061
Phone: 856-423-0043
Fax: 856-423-0082
Website:
americanmigrainefoundation.org

American Syringomyelia & Chiari Alliance Project (ASAP)
P.O. Box 1586
Longview, TX 75606-1586
Toll-Free: 800-ASAP-282
(800-2727-282)
Phone: 903-236-7079
Fax: 903-757-7456
Website: www.asap.org

Amyotrophic Lateral Sclerosis (ALS) Association
1275 K St. N.W.
Ste. 250
Washington, DC 20005
Toll-Free: 800-782-4747
Phone: 202-407-8580
Fax: 202-464-8869
Website: www.alsa.org
E-mail: alsinfo@alsa-national.org

Angioma Alliance (AA)
520 W. 21st St.
Ste. G2-411
Norfolk, VA 23517
Fax: 757-623-0616
Website: www.angiomaalliance.
org

Antiepileptic Drug (AED)
Pregnancy Registry
Massachusetts General Hospital
125 Nashua St.
Ste. 8438
Boston, MA 02114
Toll-Free: 888-233-2334
Fax: 617-643-0071
Website: www.
aedpregnancyregistry.org

ARCH National Respite
Network and Resource
Center
4016 Oxford St.
Annandale, VA 22003
Phone: 703-256-2084
Website: archrespite.org

Association for
Frontotemporal Degeneration
(AFTD)
290 King of Prussia Rd.
Radnor Stn Bldg. 2 Ste. 320
Radnor, PA 19087
Toll-Free: 866-507-7222
Phone: 267-514-7221
Website: www.theaftd.org

Batten Disease Support
and Research Association
(BDSRA)
2780 Airport Dr.
Ste. 342
Columbus, OH 43219
Toll-Free: 800-448-4570
Toll-Free Fax: 866-648-8718
Website: www.bdsra.org

Birth Defect Research for
Children, Inc. (BDRC)
976 Lake Baldwin Ln.
Ste. 104
Orlando, FL 32814
Phone: 407-895-0802
Website: www.birthdefects.org

Brain Aneurysm Foundation
(BAF)
269 Hanover St.
Hanover, MA 02339
Toll-Free: 888-272-4602
Phone: 781-826-5556
Fax: 781-826-5566
Website: www.bafound.org

Brain Attack Coalition
(BAC)
31 Center Dr. MSC 2540
Bldg. 31 Rm. 8A-07
Bethesda, MD 20892
Phone: 301-496-5751
Website: www.
brainattackcoalition.org

Brain Injury Association of America, Inc. (BIAA)
1608 Spring Hill Rd.
Ste. 110, Vienna, VA 22182
Toll-Free: 800-444-6443
Phone: 703-761-0750
Fax: 703-761-0755
Website: www.biausa.org

Brain Injury Resource Center
P.O. Box 84151
Seattle, WA 98124-5451
Phone: 206-621-8558
Website: www.headinjury.com
E-mail: brain@headinjury.com

Brain Trauma Foundation (BTF)
708 Third Ave., Ste. 1810
New York, NY 10017
Phone: 212-772-0608
Fax: 212-772-0357
Website: www.braintrauma.org

BrightFocus Foundation
22512 Gateway Center Dr.
Clarksburg, MD 20871
Toll-Free: 800-437-2423
Fax: 301-258-9454
Website: www.brightfocus.org/alzheimers
E-mail: info@brightfocus.org

Caregiver Action Network (CAN)
1150 Connecticut Ave. N.W.
Ste. 501
Washington, DC 20036-3904
Phone: 202-454-3970
Website: www.caregiveraction.org
E-mail: info@caregiveraction.org

Center for Parent Information and Resources (CPIR)
c/o Statewide Parent Advocacy Network (SPAN)
35 Halsey St.
Fourth Fl.
Newark, NJ 07102
Phone: 973-642-8100
Website: www.parentcenterhub.org

Center on Technology and Disability (CTD)
Family Health International (FHI) 360
1825 Connecticut Ave. N.W.
Washington, DC 20009
Website: www.ctdinstitute.org
E-mail: ctd@fhi360.org

Cerebral Palsy International Research Foundation (CPIRF)
186 Princeton Hightstown Rd.
Bldg. 4, Second Fl.
Princeton Junction, NJ 08550
Phone: 609-452-1200
Fax: 609-452-1201
Website: www.cpirf.org
E-mail: cpirf@cpirf.org

Charcot-Marie-Tooth Association (CMTA)
P.O. Box 105
Glenolden, PA 19036
Toll-Free: 800-606-2682
Phone: 610-499-9264
Fax: 610-499-9267
Website: www.cmtausa.org
E-mail: info@cmtausa.org

The Charlie Foundation
515 Ocean Ave.
Ste. 602N
Santa Monica, CA 90402
Phone: 310-393-2347
Website: www.charliefoundation.
org

Chiari & Syringomyelia Foundation (CSF)
29 Crest Loop
Staten Island, NY 10312
Phone: 718-966-2593
Website: www.csfinfo.org

Children's Hemiplegia and Stroke Association (CHASA)
4101 W. Green Oaks
Ste. 305-149
Arlington, TX 76016
Website: www.chasa.org

Citizens United for Research in Epilepsy (CURE)
430 W. Erie
Ste. 210
Chicago, IL 60654
Toll-Free: 844-231-2873
Phone: 312-255-1801
Website: www.cureepilepsy.org
E-mail: info@CUREepilepsy.org

CJD (Creutzfeldt-Jakob disease) Aware!
Phone: 504-861-4627
Website: www.cjdaware.com
E-mail: info@cjdaware.com

Creutzfeldt-Jakob Disease (CJD) Foundation Inc.
3610 W. Market St.
Ste. 110 East Entrance
Fairlawn, OH 44333
Toll-Free: 800-659-1991
Fax: 234-466-7077
Website: www.cjdfoundation.org
E-mail: help@cjdfoundation.org

CurePSP
404 Fifth Ave.
Third Fl.
New York, NY 10018
Toll-Free: 800-457-4777
Phone: 347-294-CURE
(347-294-2873)
Fax: 410-785-7009
Website: www.psp.org
E-mail: info@curepsp.org

Dana Alliance for Brain Initiatives (DABI)
505 Fifth Ave.
Sixth Fl.
New York, NY 10017
Phone: 212-223-4040
Fax: 212-317-8721
Website: www.dana.org/
danaalliances
E-mail: dabiinfo@dana.org

Easter Seals
141 W. Jackson Blvd.
Ste. 1400 A
Chicago, IL 60604
Toll-Free: 800-221-6827
Phone: 312-726-6200
Fax: 312-726-1494
Website: www.easterseals.com
E-mail: info@easterseals.com

Elizabeth Glaser Pediatric AIDS Foundation (EGPAF)
1140 Connecticut Ave. N.W.
Ste. 200
Washington, DC 20036
Phone: 202-296-9165
Fax: 202-296-9185
Website: www.pedaids.org
E-mail: info@pedaids.org

Epilepsy Foundation
8301 Professional Pl. E.
Ste. 200
Landover, MD 20785-2353
Toll-Free: 800-332-1000
Phone: 301-459-3700
Fax: 301-577-2684
Website: www.epilepsy.com
E-mail: contactus@efa.org

Family Caregiver Alliance (FCA)
National Center on Caregiving (NCC)
285 Montgomery St.
Ste. 950
San Francisco, CA 94104
Toll-Free: 800-445-8106
Phone: 415-434-3388
Website: www.caregiver.org

Fibromuscular Dysplasia Society of America (FMDSA)
26777 Lorain Rd.
Ste. 408
North Olmsted, Ohio 44070
Toll-Free: 888-709-7089
Phone: 216-834-2410
Website: www.fmdsa.org
E-mail: admin@fmdsa.org

The Foundation for Peripheral Neuropathy
485 Half Day Rd., Ste. 350
Buffalo Grove, IL 60089
Toll-Free: 877-883-9942
Fax: 847-883-9960
Website: www.foundationforpn.org
E-mail: info@tffpn.org

Friedreich's Ataxia Research Alliance (FARA)
533 W. Uwchlan Ave.
Downingtown, PA 19335
Toll-Free: 800-457-4777
Phone: 484-879-6160
Fax: 484-872-1402
Website: www.curefa.org
E-mail: info@curefa.org

Genetic Alliance
4301 Connecticut Ave. N.W.
Ste. 404
Washington, DC 20008-2369
Phone: 202-966-5557
Fax: 202-966-8553
Website: www.geneticalliance.org

Hazel K. Goddess Fund for Stroke Research in Women
4801 Courthouse St., Ste. 220
Williamsburg, VA 23188
Website: www.guidestar.org
E-mail: info@guidestar.org.

Heart Rhythm Society (HRS)
1325 G St. N.W.
Ste. 400, Washington, DC 20005
Phone: 202-464-3400
Fax: 202-464-3401
Website: www.hrsonline.org
E-mail: info@HRSonline.org

Hereditary Disease Foundation (HDF)
3960 Bdwy.
Sixth Fl.
New York, NY 10032
Phone: 212-928-2121
Fax: 212-928-2172
Website: www.hdfoundation.org/home.php
E-mail: cures@hdfoundation.org

Hide and Seek Foundation / SOAR
6475 E. Pacific Coast Hwy
Ste.466
Long Beach, CA 90803
Toll-Free: 844-762-7672
Website: www.hideandseek.org

Hope for Hypothalamic Hamartomas (Hope for HH)
P. O. Box 721
Waddell, AZ 85355
Website: www.hopeforhh.org
E-mail: info@hopeforhh.org

Huntington's Disease Society of America (HDSA)
505 Eighth Ave.
Ste. 902
New York, NY 10018
Toll-Free: 800-345-HDSA
(800-345-4372)
Phone: 212-242-1968
Website: hdsa.org
E-mail: hdsainfo@hdsa.org

Hydrocephalus Association
4340 East West Hwy.
Ste. 905
Bethesda, MD 20814-4447
Toll-Free: 888-598-3789
Phone: 301-202-3811
Fax: 301-202-3813
Website: www.hydroassoc.org
E-mail: info@hydroassoc.org

Indiana University School of Medicine
Indiana Alzheimer's Disease Center
340 W. Tenth St.
Fairbanks Hall Ste. 6200
Indianapolis, IN 46202-3082
Phone: 317-274-8157
Fax: 317-963-7547
Website: medicine.iu.edu
E-mail: iusm@iu.edu

International RadioSurgery Association (IRSA)
P.O. Box 5186
Harrisburg, PA 17110
Website: www.irsa.org

Intracranial Hypertension Research Foundation (IHRF)
6517 Buena Vista Dr.
Vancouver, WA 98661
Phone: 360-693-IHRF
(360-693-4473)
Fax: 360-694-7062
Website: www.IHRFoundation.org
E-mail: contact@ihrfoundation.org

John Douglas French
Alzheimer's Foundation
(JDFAF)
6320 Canoga Ave.
Ste. 1500
Woodland Hills, CA 91367
Phone: 310-445-4652
Website: www.jdfaf.org

Johns Hopkins University
School of Medicine
733 N. Bdwy.
Ste G-49
Baltimore, MD 21205-2196
Phone: 410-955-3182
Website: www.hopkinsmedicine.
org
E-mail: somadmiss@jhmi.edu

Les Turner ALS Foundation
5550 W. Touhy Ave.
Ste. 302
Skokie, IL 60077-3254
Toll-Free: 888-679-3311
Fax: 847-679-9109
Website: www.lesturnerals.org
E-mail: info@lesturnerals.org

Lewy Body Dementia
Association (LBDA)
912 Killian Hill Rd. S.W.
Lilburn, GA 30047
Fax: 480-422-5434
Website: www.lbda.org

LGS Foundation
80 Orville Dr.
Ste. 100
Bohemia, NY 11716
Phone: 718-374-3800
Website: www.lgsfoundation.org
E-mail: info@lgsfoundation.org

March of Dimes
1275 Mamaroneck Ave.
White Plains, NY 10605
Toll-Free: 888-663-4637
Phone: 914-997-4488
Fax: 914-997-4532
Website: www.marchofdimes.
com

Massachusetts General
Hospital (MGH)
55 Fruit St.
Boston, MA 02114
Phone: 617-726-5571
Website: www.ftd-boston.org

Mayo Clinic
13400 E. Shea Blvd.
Scottsdale, AZ 85259
Toll-Free: 800-446-2279
Phone: 480-301-8000
Website: www.mayoclinic.org

Meningitis Foundation of
America, Inc. (MFA)
P.O. Box 1818
El Mirage, AZ 85335
Phone: 480-270-2652
Website: www.musa.org
E-mail: info@musa.org

Michael J. Fox Foundation
for Parkinson's Research
P.O. Box 4777
New York, NY 10163-4777
Toll-Free: 800-708-7644
Website: www.michaeljfox.org

Migraine Research Foundation
300 E. 75th St., Ste. 3K
New York, NY 10021
Phone: 212-249-5402
Website: www.
migraineresearchfoundation.org
E-mail: contactmrf@
migraineresearchfoundation.org

Multiple Sclerosis Association of America (MSAA)
375 Kings Hwy N.
Cherry Hill, NJ 08034
Toll-Free: 800-532-7667
Fax: 856-661-9797
Website: www.mymsaa.org
E-mail: CommDept@mymsaa.org

Multiple Sclerosis Foundation (MS Focus)
6520 N. Andrews Ave.
Ft. Lauderdale, FL 33309-2132
Toll-Free: 888-MSFOCUS
(888-673-6287)
Fax: 954-351-0630
Website: www.msfocus.org
E-mail: support@msfocus.org

Muscular Dystrophy Association (MDA)
222 S. Riverside Plaza
Ste. 1500, Chicago, IL 60606
Toll-Free: 800-572-1717
Website: www.mda.org
E-mail: mda@mdausa.org

Myelin Repair Foundation (MRF)
Phone: 408-871-2410
Website: www.myelinrepair.org
E-mail: info@myelinrepair.org

Narcolepsy Network
P.O. Box 2178
Lynnwood, WA 98036
Toll-Free: 888-292-6522
Phone: 401-667-2523
Fax: 401-633-6567
Website: www.
narcolepsynetwork.org
E-mail: narnet@
narcolepsynetwork.org

Nathan's Battle Foundation
459 S. State Rd. 135
Greenwood, IN 46142
Phone: 317-888-7396
Fax: 317-888-0504
Website: www.nathansbattle.com

National Academy of Elder Law Attorneys, Inc. (NAELA)
1577 Spring Hill Rd.
Ste. 310
Vienna, VA 22182
Phone: 703-942-5711
Fax: 703-563-9504
Website: www.naela.org

National Ataxia Foundation (NAF)
600 Hwy 169 S., Ste. 1725
Minneapolis, MN 55426
Phone: 763-553-0020
Fax: 763-553-0167
Website: www.ataxia.org
E-mail: naf@ataxia.org

National Council on Patient Information and Education (NCPIE)
9710 Traville Gateway Dr.
Ste. 272
Rockville, MD 20850
Phone: 301-340-3940
Fax: 301-340-3944
Website: www.bemedwise.org
E-mail: ncpie@ncpie.info

National Headache Foundation (NHF)
820 N. Orleans
Ste. 201
Chicago, IL 60610-3131
Phone: 312-274-2650
Website: www.headaches.org
E-mail: info@headaches.org

National Hospice and Palliative Care Organization (NHPCO)
1731 King St.
Ste. 100
Alexandria, VA 22314
Toll-Free: 800-658-8898
Phone: 703-837-1500
Fax: 703-837-1233
Website: www.nhpco.org
E-mail: nhpco_info@nhpco.org

National Meningitis Association (NMA)
P.O. Box 60143
Ft. Myers, FL 33906
Toll-Free: 866-FONE-NMA
(866-366-3662)
Website: www.nmaus.org

National Multiple Sclerosis Society (NMSS)
733 Third Ave.
Third Fl.
New York, NY 10017
Toll-Free: 800-344-4867
Phone: 212-463-7787
Fax: 212-986-7981
Website: www.
nationalmssociety.org

National NeuroAIDS Tissue Consortium (NNTC)
401 N. Washington St.
Rockville, MD 20850
Toll-Free: 866-668-2272
Phone: 301-251-1161
Fax: 301-576-4597
Website: www.nntc.org
E-mail: nntc@emmes.com

National Organization for Rare Disorders, Inc. (NORD)
55 Kenosia Ave.
Danbury, CT 06810
Toll-Free: 800-999-NORD
(800-999-6673)
Phone: 203-744-0100
Fax: 203-263-9938
Website: www.rarediseases.org
E-mail: orphan@rarediseases.org

National Rehabilitation Information Center (NARIC)
8400 Corporate Dr.
Ste. 500
Landover, MD 20785
Toll-Free: 800-346-2742
Fax: 301-459-4263
Website: www.naric.com
E-mail: naricinfo@
heitechservices.com

National Sleep Foundation (NSF)
1010 N. Glebe Rd.
Ste. 420
Arlington, VA 22201
Website: www.sleepfoundation.org
E-mail: nsf@sleepfoundation.org

National Stroke Association
9707 E. Easter Ln., Ste. B
Centennial, CO 80112
Toll-Free: 800-STROKES
(800-787-6537)
Website: www.stroke.org
E-mail: info@stroke.org

Neurologic AIDS Research Consortium
Department of Neurology,
Washington University School of Medicine
660 S. Euclid Ave.
Campus Box 8111
St. Louis, MO 63110
Phone: 314-747-8423
Fax: 314-747-8177
Website: www.neuro.wustl.edu

Northwestern University Feinberg School of Medicine
Cognitive Neurology and Alzheimer's Disease Center
320 E. Superior
Searle 11
Chicago, IL 60611
Phone: 312-908-9339
Fax: 312-908-8789
Website: www.brain.northwestern.edu
E-mail: medcommunications@northwestern.edu

Paralyzed Veterans of America (PVA)
801 18th St. N.W.
Washington, DC 20006-3517
Toll-Free: 800-424-8200
Toll-Free TTY: 800-795-HEAR
(800-795-4327)
Toll-Free Fax: 800-795-4327
Website: www.pva.org
E-mail: info@pva.org

Parkinson's Foundation
200 S.E. First St., Ste. 800
Miami, FL 33131
Toll-Free: 800-4PD-INFO
(800-473-4636)
Website: www.parkinson.org
E-mail: contact@parkinson.org

Pathways
150 N. Michigan Ave.
Chicago, IL 60601
Toll-Free: 800-955-CHILD
(800-955-2445)
Website: www.pathways.org
E-mail: friends@pathways.org

Pedal-with-Pete
P.O. Box 1233
Worthington, OH 43085
Phone: 614-527-0202
Website: www.pedal-with-pete.org
E-mail: pwp@pedal-with-pete.org

Pediatric Brain Foundation
2144 E. Republic Rd. Bldg. B
Ste. 201
Springfield, MO 65804
Phone: 417-887-4242
Website: www.pediatricbrainfoundation.org

613

Pediatric Hydrocephalus Foundation, Inc. (PHF)
10 Main St.
Woodbridge, NJ 07095
Phone: 732-634-1283
Fax: 847-589-1250
Website: www. hydrocephaluskids.org/ wordpress

The Penn Frontotemporal Degeneration (FTD) Center
University of Pennsylvania Health System
3 W. Gates
3400 Spruce St.
Philadelphia, PA 19104
Phone: 215-349-5863
Fax: 215-349-8464
Website: www.ftd.med.upenn. edu

Prize4Life
P.O. Box 578835
Chicago, IL 60657
Phone: 617-545-4882
Website: www.prize4life.org
E-mail: contact@prize4life.org

Project ALS
801 Riverside Dr.
Ste. 6G
New York, NY 10032
Toll-Free: 855-900-2ALS (855-900-2257)
Phone: 212-420-7382
Fax: 646-559-9290
Website: www.projectals.org
E-mail: info@projectals.org

Radiological Society of North America (RSNA)
820 Jorie Blvd.
Oak Brook, IL 60523-2251
Toll-Free: 800-381-6660
Phone: 630-571-2670
Fax: 630-571-7837
Website: www.rsna.org
E-mail: membership@rsna.org

The RE Children's Project
79 Christie Hill Rd.
Darien, CT 06820
Website: www.rechildrens.org

Restless Legs Syndrome (RLS) Foundation
3006 Bee Caves Rd.
Ste. D206
Austin, TX 78746
Phone: 512-366-9109
Fax: 512-366-9189
Website: www.rls.org
E-mail: info@rls.org

Spina Bifida Association (SBA)
1600 Wilson Blvd.
Ste. 800
Arlington, VA 22209
Toll-Free: 800-621-3141
Phone: 202-944-3285
Fax: 202-944-3295
Website: www. spinabifidaassociation.org
E-mail: sbaa@sbaa.org

United Cerebral Palsy (UCP)
1825 K St. N.W.
Ste. 600
Washington, DC 20006
Toll-Free: 800-872-5827
Phone: 202-776-0406
Website: www.ucp.org

United Leukodystrophy Foundation (ULF)
224 N. Second St.
Ste. 2
DeKalb, IL 60115
Toll-Free: 800-728-5483
Phone: 815-748-3211
Fax: 815-748-0844
Website: www.ulf.org
E-mail: office@ulf.org

University of California, Los Angeles (UCLA)
Frontotemporal Dementia
(FTD) & Neurobehavior Clinic
and Research
300 UCLA Medical Plaza
Ste. B200
Los Angeles, CA 90095
Phone: 310-794-1195
Fax: 310-794-7491
Website: neurology.ucla.edu

University of California, San Francisco (UCSF)
Memory and Aging Center
(MAC)
675 Nelson Rising Ln.
Ste. 190
San Francisco, CA 94143
Phone: 415-353-2057
Website: www.memory.ucsf.edu

Wake Up Narcolepsy
P.O. Box 60293
Worcester, MA 01606
Phone: 978-751-DOZE
(978-751-3693)
Website: www.
wakeupnarcolepsy.org
E-mail: info@wakeupnarcolepsy.
org

Well Spouse Association
63 W. Main St.
Freehold, NJ 07728
Toll-Free: 800-838-0879
Website: www.wellspouse.org
E-mail: info@wellspouse.org

YoungStroke, Inc.
Website: www.youngstroke.org
E-mail: info@youngstroke.org

Index

Index

children, *continued*
hydranencephaly 245
infantile neuroaxonal
dystrophy 218
LaCrosse encephalitis 295
lead exposure 36
lissencephaly 246
manganese 43
memories 15
mercury exposure 33
Moebius syndrome 236
myelomeningocele 262
pneumococcal meningitis 292
shaken baby syndrome 356
spina bifida 260
vacuolar myelopathy 277
Zika 240
Children's Hemiplegia and Stroke
Association (CHASA), contact 611
cholesterol
atherosclerosis 447
CADASIL 205
defined 588
dementia 63
obesity 392
stroke 391
vascular dementia 456
cholesterol levels
obesity 392
stroke 395
chorionic villus sampling,
described 103
chromosome, defined 588
chronic headache, defined 588
Citizens United for Research in
Epilepsy (CURE), contact 611
CJD *see* Creutzfeldt-Jakob disease
CJD (Creutzfeldt-Jakob disease)
Aware!, contact 611
Creutzfeldt-Jakob Disease (CJD)
Foundation Inc., contact 611
classic CM, described 259
cleft palate
antiseizure medications 556
Moebius syndrome 236
clinical trial, defined 588
clipping
cerebral aneurysms 374
defined 588

clonazepam
benzodiazepines 579
Creutzfeldt-Jakob disease (CJD) 496
myoclonus 571
sleep disorder 470
clozapine, Lewy body dementia
(LBD) 471
cluster headache, defined 588
codeine, restless legs syndrome
(RLS) 579
cognitive ability, Lewy body dementia
(LBD) 461
cognitive changes
aging 22
cancer 126
multiple sclerosis (MS) 521
cognitive decline
cancer survivors 127
cerebral vasculitis 57
multiple sclerosis (MS) 521
cognitive dysfunction, delirium 95
cognitive functions, defined 588
cognitive impairment
Aicardi syndrome 224
chemobrain 126
microcephaly 247
postconcussion syndrome 341
schizencephaly 248
treatment-resistant epilepsy 554
"Cognitive Impairment in Adults
with Non-Central Nervous
System Cancers (PDQ®)–Health
Professional Version" (NCI) 165n
cognitive rehabilitation therapy
(CRT), overview 165–74
cognitive training, cognitive
rehabilitation Interventions 167
coloboma, Aicardi syndrome 212
colpocephaly, described 243
coma
assessment 337
brain aneurysm 372
defined 588
nervous system complications 274
nonconvulsive status epilepticus 543
overview 97–8
Powassan encephalitis 294
see also minimally conscious state;
vegetative state

functional magnetic resonance
imaging (fMRI), *continued*
neurological complications
associated with AIDS 278
neurological imaging 114
see also magnetic resonance imaging
fungal meningitis, meningitis and
encephalitis 293
fusiform aneurysm, cerebral
aneurysm 371

G

GABA *see* gamma-aminobutyric acid
gabapentin
defined 590
multiple sclerosis (MS) 520
restless legs syndrome (RLS) 578
gadolinium
central nervous system tumor 412
childhood brain tumors 428
galantamine, dementias 449
Galen defect, arteriovenous
malformations (AVMs) 227
gamma-aminobutyric acid (GABA)
brain basics 10
myoclonus 571
gamma rays, neurological tests and
procedures 112
gastroesophageal reflux disease
(GERD), Aicardi syndrome 213
gastrointestinal problems, Aicardi
syndrome 213
"Gateway to Health Communication—
Shaken Baby Syndrome" (CDC) 355n
gender factor
agenesis of the corpus callosum
(ACC) 224
amyotrophic lateral sclerosis
(ALS) 482
megalencephaly 246
toxins effect on brain 29
generalized seizures
described 538
seizures 64, 537
genes
adolescent brain 17
amyotrophic lateral sclerosis
(ALS) 483

genes, *continued*
cerebral cavernous malformations
(CCMs) 377
chemotherapy and the brain 129
Creutzfeldt-Jakob disease (CJD) 497
defined 590
dementias 453
epilepsies 65
genetic brain disorders 207
multiple sclerosis (MS) 514
neurological tests and
procedures 103
neuronal ceroid lipofuscinoses
(NCL) 198
neuronal migration disorders 238
pituitary tumors 421
stroke 393
toxins effect on brain 29
traumatic brain injury (TBI) 342
Genetic Alliance, contact 612
Genetic and Rare Diseases
Information Center (GARD)
publications
agnosia 365n
CADASIL 203n
cerebral cavernous
malformation 377n
Friedreich ataxia 501n
Gerstmann-Straussler-
Scheinker disease 215n
X-linked adrenoleukodystrophy
(X-ALD) 193n
genetic mutation
arteriovenous malformations and
other vascular lesions 232
Creutzfeldt-Jakob disease
(CJD) 493
genetic brain disorders 208
genetic testing
dementia 448
Gerstmann-Straussler-Scheinker
(GSS) 217
neurological tests and
procedures 103
X-linked adrenoleukodystrophy
(X-ALD) 195
genetic testing registry (GTR),
Gerstmann-Straussler-Scheinker
(GSS) 217

Indiana University School of
Medicine, contact 613
infantile neuroaxonal dystrophy
(INAD), overview 218–9
"Infantile Neuroaxonal Dystrophy"
(GHR) 218n
"Infantile Neuroaxonal Dystrophy
Information Page" (NINDS) 218n
infantile neuronal ceroid
lipofuscinosis, Batten disease 202
infantile spasms
Aicardi syndrome 212
cephalic disorders 248
epilepsy 540
infants
brain development 15
cephalic disorders 242
cerebral cavernous malformations
(CCMs) 378
concussion 321
electronystagmography 109
epilepsies 65
febrile seizures 563
Leigh disease 220
manganese and brain damage 43
meningitis and encephalitis 300
Moebius syndrome 237
traumatic brain injury (TBI) 343
infarcts
defined 592
multi-infarct dementia (MID) 445
infections
brain abscess 281
delirium 93
epilepsies 69
headache 54
hydranencephaly 245
meningitis and encephalitis 291
multiple sclerosis (MS) 516
neurological complications
associated with AIDS 274
inflammation
dementias 453
manganese and brain damage 42
meningitis and encephalitis 291
multiple sclerosis (MS) 515
neurological complications
associated with AIDS 273
stroke 79

iniencephaly, described 245
inorganic mercury compounds,
mercury and neuro-development 31
insomnia
Chiari malformation 258
Creutzfeldt-Jakob disease (CJD) 494
dementias 464
polysomnogram 112
rabies 305
restless legs syndrome (RLS) 579
intellectual impairment
agenesis of the corpus callosum
(ACC) 224
epilepsies 66
intentional self-harm, traumatic brain
injury (TBI) 327
internal radiation therapy
brain and spinal cord tumors 414
described 149
International RadioSurgery
Association (IRSA), contact 613
intracerebral hematoma, defined 592
intracerebral hemorrhage (ICH),
defined 592
intracranial hemorrhage
arteriovenous malformations
(AVMs) 228
subarachnoid hemorrhage 87
Intracranial Hypertension Research
Foundation (IHRF), contact 613
intracranial pressure
anticonvulsants 89
brain abscess 284
brain herniation 82
brain tumors 49
cerebrospinal fluid analysis 106
intracranial pressure monitoring,
overview 122–4
intractable epilepsy, Alpers-
Huttenlocher syndrome (AHS) 214
intrathecal contrast enhanced
CT scan (cisternography),
described 107
ionizing radiation, neurological tests
and procedures 107
ischemia
defined 592
ischemic stroke and transient
ischemic attack 79

metastatic brain tumors
adult central nervous system
tumors 405
brain tumor 399
adult central nervous system
tumors 405
methylmercury
mercury 31
neurodevelopmental effects 33
toxic effects 34
Michael J. Fox Foundation for
Parkinson's Research, contact 614
micrencephaly, described 249
microbleeds, described 228
microcephaly
colpocephaly 243
described 247
lissencephaly 245
porencephaly 248
schizencephaly 248
Zika 239
micrognathia, Moebius
syndrome 236
microgyria, neuronal migration
disorders 238
microphthalmia, Aicardi
Syndrome 212
micropolygyria, neuronal migration
disorders 238
microstomia, Moebius syndrome 236
microtubule, defined 593
midbrain
brain architecture 4
defined 593
Lewy bodies 460
newborn brain 12
migraine
Alpers-Huttenlocher syndrome
(AHS) 214
CADASIL 203
defined 593
primary headaches 52
seizures 59
migraine headaches
Alpers-Huttenlocher syndrome
(AHS) 214
CADASIL 203
Migraine Research Foundation,
contact 614

mild cognitive impairment (MCI)
Alzheimer disease 451
defined 593
minimally conscious state,
neurological imaging 116
mitochondria
defined 593
Leigh disease 220
mitoxantrone, disease modifying
drugs 517
mixed dementia
defined 593
overview 479–80
mixed glioma, described 407
"Moderate to Severe Traumatic Brain
Injury Is a Lifelong Condition"
(CDC) 345n
Moebius syndrome, overview 235–7
"Moebius Syndrome" (GHR) 235n
"Moebius Syndrome Information
Page" (NINDS) 235n
monoclonal antibody, targeted
therapy 415
mood disorders
CADASIL 457
deep brain stimulation 142
mood swing
cognitive problems 91
emotional disorders 51
mental disorders 50
mild traumatic brain injury 340
psychogenic nonepileptic seizures 560
motor area, brain architecture 6
motor coordination
agenesis of the corpus callosum
(ACC) 224
cerebral hypoxia 86
motor neuron
amyotrophic lateral sclerosis 481
cellular defects 490
defined 593
motor vehicle crashes, traumatic
brain injury (TBI) 327
MRA *see* magnetic resonance
angiography
MRI *see* magnetic resonance imaging
multi-infarct dementia
CADASIL 457
defined 593

649

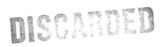